SUPERVISION & MENTORING IN HEALTHCARE

Sara Miller McCune founded SAGE Publishing in 1965 to support the dissemination of usable knowledge and educate a global community. SAGE publishes more than 1000 journals and over 800 new books each year, spanning a wide range of subject areas. Our growing selection of library products includes archives, data, case studies and video. SAGE remains majority owned by our founder and after her lifetime will become owned by a charitable trust that secures the company's continued independence.

Los Angeles | London | New Delhi | Singapore | Washington DC | Melbourne

NEIL GOPEE

SUPERVISION & MENTORING IN HEALTHCARE

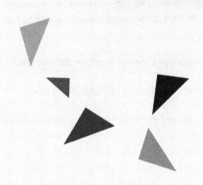

4TH EDITION

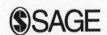

Los Angeles | London | New Delhi
Singapore | Washington DC | Melbourne

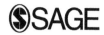

Los Angeles | London | New Delhi
Singapore | Washington DC | Melbourne

SAGE Publications Ltd
1 Oliver's Yard
55 City Road
London EC1Y 1SP

SAGE Publications Inc.
2455 Teller Road
Thousand Oaks, California 91320

SAGE Publications India Pvt Ltd
B 1/I 1 Mohan Cooperative Industrial Area
Mathura RoadA
New Delhi 110 044

SAGE Publications Asia-Pacific Pte Ltd
3 Church Street
#10-04 Samsung Hub
Singapore 049483

Editor: Alex Clabburn
Editorial assistant: Jade Grogan
Assistant editor, digital: Chloe Statham
Production editor: Katie Forsythe
Copyeditor: Christine Bitten
Indexer: Author
Marketing manager: Tamara Navaratnam
Cover design: Wendy Scott
Typeset by: C&M Digitals (P) Ltd, Chennai, India
Printed in the UK

Chapters 1, 2, 3, 4, 5, 6, 7, 9 © Neil Gopee 2018

Chapter 8 © Natasha Taylor, Collette Clay and
Neil Gopee 2018

First edition published 2007. Reprinted in 2008 twice, 2009
and 2010

Second edition published 2011. Reprinted in 2011

Third edition published 2015. Reprinted 2015, 2016 and 2017

This fourth edition first published 2018

Library of Congress Control Number: 2018935663

British Library Cataloguing in Publication data

A catalogue record for this book is available from the
British Library

ISBN 978-1-5264-2450-1
ISBN 978-1-5264-2451-8 (pbk)

At SAGE we take sustainability seriously. Most of our products are printed in the UK using responsibly sourced
papers and boards. When we print overseas we ensure sustainable papers are used as measured by the PREPS
grading system. We undertake an annual audit to monitor our sustainability.

CONTENTS

LIST OF BOXES, TEMPLATES, FIGURES AND TABLES

BOXES

CONTENTS

LIST OF BOXES, TEMPLATES, FIGURES AND TABLES

BOXES

TEMPLATES

FIGURES

TABLES

ABOUT THE AUTHOR

I am currently employed as Lecturer at the Faculty of Health and Life Sciences at Coventry University, and have previously also been Associate Lecturer at the Open University for mentorship and Post-Graduate Certificate in Academic Practice (Education) courses. My role as external examiner at various higher education institutions in my subject areas has further broadened my insights into the two subject areas that I teach and research: first, learning, teaching and assessment in relation to undergraduate and postgraduate students; and, second, leadership and management in healthcare settings.

I first qualified as a nurse a few decades ago and worked in general surgical nursing for a year before moving on to complete the registered mental health nurse course. Through my nursing career, a combination of clinical experiences in primary care and general intensive care nursing was also complemented by attendance at numerous professional development short and long courses, including various workshops on writing for publication, and also completing my doctorate in continuing professional education at the University of Warwick.

My first peer-reviewed article was related to the evaluation of a novel mode of delivery of the enrolled nurse Conversion Course based on my then nurse tutor role. By the turn of the millennium nurse education programmes became established in UK universities, which further opened up authoring opportunities, and I negotiated with Alison Poyner, Commissioning Editor at SAGE Publications, to write the *Mentoring and Supervision in Healthcare* book, the first edition of which was published in 2007. Along the way, I also worked with SAGE Publications to write *Leadership and Management in Healthcare* (now third edition) and *Practice Teaching in Healthcare* textbooks. I have also had chapters published in edited books and a range of peer-reviewed articles.

Neil Gopee, August 2018

ACKNOWLEDGEMENTS

I would like to acknowledge the constructive comments provided by the reviewers for this edition, and the support and guidance provided by the editors at SAGE Publications, especially Alex Clabburn and Katie Forsythe. I am also thankful to my daughters Hema, Sheila and Neeta for their recognition of my scholarly work.

I would like to say a further thank you to:

David Hopkins, Senior Lecturer for Operating Department Practitioners (ODP) programmes, Coventry University – for a case study related to an underachieving ODP student, presented in Chapter 7.

Natasha Taylor, Principal Lecturer and Lead for Simulation, Coventry University, and Collette Clay, Principal Lecturer (Masters in Research programme) and Senior Lecturer in Midwifery, Coventry University, for co-authoring Chapter 8.

PUBLISHER'S ACKNOWLEDGEMENTS

The author and publishers would like to thank Claire McGuinness, Lecturer and Mentorship Lead at Glasgow Caledonian University, and Su Everett, Senior Lecturer, Middlesex University, for providing scenario suggestions for the Online Resources.

We would also like to thank the reviewers who provided feedback on the proposal for the fourth edition of this textbook, and for their comments on draft chapters:

Maria Pearson, University of Nottingham

Andrew Southgate, Canterbury Christ Church University

Mary Collins, Kingston and St. George's University of London

Louise Lawson, University of Hertfordshire

Adele Kane, Plymouth University

Janette Barker, Grimsby Institute of Further and Higher Education

Kathryn Steele, Northumbria University

Deb Hearle, Cardiff University

LIST OF ABBREVIATIONS

AHP	Allied health professions
BACP	British Association for Counselling and Psychotherapy
CAIPE	Centre for Advancement of Inter-Professional Education
CATS	Credit accumulation and transfer scheme
CCG	Clinical commissioning group
CHEF	Care Home Education Facilitator
CINAHL	Cumulative Index to Nursing and Allied Health Literature
CIPD	Chartered Institute of Personnel and Development
CLE	Clinical Learning Environment
CLEI	Clinical Learning Environment Inventory
CLES+T	Clinical Learning Environment, Supervision and Nurse Teacher
CLiP	Collaborative Learning in Practice
CNO	Chief Nursing Officer
CODP	College of Operating Department Practitioners
COPD	Chronic Obstructive Pulmonary Disease
CPD	Continuing professional development
CPS	Crown Prosecution Service
CQC	Care Quality Commission
CSP	Chartered Society of Physiotherapy
DDA	Disability Discrimination Act
DH	Department of Health
EBHC	Evidence-based healthcare
EBM	Evidence-based medicine
EBP	Evidence-based practice
ESC	Essential skills clusters
GMC	General Medical Council
GP	General Practitioner

GROW	Goal, Reality, Options, Will/Wrap up (model)
HCPC	Health and Care Professions Council
HEE	Health Education England
HEI	Higher education institute
HMSO	Her Majesty's Stationery Office
HoM	Head of Midwifery
IPE	Inter-professional education
IPL	Inter-professional learning
LETB	Local Education and Training Boards
LSQ	Learning Style Questionnaire
LWAB	Local Workforce Action Board
MDT	Multidisciplinary team
NCIHE	National Committee of Inquiry into Higher Education
NEWS	National Early Warning Score
NHS KSF	NHS Knowledge and Skills Framework
NICE	National Institute for Health and Care Excellence
NMC	Nursing and Midwifery Council
NQB	National Quality Board (NHS)
NVQ	National Vocational Qualification
OAR	Ongoing Achievement Record (also referred to as ORA – Ongoing Record of Achievement)
ODP	Operating department practitioner
OSCE	Objective Structured/Simulated Clinical Examination (at times referred to as OSCA, with the substituted alphabet A signifying Assessment)
PAD	Practice Assessment Document
PARE	Practice Assessment Record and Evaluation
PCA	Patient-controlled analgesia
PDP	Personal development plan
PDSA	Plan–Do–Study–Act
PEF	Practice education facilitator
QAA	Quality Assurance Agency for Higher Education
RAPSIES	Recognition, Analysis, Preparation, Strategies, Implementation, Evaluation, Sustaining (framework)
RCN	Royal College of Nursing
RCT	Randomised controlled trial

RM	Registered midwife
RN	Registered nurse
SCPHN	Specialist community public health nurse
SDL	Self-directed learning
SEND	Special education needs and disability
SMART	Specific, measurable, achievable, realistic and time-limited
SMS	Short message service (texting)
SOLER	Sit squarely, open posture, lean towards the other, eye contact, relax
SOP	Standards of proficiency
STEP	Social, technological, economic and political
SURETY	Sit at an angle, uncross legs and arms, relax, eye contact, touch, your intuition
SWOT	Strengths, weaknesses, opportunities and threats
VARK	Visual, aural, read–write and kinaesthetic
WBL	Work-based learning

HOW TO USE THE ONLINE RESOURCES

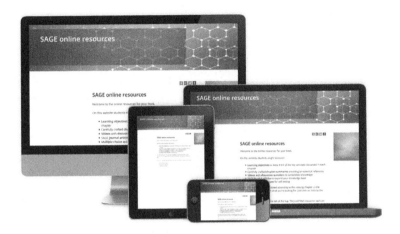

The 4th edition of *Supervision and Mentoring in Healthcare* is supported by a variety of online resources for both students and lecturers, to aid you in your involvement in practice learning: as a learner, supervisor/mentor and as a lecturer. All resources are available at: https://study.sagepub.com/gopee4e.

RESOURCES FOR STUDENTS:

- A video of Neil Gopee introducing the book and its key themes.
- An interactive glossary that allows you to check your knowledge of important concepts.
- Examples of evidence you can give to show you meet the NMC Mentor Outcomes.

JOURNAL ARTICLES:

- Read more widely! A selection of free SAGE journal articles that support each chapter to help deepen your knowledge and reinforce your learning of key topics. An ideal place to start for literature reviews/ dissertations/ assignments. Preceding each article is an annotation from the book's author, Neil Gopee, introducing its relevance for practice and/ or supervision.

RESOURCES FOR LECTURERS:

- A lesson plan for teaching a component of knowledge or healthcare theory.
- Extra case studies, not available in the book, for use in your teaching.
- Videos of Neil Gopee giving his response to case scenarios (Neil's videos are not exhaustive answers to the scenarios, your students can discuss them in class and come up with other ideas).

WEBLINKS:

- Weblinks direct you to relevant resources to broaden your understanding of chapter topics and expand your knowledge by linking to real world organizations and/or conversations on supervision and mentoring. Preceding each article is an annotation from the book's author, Neil Gopee, introducing its relevance for practice and/ or supervision.

INTRODUCTION

THE RATIONALE AND SCOPE OF THIS BOOK

Supervision of practice-based learning, mentoring and practice assessment have become significant dimensions of professional life in nursing, midwifery and allied healthcare professions, in particular in relation to supporting the educational preparation of pre-registration students. The practice learning supervisor role is also known by other titles such as clinical educator, practice educator, clinical instructor, etc., in different healthcare professions, and in non-UK countries, appropriate educational preparation for such roles is required in nursing and midwifery (be they university-based or healthcare trust based) so as to enable supervisors of learning to perform these roles competently (see Glossary at the back of this book for brief explanation of different roles).

Different versions of these roles have evolved over the years and various research findings on facilitation of practice learning and student assessment have been published. The roles, responsibilities and educational preparation of supervisors of practice-based learning and assessors of practice competencies for nursing and midwifery students are delineated in *Standards for Student Supervision and Assessment* (NMC, 2018a). The mentor role is thereby replaced by 'practice supervisor' and 'practice assessor' roles, and a new 'academic assessor' role is also identified, with the requirement for all to work in collaboration.

For mentoring nursing and midwifery students, up to very recently, in *Standards to Support Learning and Assessment in Practice* the NMC (2008) identified a mentor as a registrant who facilitates learning, supervises, and also assesses students in practice settings. Additionally, the standards provided details of the specific competencies that were required to fulfil the role effectively.

Although the standards for mentors in the NMC publication were for registered nurses (RN) and registered midwives (RM) (from here on all healthcare professionals registered with the NMC or the Health and Care Professions Council [HCPC] will be referred to as 'registrants'), they were based on general principles of facilitation of learning and student assessment in healthcare settings so that they were fully applicable to the other groups of health and social care professions, such as allied health professions (AHP), social work and medicine. In the current scene of interprofessional learning, reciprocal supervision of learning and student assessment between health professions has already been happening, where permissible, for at least a decade.

This book explores in detail the necessary standards, competence areas and outcomes for effective supervision of practice-based learning and practice assessment. To do so, the book draws on the wider contemporary and previous knowledge of the dynamics of practice supervision and mentoring across different professions, as well as research and current policies, and aims to support registrants to acquire the knowledge and skills that are necessary to fulfil all NMC's (2018a) standards for practice supervision and practice assessment. It thus brings together and builds on existing knowledge of principles and practices of enabling and supporting learning and student assessment in various current health and social care arenas. Thereby it also constitutes a firm backdrop for healthcare professionals to further develop and enhance their expertise in teaching and assessment.

The NMC indicates that all health and social care registrants should be able to fulfil the role of practice supervisor for nursing and midwifery students as long as it is within their areas of competence. Both recently qualified registrants and those who are more experienced, as well as previously qualified mentors should find this book useful, as also should those who were prepared for these roles through the older 'teaching and assessing' courses.

This book is a direct result of my numerous years of experience of teaching and examining on mentoring and 'teaching and assessing' courses, as well as my experience as a registered nurse in adult nursing and mental health nursing, along with the need for a textbook that reflects current policies and research findings on practice learning supervision comprehensively. In addition to current knowledge in the field, this textbook also recognises the challenges encountered by both newly qualified and more experienced practice learning supervisors, often doing so within resource constraints, role changes and changing healthcare workforce profiles. It confronts the day-to-day and longer-term issues and challenges in the supervision of practice learning, and explores potential solutions, where possible supporting them with relevant theories, frameworks and contemporary research findings. The ensuing implications with regard to responsibility and accountability are also necessarily explored.

THE STRUCTURE OF THIS BOOK

As just indicated, this book is firmly based on current knowledge in the field and is structured to ensure that it also addresses all NMC's (2018a; 2018c) standards and framework for student supervision and assessment. These standards, which can be easily applied to other healthcare professions as well, are based on the recognition that all registrants' roles include teaching and supporting learning, along with being role models for the highest standards of care for health and social care service users.

Standards for mentors and other teachers of practice-based learning have been available for almost two decades, and they have been revised a few times, leading up to the current NMC's (2018a) *Standards for Student Supervision and Assessment* directive.

This textbook focuses on the wider principles and practice of effective supervision of practice learning and student assessment in health and social care, and also addresses the NMC's (2018a; 2018c) standards for practice learning supervision and practice assessment, examining and analysing these roles, and supporting them with relevant research related to these roles.

Chapter 1 begins by examining practice learning supervision as a concept in its own right. It starts by unravelling the exact nature of the terms practice supervisor and supervision, and differentiates them from other similar or overlapping roles, such as preceptors, clinical supervisors, practice teachers, link lecturers, practice education facilitators (PEF), and practice educators. The common aim of all these roles is to facilitate healthcare profession students and learners to acquire clinical intervention skills and knowledge, especially during practice placements.

A range of different rationales for these roles is then identified, which is followed by the factors that enable practice learning supervisors to fulfil their role effectively, including the modes of communication that enable them to build effective working relationships with their learners. Subsequently, the necessary personal and professional attributes of effective practice supervisors, including being role models, are explored. The nature and detrimental effects of poor or adverse forms of supervision are also discussed, followed by an examination of different models and approaches to practice learning supervision.

Then, *Chapter 2* takes a detailed look at how learning occurs. It examines why and what learners learn, significant different perspectives on learning, teaching and education, and learning theories, styles and approaches in healthcare professions, including use of learning contracts and learning agreements.

Chapter 3 builds on how learners learn and explores the principles of teaching and facilitation of learning. The chapter starts by ascertaining the range of people whom healthcare professionals teach, followed by the reasons for teaching and learning. It then focuses on various ways in which healthcare students learn healthcare delivery skills, and how practice learning supervisors utilise opportunities for informal teaching.

Analysis of the concept of facilitation of learning, as distinct from teaching, is followed by key perceptions and major views and approaches in teaching, including andragogy. The levels and stages of skill acquisition (taxonomy levels) are explored, and the types of knowledge associated with skills are considered, along with levels of knowledge acquisition.

Steps in lesson planning for structured short teaching sessions for teaching skills and knowledge are then discussed, followed by an examination of different teaching methods and the use of different teaching aids, including those for special education needs of students with disabilities.

Following on from facilitation of learning, *Chapter 4* focuses on the attributes that are important to make healthcare settings effective learning environments, and on ways in which practice supervisors can maintain and enhance the learning ethos. Students' perspectives on practice placements such as their own expectations and their practice objectives are considered, and then an examination is made of the part played by national guidelines and current policy documents on practice placements. Issues related to practice placements are also examined.

Research related to clinical learning environments, which underpins the development of the tool for regular educational audits of practice placement areas, is then discussed. The audits aim to ascertain the psychosocial factors and learning resources (human and material) for facilitation of the acquisition of practice competencies by healthcare profession students. The utilisation of learning pathways (based on patients' journeys through healthcare provision), which can be incorporated into learning contracts and can play an important role in ensuring the success of the placement, is also explored, as well as the concept of work-based learning.

Fundamental to practice learning supervision are safe, compassionate and effective clinical practice, evidence-based practice (EBP), implementation of research findings, and practice development, together with leadership in these. How the practice supervisor engages with these activities constitutes the focus of *Chapter 5*, as the practice supervisor has to exercise leadership, to be a role model for learners, to practise evidence-based care, which may also be followed by practice development and dissemination of innovations. Hierarchies of evidence and systematic reviews are also considered.

One of the principal purposes of practice assessor education programmes is to equip course participants with the capability of assessing students' clinical competence, with practice supervisors having a contributory role in continuous assessment. Ongoing assessment of competence of healthcare students is a fundamental component of this role, as well as a component of all educational programmes for skill-based healthcare professions, which are the areas that *Chapter 6* focuses on.

To fulfil the practice assessor role effectively, it is important to know and understand the principles and processes of assessment – i.e. what assessments are, the various reasons for assessment of competence, who assesses and when, and differing ways in which they are conducted – and also have a comprehensive understanding of the student's pre-registration programme and how to utilise the different methods of student assessment in care settings.

Under how to assess, in addition to different methods of assessment, the chapter explores key principles of assessments, such as levels of assessment and fairness of assessments. Student self-assessment and peer-assessment are also explored. Validity and reliability as crucial attributes of assessments are then explored in some detail, the aim being to ascertain the student's fitness to practise and purpose.

Consequently, the management of assessments is explored in *Chapter 7*, along with techniques for giving useful feedback and the documentation of assessments. Pass or fail criteria are examined, followed by the academic assessor's role in ascertaining proficiency at the point of registration.

Recent research findings have highlighted various day-to-day problems encountered by both assessors and students in relation to assessment of competence during practice placements. Therefore, practice assessors and practice supervisors need to exercise leadership in planning students' assessment of competence proactively, and also in averting problems of assessment. The ethical implications of assessments are also examined, along with the assessor's accountability, responsibility and the use of 'professional judgement', and includes the use of action plans, and also reassessment of the learner. Monitoring ways in which intra- and inter-assessor reliability are achieved, is also explored.

Although aspects of practice-based supervision and assessment of AHP students will have been noted in earlier chapters of this textbook, *Chapter 8* specifically examines the practice competencies that AHP students have to pass during practice placement (or internship) experience as part of their education to attain registrant status in their specific healthcare professions. In particular, the chapter examines in fair detail the competencies that paramedic students, and then midwifery students, have to achieve, and how these are facilitated and assessed.

Chapter 9 concentrates on the evaluation of learning facilitation by practice supervisors. The nature and purpose of evaluation amount to practice supervisors self-monitoring the quality of their work with students. The chapter therefore considers what evaluation is, who is involved in evaluation of learning facilitation and assessment, and how it is performed, including the use of models of evaluation.

Consideration of the results of evaluations might trigger the need for further learning for care professionals, and consequently this chapter also examines ongoing professional development for practice supervisors, incorporating details of regular updates for practice supervisors and practice assessors, along with lifelong learning and revalidation requirements.

Each chapter in the book begins with an Introduction to key concepts in the chapter and the chapter objectives, which is followed by the main text, a chapter summary and suggestions for further reading. A logical combination of text, illustrations, activities, reflection points and case studies is incorporated to engage the reader fully with the material in the book.

HOW TO USE THIS BOOK

To examine the knowledge base, skills and attitudes required for effective practice supervision, mentoring and practice assessment, and achievement of care professions' standards for supervision and assessment, this textbook adopts an analytical and interactive style throughout, with a clear focus on the means of application of principles and theories of supervision of learning to various practice settings, and assessment of students' practice competencies. Therefore, through activities and reflection points, the reader is encouraged to explore and apply concepts to their own practice and roles.

The activities usually ask the reader to consider a particular point or component and make some notes, whilst reflection points ask the reader to reflect on their own experience and knowledge prior to moving on to the next theme in the text. They thus allow practice supervisors and practice assessors to exercise the freedom and scope to be creative in enabling students' learning and assessment of their competence.

A number of case studies have been incorporated into the text as examples of situations that practice supervisors and practice assessors might encounter, so that the reader can explore ways in which they can manage the situation satisfactorily. Furthermore, the information in some of the boxes, for example in Chapter 4's box titled 'Attributes of effective practice-based healthcare learners', is derived from a number of workshops on the previous mentor preparation programmes. As events evolve, and because different practice settings have their own specific requirements and strengths, feel free to make further notes of your own on other components in addition to those in the boxes.

To summarise:

CHAPTER OBJECTIVES

These identify briefly the key theories and concepts covered in the chapter.

ACTIVITIES

These ask you to consider a particular point and make some notes. They are not compulsory, but they endeavour to enable you to apply or explore the theories or concepts inherent within student supervision and assessment in your own practice setting.

REFLECTION POINTS

Ask you to reflect on your own personal experience and potential actions, but can also be discussed with a peer or in a small group.

TEXT BOXES

These highlight multiple aspects of a key theme.

TEMPLATES

These are examples of tools that you can use with your own students in your role as a practice supervisor or practice assessor.

CASE STUDIES

Are examples of situations that you may encounter when you become a practice supervisor or practice assessor, as they are based on previous actual supervision of learning and student assessment situations.

CHAPTER SUMMARIES

These remind you of the key points addressed in the chapter that you have just read or worked through.

FURTHER OPTIONAL READING

Carefully selected learning material that will enable you to expand your knowledge further with regard to some of the main themes in the chapter.

ONLINE RESOURCES

Lively presentation of further aspects of the practice supervisor and practice assessor roles. Please refer to p.xv 'How to use the online resources' for further guidance.

TERMINOLOGY

The term **healthcare professional** is used in this textbook to signify all health and social care employees, that is medical and non-medical, and include nurses and allied health professionals who hold a qualification that is recognised by either their national regulatory body (that is, the NMC, HCPC, etc.) or professional body. The term **healthcare** incorporates **social care** where appropriate.

The term **learner** is used to refer to everyone who wants or needs to learn healthcare skills, whilst **students** are those learners who are actually following professional education programmes leading to university qualifications.

The term **practice learning supervisor** is used interchangeably with the NMC's **practice supervisor** role. Finally, the terms **healthcare service user, care service user** and **service user,** client and patient are all used in this book to incorporate anyone who avail themselves of health and social care provision in the UK.

The Glossary just before the Index section defines a range of other terminologies that are integral components of this book.

NMC GUIDANCE

The UK reader is strongly advised to have a good look through the NMC's (2018a) directive document *Standards for Student Supervision and Assessment* or HCPC's (2017a) *Standards of Education and Training,* which essentially provide sound guidance on effective practice learning and student assessment.

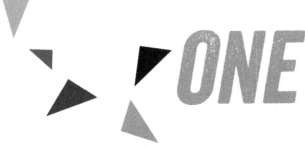

ONE

EFFECTIVE SUPERVISION OF PRACTICE LEARNING

INTRODUCTION

As in many professions, nursing, midwifery and other health and social care students on pre-registration courses acquire their clinical intervention skills predominantly in the work setting, where their learning is facilitated under supervision of appropriately qualified registrants. The first chapter of this book focuses on the supervision of students' learning in care settings, clarifies the meaning of the terms supervision and practice supervision, and differentiates them from similar and overlapping roles and titles. It then explores the various reasons for practice supervision for enabling practice-based learning, and ways of performing the role effectively.

The chapter also examines potential problematic aspects of these roles, and the steps that can be taken to avert or resolve them. Thereafter the chapter explores further perspectives on practice supervision, including models and frameworks for effective practice learning for health and social care students on practice placement, and culminates into proposing an informed framework for effective practice supervision.

In context, although practice learning supervision is not a new activity, the title 'practice supervisor' (NMC, 2018a) is, and therefore direct empirical evidence of the effectiveness of this role does not as yet exist. As Kilminster et al. (2007: 3) acknowledge, supervision is 'the least researched and supported in medical education'. Therefore, the intelligence in this chapter is based partly on the available literature on the concept supervision, and relevant research and previous policies on similar roles, such as mentoring and practice education, as long as their content is transferable to the novel practice supervisor role.

In addition, while the NMC has replaced the term and role of mentor by the practice supervisor and practice assessor roles, the mentor role still prevails in various health professions, with alternative titles being 'practice educator' and 'clinical instructor' for example. The practice assessor role is examined in full detail, particularly in Chapters 6 and 7. The HCPC, GMC and other healthcare regulators also specify certain requirements for supervising acquisition of competence and knowledge in healthcare settings, which are specifically explored in relevant sections of this book.

CHAPTER OBJECTIVES

1. Distinguish between practice supervision and similar roles that support learning for health and social care students and learners.
2. Explain a range of reasons for requiring practice supervisor-type roles, in addition to facilitating students' acquisition of professional competence.
3. Identify and evaluate a range of factors that can enable effective supervision of learning, including the personal attributes and roles of effective supervisors, and establishing stable 'working' relationships with students.
4. Analyse the likelihood and effects of poor or faulty supervision and the actions that can be taken where it is likely to occur.
5. Analyse a number of approaches, frameworks and models of informed and systematic supervision of practice learning, that enable students' acquisition of clinical skills for safe and effective practice.

PRACTICE SUPERVISION FOR PRACTICE-BASED LEARNING

For nursing and midwifery students' practice-based learning in healthcare settings, the publication of *Standards for Student Supervision and Assessment* by the Nursing and Midwifery Council (NMC, 2018a) set out the details around how the mentor role is to be replaced by two other separate roles, namely 'practice supervisor' and 'practice assessor'. The mentor role had been firmly established for facilitating learning in clinical workplaces during practice placement since the 1980s, and the successful mentoring mechanism gradually pervaded numerous other areas of learning (e.g. research mentoring, mentoring in medicine, youth rehabilitation mentoring, business mentoring, etc.).

In relation to the practice supervisor role, the NMC (2018a: 6) indicates firmly that 'practice supervision enables students to learn and safely achieve proficiency and autonomy in their professional role'. It indicates that all nurses and midwives are capable of supervising students, and that student learning can also be supervised by other health and social care registrants. The NMC consequently details its 'expectations' of operationalisation of practice supervision, along with:

- practice supervisors' roles and responsibilities
- practice supervisors' contribution to student assessment and progression

- preparation of practice supervisors and subsequent ongoing support
- the organisation of practice learning.

The practice supervisor role, as well as the concept of supervision, are examined in substantial detail in the course of this chapter.

The aim of separating the learning and assessment roles in this way is partly to make student assessment of competence more objective, fair and consistent (see also Chapter 7), particularly in the light of several years of research that have identified various problems with student assessment (e.g. Duffy, 2016; Hunt et al., 2016). This may, however, leave qualified mentors disillusioned, state Morley et al. (2017: 170), who add that dividing the role will add a further level of bureaucracy and suggest concerted investment in experienced nurse educators in practice settings.

Nonetheless, Professor Macleod-Clark, who recommended this change to the NMC, indicates that separating the opposite roles of support and supervision from assessment will mean that all registrants can be practice supervisors (Agnew, 2018: 14), and thereby 'vastly expand the pool of nurses involved in the training of students'. That student supervision and student assessment are roles that are in conflict, and which mentors struggle with, has also been documented from research by Bray and Nettleton (2007), Tweed et al. (2010), Hutchison and Cochrane (2014) and others.

DISTINGUISHING BETWEEN PRACTICE SUPERVISOR AND SIMILAR ROLES

The practice supervisor role is just one of several that support learning in practice settings and therefore there is some overlap in certain aspects of such roles, such as in the personal qualities of registrants who willingly support learning, but there are distinct boundaries as well. For instance, a study conducted by Carnwell et al. (2007) to explore the likely differences in the roles of mentors, lecturer–practitioners and link lecturers indicates that mentors tend to focus principally on individual students, lecturer–practitioners on the 'learning environment', and link lecturers on knowledge acquisition and fulfilling course requirements.

ACTIVITY 1.1   DIFFERENT EDUCATION SUPPORT ROLES AND FUNCTIONS

To begin with, make notes on what you think are the meanings and functions of the following roles: mentor, preceptor, practice educator, clinical supervisor, assessor and other similar roles that you have encountered, and the differences between them.

You are likely to have identified a variety of roles that enable or support learning for students and other learners in practice settings, which might include practice facilitator, practice educator, clinical instructor, clinical supervisor, field instructor and specialist nurse as alternative titles. Additionally, other roles, such as buddy and coach, have also emerged (the latter is discussed later in this chapter). All the same, although there are common elements in the definitions, scope and remit of practice supervisor and similar roles, there are also differences. The most popular learning support roles are examined next.

MENTOR

The mentor role has prevailed for around two decades in nursing and midwifery, and as the NMC (2008) indicated, the role incorporated facilitating of learning and student assessment in healthcare settings. Prior to this era, the mentor was identified as a registrant who facilitated learning, and the assessor was another registrant who assessed students' competencies, which is akin to the NMC's (2018a) current differentiation. The mentor would have received appropriate education preparation for the role, and be deemed competent in a set of specified mentor competencies (outcomes) that were grouped under eight domains, which essentially comprised a framework for effective mentoring. The NMC's view of the mentor was built on existing knowledge of the subject area, such as research by Kerry and Mayes (1995) that indicated that mentorship needs to include:

- nurturing
- role modelling
- functioning (as teacher, sponsor, encourager, counsellor and friend)
- focusing on the professional development of the student and
- sustaining a caring relationship over time.

A subsequent concept analysis of the mentor role by Billay and Yonge (2004: 573) across several health, non-health and social care professions indicated that its defining attributes include 'being a role model, being a facilitator, having good communication skills, being knowledgeable about the field of expertise, and needing to understand the principles of adult education'. These defining attributes of the mentor role correspondingly also apply to the practice supervisor role. A more recent concept analysis of mentoring by Hodgson and Scanlan (2013) reveals that the role is associated with increased job satisfaction and staff retention, which is beneficial for learners, supervisors of practice learning, the organisation and nursing profession, as ultimately patient care benefits. It also empowers supervisors of practice learning and learners, which 'enhances employees' motivation and professional development ... [and] ... a culture and workplace is created in which nurses want to come to work' (ibid.: 392).

In some countries, however, the formal mentor role does not exist, and also in some UK professions, for instance psychologists, the term 'protégé' is used when referring to the student receiving supervision (for example, Barnett, 2008).

PRECEPTOR

The Department of Health (2010: 6) identifies a preceptor as: 'a registered practitioner who has been given a formal responsibility to support a newly registered practitioner through preceptorship'. In the UK, the term 'preceptor' is identified by the NMC (2006) as a first-level registrant who has had at least 12 months' (or equivalent) experience within the same area of practice as the practitioner requiring support, and will normally have completed a mentor or practice teacher course through a Higher Education Institute (HEI).

Additionally, preceptorship is defined by the DH (2010: 11) as:

A period of structured transition for the newly registered practitioner during which he or she will be supported by a preceptor, to develop their confidence as an autonomous professional, refine skills, values and behaviours and to continue on their journey of lifelong learning.

The preceptor role emerged from the realisation that, for newly qualified nurses, the transition from being a student to becoming a registered healthcare professional is a major leap in responsibility and accountability, which can also cause disillusionment (e.g. Kramer, 1974; Marks-Maran et al., 2013; NHS Education for Scotland, 2017).

The DH (2010) presents a framework for effective preceptoring, within which it also identifies the 'attributes' of an effective preceptor, which are similar to those of practice supervisors, as discussed later in this chapter. The DH framework is generic for health professions and can be easily adapted as appropriate. Furthermore, Moore (2018) describes a new well-received preceptorship framework for newly qualified nurses in London, which includes a minimum of two weeks' supernumerary status, protected time for both preceptor and preceptee, etc.

COACH

Some learning supervision roles that are still developing include *practice facilitator*, *buddy*, *coach* and *clinical educator*, etc. The more developed terms 'coach' and 'coaching' tend to surface sporadically in nursing and involve instructing and supporting the coachee to perform a skilled task step-by-step. The Chartered Institute of Personnel and Development (CIPD) (2017: 1) indicates that coaching techniques are based on the use of one-to-one discussions to enhance an individual's skills, knowledge or work performance, and:

Coaching targets high performance and improvement at work and usually focuses on specific skills and goals, although it may also have an impact on an individual's personal attributes such as social interaction or confidence.

'Performance', 'specific skills' and 'goals' are key common words used in determining a common understanding of the term coaching, which in turn usually incorporates a more directive and prescriptive approach. This term, title and performance enhancement function of the coach, however, is more closely linked to sports, which involves training coachees using individually tailored programmes aimed at enhancing their physical performance, usually so that they are able to take part in competitions in specific sports. Other prominent areas include life coaching (enabling the coachee to live a healthier and more fulfilled life); health coaching (enabling individuals with long-term conditions such as chronic obstructive pulmonary disease [COPD] to self-care); and business coaching (guiding someone who is starting their own business for the first time and helping them to succeed). These arguments see coaching very much from a management speak that includes productivity and efficiency, rather than safety, effectiveness and compassion that is widely advocated by the NMC.

The Royal College of Nursing (RCN) (2016: 18), however, reports on an approach to practice learning supervision whereby the coach is one amongst other healthcare professionals who teaches learners, but it is the practice assessor who is qualified to assess students on their practice competencies. Coaching also features in Collaborative Learning in Practice (CLiP), which is another way of facilitating learning during practice placements, and is discussed later in this chapter.

Reporting on the findings of an audit of a new role termed 'clinical coach', whereby an appointed academic coaches underachieving (referred to as 'marginal' or 'at risk') student nurses during practice placements, Kelton (2014) indicates that a systematic approach to clinical coaching can significantly enhance students' successful completion of the placement. Clinical coaching entails the appointed clinical coach, that is a new resource, providing additional support and guidance to the identified student. Another application of coaching in healthcare is management coaching, as discussed under 'Supervising students to learn management skills' later in this chapter.

ASSESSOR

The term 'assessor' is often used to denote a registrant whose duties incorporate student assessment, for which they will have had appropriate educational preparation and subsequent support. It usually refers to an appropriately qualified and experienced health or social care professional whose educational preparation entailed developing skills in assessing students' level of attainment related to the stated practice competencies (for example, National Vocational Qualifications [NVQ] assessor).

PRACTICE ASSESSOR

This is a novel role of registrants, the principal remit of which is to assess students' achievement of practice competencies and NMC (2018b) standards for pre-registration education, and uses student information provided by practice supervisors and others. Practice assessors liaise directly with academic assessors to determine each student's fitness to register with the NMC. Practice assessors for nursing students will not be required to be from the same field of practice as the student they are assessing, if they have suitable equivalent experience.

ACADEMIC ASSESSOR

This is another novel role, that of a university-based lecturer who works closely with practice assessors to determine each students' fitness to register with the NMC.

PRACTICE EDUCATOR

While being largely similar to the practice supervisor role, the practice educator role entails guiding and supporting allied health professions (AHP) students during their practice placement.

The College of Social Work (2013: 20) defines a practice educator as a person who 'takes overall responsibility for the student's learning and assessment, utilising information from his/her own assessment and other sources', which suggests that the practice educator role in social work (as well as in other AHPs) is largely similar to the previous mentor role identified by the NMC (2008). Different AHPs offer different forms of training or education for the role, some more formal than others, and encourage networking. Until recently the role was known as clinical educator.

Formally, some AHPs have established the title of 'accredited practice educator', educational preparation for which can be through the taught route based at an HEI, or an experiential learning route (for example, Society and College of Radiographers, 2018).

PRACTICE EDUCATION FACILITATOR

The practice education facilitator (PEF) role in nursing and midwifery emerged largely from research by Phillips et al. (2000) that identified several problems with mentoring. The purpose of the role has been to ensure student experience during practice placements is successful by ensuring provision of support and guidance to practice learning supervisors and others who contribute to the student's learning in practice settings. An alternative title has been implemented for PEFs who are based in non-NHS nursing homes as Care Home Education Facilitator (CHEF) (NHS Education for Scotland, 2014).

This is a very important role as PEFs are also called upon to advise practice learning supervisors when students are struggling or are failing to make progress with achievement of their practice placement competencies. For students on practice placements, PEFs also organise dedicated group discussion sessions away from the practice setting for particular categories of students for reflection and peer support purposes.

The study by Carlisle et al. (2009: 715) on the impact of the PEF role in Scotland revealed that the PEF role is 'accepted widely across Scotland and is seen as valuable to the development of quality clinical learning environments, providing support and guidance for practice-based learning supervisors when dealing with "failing" students, and encouraging the identification of innovative learning opportunities'. However, more recently Scott et al. (2017) examined the PEF role in healthcare trusts in London and the surrounding area and concluded that there is a lack of consistency in the job definition of the role across the trusts, and that PEFs feel undervalued and vulnerable to budget cuts. However, in the context of the Collaborative Learning in Practice (CLiP) model of mentoring, PEFs are seen as key facilitators of practice education, along with the new 'clinical educator' who is appointed specifically for this mode of facilitation of learning.

PRACTICE TEACHER

The title or role of practice teacher was initially specifically adopted in recognition of the additional educational preparation required for supervision of learning for students on specialist community public health nurses (SCPHN) courses. A practice teacher is therefore a registrant who has gained knowledge, skills and competencies as well as qualifications in both their specialist area of practice and in their teaching role, and for assessment of students on specialist or advanced practice courses (NMC, 2008). However, practice teachers can only supervise learning and assess students who are on courses on the same specialism as the practice teacher (for example in health visiting, school nursing, occupational health nursing, etc.).

An extensive analysis of the application of the practice teacher role is provided in detail by Gopee (2010) in *Practice Teaching in Healthcare*.

PERSONAL TUTOR

Each pre-registration student is allocated to a nurse lecturer who acts as a personal tutor to the student. This role normally lasts for the duration of the three-year pre-registration course, is also known by other terms such as 'academic adviser', and involves:

- supporting, advising and monitoring students' progress throughout the educational programme
- accessing students' practice records for required information, within an ethos of confidentiality and professional accountability
- liaising with practice supervisors, link lecturer, practice assessors and the student and, where concern is expressed, considering evidence and developing an action plan with the student.

LINK LECTURER

The link lecturer is usually a university lecturer whose responsibility is to assist clinicians with supervising students' practice-based learning in named practice settings. Also known at some institutions as 'academic in practice', link lecturers assist practice supervisors to interpret students' practice competencies and are available to support practice supervisors when required. They might also assist in the development of the practice setting as a more effective learning environment for all learners. Students tend to receive a visit by the link lecturer early in the placement, especially first-year students, to ascertain which learning objectives are realistically achievable. Further visits are arranged as required.

Some of the functions of the personal tutor and the link lecturer have increasingly become part of the PEF's remit but they continue to provide an essential complementary function. Practice learning supervision activities, specifically in allied health and social care professions, is examined in fair detail in Chapter 8.

CLINICAL SUPERVISOR AND CLINICAL SUPERVISION

Clinical supervisor is a term used in the context of clinical supervision signifying the provider of peer support to the clinical supervisee, which is performed in a structured way through regular meetings. However, it is also used to signify a practice-based teaching role in some healthcare professions or vocations, as for internship in clinical psychology (Johnson, 2017), and in medical education for doctors who facilitate medical students' learning during practice placements.

Clinical supervision for peer-support role is based on a clinically focused professional relationship between healthcare professionals in which one party is the clinical supervisor and the other the supervisee. The clinical supervisor undergoes educational preparation for this role and utilises clinical knowledge and experience to assist peers to develop their own knowledge, competence, values and practices further. Kumar et al.'s (2015) research revealed that AHPs value receiving clinical supervision, which consequently results in positive effects on their care delivery and improvement in their clinical skills.

However, Kumar's study also noted barriers to clinical supervision, including organisational issues such as time for clinical supervision and heavy workload.

Waskett (2010: 12) also notes that 'many nurses do not have regular, protected access to confidential conversations about the everyday challenges of their work', and amongst the various models of clinical supervision that are available for a systematic approach to this activity is Waskett's 4S model of clinical supervision, comprising: structure, skills, support and sustainability.

In summarising this section on practice learning supervisor and similar roles, it is clear that there are areas within these roles that overlap, and there are distinctions between them when current national policy and professional bodies' definitions are considered. However, as these roles evolve, and different models of implementation are applied in different settings, endeavouring to disentangle the educational philosophy underlying these roles – such as differentiating between coaching and mentoring – is seen by Megginson et al. (2006: 5) as a 'sterile debate'.

UNRAVELLING SUPERVISION AND THE SUPERVISOR ROLE

The term 'supervisor' tends to be used in the context of management of workers to ensure designated tasks are completed, and to a specified standard. It also refers to individuals in the organisation who have authority in the interest of the employer to recruit staff for specified posts, assign duties, oversee the quality of their work and provide relevant training or professional development, or take disciplinary actions when appropriate.

However, in the context of the recently implemented 'nursing associate' role, Health Education England (HEE) (2017a: 10) indicates that a supervisor is a 'suitably prepared professional trained to support students in practice', which is somewhat similar to the NMC's (2018a) practice supervisor role, but in the context of nursing associate training the supervisor can also be an appropriate manager.

In a comprehensive exploration of the concept and applications of supervision in health and social care professions, Hawkins and Shohet (2012) refer to supervision as a joint endeavour in which the identified supervisor helps the supervisee to improve the quality of their work and continuously develop themselves and their practice.

The term does, however, have a very specific meaning in the field of counselling, in which it refers to counselling activities, whereupon one or more highly experienced counsellors help a less experienced or more junior counsellor develop their practice. The British Association for Counselling and Psychotherapy (BACP) (2016) recommends supervision to anyone providing therapeutically based services, working in roles that require regularly giving or receiving emotionally challenging communications, or engaging in relationally complex and challenging roles.

Furthermore, the BACP (2016: 12) notes that 'Supervisors and supervisees will periodically review how responsibility for work with clients is implemented in practice and how any difficulties or concerns are being addressed.' An effective interpersonal relationship is essential in both above-mentioned aspects of supervision.

The dictionary (Brookes and O'Neill, 2017: 808) indicates that to supervise means: (1) to direct or oversee the performance, action or work of another; and (2) to watch over (people) to ensure appropriate behaviour. In the context of supervision of practice-based learning, Johnson (2017: 6) asserts that supervision is a formal provision, by approved supervisors, of a relationship-based, work-focused education and training. Johnson adds that 'supervisors bear clinical, ethical, and legal responsibility for their supervisees' work'.

Many elements of the above explanations of supervise, supervisor and supervision apply to overseeing the facilitation of students' learning, and to support functions of the practice supervisor role currently being implemented in nursing and midwifery pre-registration education. Implicit in the meanings of the word supervision is the implication that the supervisee (e.g. student nurse) is likely to have training needs, and presumably motivated to learn to perform healthcare interventions to a very high standard.

Additionally, on examining the multiple approaches to learner supervision within healthcare professions, Nancarrow et al. (2014) perused several definitions of the term supervision related to placement learning, and note that they all tend to refer to working relationships, and intentional support for learning that enables sharing and enhancing knowledge and skills. They note that definitions of supervision also apply to support mechanisms for practising professionals within which they can share clinical, organisational, and developmental experiences with others in order to enhance knowledge and skills (p. 240).

Furthermore, from a study of student nurses' satisfaction with practice settings as effective learning environments, Papastavrou et al. (2016) conclude that the 'supervisory relationship' between supervisor and student is the most influential factor on student learning during practice placements; the teaching and learning atmosphere is also 'pivotal'. Effective supervision is thus dependent upon a strong relationship between student and supervisor, and also on the amount and content of feedback to students, according to research on students' expectations and perceptions by Gratrix and Barrett (2017).

However, research on student social workers' 'field supervision' conducted by Cleak and Smith (2012) conclude that when the field supervisor is based on-site, this resulted in superior quality student supervision, while off-site, or external supervision, (also known as distant supervision or long-arm mentoring) was found to be the least effective. Nonetheless, Maynard et al.'s (2015) research demonstrate how off-site supervision can be very effective, by:

- careful planning and preparation for the placement
- selection of an appropriately motivated 'task supervisor' on-site
- communication among all involved
- knowledge of roles and expectations.

A popular framework for effective clinical supervision by Proctor (2011) provides another perspective on a more holistic model of learning supervision, as also advocated by Johnson (2017). Proctor's model comprises addressing the formative, normative and restorative aspects of supervision. *Formative* refers to the educational aspect of supervisor–student relationship; *normative* addresses the clinical guidelines and procedures that must be adhered to; and *restorative* whereby the practitioner develops resilience to be able to resolve challenging encounters, engages in reflective conversation, etc. In addition to all three aspects needing to be addressed for effective appropriate supervision, Proctor indicates that their supportive function underpins the model, which incorporates attitude, skill and intentions in the relationship (more later in this chapter).

Another shade of the term supervision is 'academic supervision', which refers to the support available to students when writing assignments. The mechanism for effective practice supervision in nursing and midwifery is detailed by the NMC (2018a), which include components such as:

2.1 all students on an NMC approved programme are supervised while learning in practice

2.4 practice supervision ensures safe and effective learning experiences that uphold public protection and the safety of people

3.1 serve as role models for safe and effective practice in line with their code of conduct

3.2 support learning in line with their scope of practice to enable the student to meet their proficiencies and programme outcomes

4.2 contribute to student assessments to inform decisions for progression

These aspects of the practice supervisor role clearly indicate that it is a collaborative role, which is focused on students' learning competencies that are set jointly between healthcare providers and the partner HEI based on the NMC's standards for nursing and midwifery education. The NMC also indicates that all NMC registered nurses and midwives are capable of supervising students, serving as role models for safe and effective practice, and students may be supervised by other registered health and social care professionals as well. This is fine and a healthy multi-professional perspective, except it must be ascertained that the registrant from the other profession is fully proficient in their area of practice prior to teaching students. Additionally, each healthcare profession is distinct and different care professionals can be protective of their cognate areas, and therefore provide selective and superficial perspectives of their areas of competence. Furthermore, Fallender (2014) suggests that 'piecemeal' (p. 8) facilitation of students' learning risks being fractional and incomplete, and indicates that the role of supervision 'requires specific training'.

The characteristics of effective practice supervisors are examined later in this chapter (p. 21). However, Macneil (2001) highlights the significance of the impact of line managers as supervisors in enhancing informal facilitation of learning through their interpersonal skills to encourage a positive learning environment, with knowledge sharing within work teams. The principles of effective practice supervisor leadership, which also comprise being emotionally intelligent and resilient, are examined in fair detail in Chapter 5, and then in Chapter 7, where the qualities of a good supervisor are also identified.

Having analysed the nature of the concept of supervision and the practice supervisor role, we now explore further reasons for the role, in addition to that of facilitation of students' learning in practice settings.

RATIONALES FOR THE PRACTICE LEARNING SUPERVISOR ROLE

Not only is practice learning supervision a requirement for supporting learning for nursing and midwifery students, but also for students on more novel programmes such as student nursing associates, and apprenticeship students in nursing and allied health professions (Council of Deans of Health, 2017a; NMC, 2017a; Institute for Apprenticeships, 2016a), and on well-established programmes such as medical education. A more detailed examination of why we need practice supervisors for learners reveals a number of reasons for this.

ACTIVITY 1.2   WHY PRACTICE SUPERVISORS AND MENTORS?

The idea of this activity is to explore in more detail a wider range of reasons why practice supervisors are required in healthcare professionals' education. Therefore, consider and make notes on the question, What are the various reasons for which we need practice learning supervisors (and preceptors) in nursing, midwifery and allied health professions?

When students on the previous mentoring courses were asked to cite as many reasons as they could think of for requiring mentors, they tended to be able to identify several, almost all of which apply to today's practice supervisor role. The reasons given include the need to ensure safe practice by learners, to enable students to achieve their course practice competencies, and to listen and act as a sounding board for any worries or fears that students might have on care delivery. Further reasons cited for practice learning supervision in nursing, midwifery and AHPs are listed in the box below.

WHY WE NEED PRACTICE SUPERVISORS

In nursing and other health professions:

- for guidance and support
- to structure working environment for learning
- for constructive and honest feedback
- for debriefing related to good/bad experience during placement
- as a link person with other areas
- as a role model
- to monitor achievement of competencies
- as a friend and counsellor
- for encouragement
- to provide the appropriate knowledge base for nursing interventions
- for questioning
- for protection from poor practice
- to build confidence
- for sharing learning, i.e. learning from each other
- it is an NMC requirement
- to keep your own skills and knowledge up to date
- for linking theory to practice
- for developing one's work skills in teaching and explaining
- to provide structured learning programmes during practice placements

Personal mentorship also has various benefits, and is recommended. Furthermore, it could be argued that everyone could benefit from having a 'mentor' in their personal lives, at times referred to as a 'soulmate'. This privileged role is self-selected by both parties and could be fulfilled by a friend, partner, parent or senior peer.

One of the advantages of practice supervision is that students who have been on placement in the particular practice setting might apply for a post in that setting after qualifying, so it can have recruitment benefits. Furthermore, in healthcare and non-healthcare professions, mentoring has been implemented quite effectively, including management mentoring, as well as in social contexts. For instance, mentoring has worked successfully in initial teacher training (see, for example, Kerry and Mayes, 1995) for some time.

Barnett (2008: 3) also notes that mentoring new teachers results in benefits for the student teacher, as well as the mentor, whereupon the latter experiences professional stimulation and collaboration, personal fulfilment, friendship and support, motivation to remain current in one's field and networking opportunities; and benefits to the institution include more satisfied staff and greater scholarly productivity.

As for medical mentoring, this consists in a relationship that is confidential between two qualified doctors (Viney and McKimm, 2010), and is more akin to clinical supervision in nursing, midwifery and AHPs, which was explained earlier in this chapter.

Other than the benefits of practice learning supervision-type roles, it is useful to note that when nurse education moved into the higher education sector *en masse* during the 1980s and 1990s with the restructured Project 2000 pre-registration curricula and a change in emphasis in certain aspects, the findings of various research studies on those novel programmes documented the strengths of these programmes as well as weaknesses. One of the prominent findings was that at the point of registration students were not clinically as skilled as those who emerged from pre-Project 2000 programmes (e.g. Elkan and Robinson, 1995; Clark et al., 1997). This reinforced the need for wider availability of competent clinically based supervisors of learning to enable students to learn clinical skills 'in the real world' of nursing so that they are 'fit for practice' (as noted by the National Committee of Inquiry into Higher Education [NCIHE], 1997).

Furthermore, the findings of Kramer's (1974) study mentioned earlier indicated the need for preceptors for newly qualified nurses. The notion was extrapolated to pre-registration students and is also a reason for the introduction of mentors as a means of supporting student nurses with their learning during practice placements.

Another reason for practice learning supervision is stated in the codes of professional practice for nurses, doctors, social workers and AHPs, which usually indicate that qualified practitioners have a duty to teach and facilitate students' learning during practice placements so that students develop their competence under supervision (for example, NMC, 2015a: Clause 9.4). Similar requirements feature in healthcare professionals' job descriptions, which are also guided by the NHS Knowledge and Skills Framework (KSF) (NHS Employers, 2010). This is one of the reasons for the NMC arguing that all registrants can take the role of practice supervisor, following appropriate preparation for the role.

Practice supervision of course also provides registrants with opportunities to practise their teaching skills, which in itself is a feature of their own professional development and can constitute a stepping stone in their own career trajectories.

Yet another basis for practice supervision is the concept of work-based learning, which constitutes practice-based development of skills and (practical) knowledge. Its main features are reflected in the social learning theory that was advocated by Bandura (1996, 1997), and which centres on learning skills by observing skilled professionals perform them first. Social learning theory therefore also involves practice supervisors being role models and comprises a four-step process of learning (see Figure 1.1).

In more detail, the four processes of learning that the learner goes through are:

1. Observation of skilled performance

   o The individual observes a skilled performance ('modelling stimulus').
   o The observed behaviour is seen as useful and distinctive.
   o Observer's level of arousal pertaining to the skill is raised.
   o Observer is keen to learn the skill.
   o Observer has previously felt positive reinforcement for learning skills.

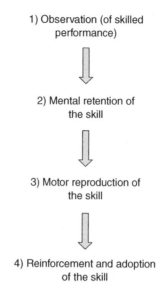

Figure 1.1   The four-step process of learning

2. Mental retention of the skill

   o   Step-by-step performance of the skill is mentally assimilated.
   o   Mental rehearsal of modelled behaviour.

3. Motor reproduction of the skill

   o   Observer carries out observed behaviour or skill and self-evaluates it in terms of performance.

4. Reinforcement and adoption of the skill

   o   The behaviour is reinforced by external reward such as praise or through self-reinforcement, and is likely to be adopted.

According to Bandura (1996), we do not possess any inherent behaviour patterns at birth except reflexes, and therefore learning occurs by observing other people, which is the essence of social learning theory and which therefore includes learning from social situations. In healthcare, learners (students and preceptees) learn and acquire practical skills by observing practice supervisors, and then following through the four processes identified in Figure 1.1.

Bandura's (1996) social learning theory had previously been termed 'observational learning' or 'modelling' and was built on behaviourist learning theory (see Chapter 2). It is a component of work-based learning, a concept that is examined in some detail in Chapter 4 in the context of learning in practice settings.

SUPERVISING STUDENTS TO LEARN MANAGEMENT AND LEADERSHIP

There is a requirement to institute management and leadership development for healthcare students on their final practice placement near the end of their course when, in addition to consolidating their care intervention skills, they also learn the practicalities of organising, managing and leading care in the practice setting (for example, NMC, 2010a, 2018b).

There have also been several endeavours to implement management coaching in various organisations, whereby trainee managers' learning is supervised by named highly experienced managers to enable those less experienced to develop their management skills (for example, Megginson et al., 2006; Brooke and Ham, 2003). A small number of healthcare professionals have had experience of management coaching, but this is a longer-term role than supervision of learning for pre-registration students on practice placement. The management coach role can initially involve advising the student to explore utilisation of particular management techniques and takes a more directive approach. Then, when the learner has developed substantial management skills, the role can become less directive; and much later coach–learner activities become more akin to those of 'buddies', i.e. equals.

As noted earlier in this chapter, clinical coaching has its benefits, and management coaching in healthcare entails guiding more junior registrants to develop their management and leadership skills, through one-to-one guidance and support that can enhance their organisational skills, as also noted by Coleman and Glover (2010). It also applies to more senior managers, such as the Executive Nurse, receiving coaching from independent appropriate personnel.

For finalist healthcare students, learning organisational skills entails taking charge of a small group of service users' care, for example those in a bay in a hospital ward, and manage all their care during one shift of work. Managing care involves dealing with changes in the service user's condition, delegating tasks to other members of staff, risk assessment, etc., and all under watch of their practice supervisor. Management activities that third-year students can learn have been identified by Gopee and Galloway (2017: 29), and include:

- delegation of duties
- supervising care delivery
- organising transfers of patient care
- receiving/giving reports on patient/service users care needs and progress
- working with multidisciplinary team (MDT) members
- doing the off-duty/facilitating self-rostering
- managing space, i.e. extra beds/patients on trolleys
- ensuring the health and safety of staff/patients/visitors.

For coaching, the GROW model (also referred to as: GROWing – which stands for Goal, Reality, Options, Will/Wrap up) is advocated (for example, Connor and

Pokora, 2012) as a framework for effective coaching. There are several other books on coaching, and short courses and modules are available from various organisations.

As should be obvious from the above reasons for the practice learning supervisor role, there are coincidentally also several possible benefits in undertaking the role, in addition to it being an NMC (2018a) requirement.

WHO CAN BE A PRACTICE SUPERVISOR?

Practice learning supervision is required for student nurses, student midwives and AHP students, the common goals for all being to facilitate practice-based learning for healthcare students. It is also required for nursing associates, medical students and students on various other healthcare profession programmes.

However, despite all the reasons for the practice supervisor role discussed so far, it should not be presumed that all qualified healthcare professionals wish to undertake practice supervision work, for all or even some of the time. Some healthcare professionals feel that continual allocation of students to them all year round can be detrimental to their own effectiveness with their workloads, and they would like some space for reflection and to focus on their own professional development.

In the selection of practice supervisors, it is important to ensure that healthcare professionals have the motivation and the necessary skills and expertise for the facilitation of students' learning in practice settings, which include establishing an effective working relationship, coaching, giving feedback, maintaining standards and continuous assessment. Other writers and researchers identify similar lists of skills. Such lists initially appear simplistic but a whole range of micro-skills are required to undertake the practice supervisor role, and this can usually be developed through appropriate educational preparation followed by experience.

The NMC (2018a) indicates that practice supervisors have to undergo preparation for the role, whereby HEIs together with practice learning partners must ensure that practice supervisors have an understanding of the proficiencies and programme outcomes they are supporting students to achieve, and that they should receive ongoing appropriate support for effective supervision and contribution to student learning, and assessment. Nursing and midwifery students can be supervised in practice by NMC registered nurses, midwives, nursing associates or other registered health and social care professionals.

SYSTEMATIC SUPERVISION OF LEARNING IN PRACTICE SETTINGS

A number of factors need to be considered to ensure a comprehensive and systematic approach to supervision of practice-based learning. This section therefore considers supervisory relationships, supervisor–learner communication (including specialist communication skills), the attributes of effective practice supervisors and a number of ways in which they enable learning, including role modelling.

In a systematic review of supervision of practice-based learning, Jokelainen et al. (2011) concluded that the activity comprises two main themes. These are, first, facilitating student learning and, second, strengthening students' professionalism (professional attributes and identities). Four subthemes were identified as well as a number of categories under each sub-theme. Therefore, practice supervision activities incorporate a number of factors that enable effective student learning, which include establishing effective working relationships, creating an environment for learning, evaluation of learning during the practice placement, etc'.

Of primary significance is the need to establish an effective supervisor–student relationship, which encompasses the multiple concerted ways by which such relationships are developed and maintained, including continuing effective supervisor–student communication, the personal characteristics of practice supervisors and the actions that they take to support learning.

EFFECTIVE SUPERVISORY RELATIONSHIPS

In a study conducted by Johansson et al. (2010) to measure the quality of teaching and learning in practice settings, it emerged that the supervisory relationship between practice learning supervisor and learner is the most important factor contributing to effective clinical learning experiences, as also found by Bennett et al. (2012) and others. Eller et al.'s (2014) study of effective supervisor–student relationships concluded that there are eight components to this, including open communication and accessibility, mutual respect and trust, and role modelling.

'Establishing effective working relationships' is one of the areas in which practice supervisors have to be competent to enable students to integrate into practice settings and to support practice-based learning. However, for two individuals who are usually initially unknown to each other, adopting the supervisor–learner roles presupposes that they are able to communicate with each other, develop a rapport and cultivate a 'working' relationship at the very least. The word *rapport* means 'a sympathetic relationship or understanding' or 'a close and harmonious relationship in which the people or groups concerned understand each other's feelings or ideas and communicate well' (e.g. Brookes and O'Neill, 2017: 778); and *relationship* refers to 'the dealings or feelings that exist between people or groups' and 'an emotional association between two people' (e.g. Brookes and O'Neill, 2017: 790).

So how are relationships formed between the two designated parties? According to Rogers and Freiberg (1994), counsellors and helpers build a trusting and working relationship by ensuring first of all that certain key conditions prevail. These conditions are:

- *acceptance (or unconditional positive regard)* – of the individual for who they are (for example, for their individual strengths and weaknesses) and through mutual respect

- *genuineness* – as a person, honesty
- *empathic understanding* – being able and willing to view situations from the other person's perspectives.

These key conditions are explored in some detail in the context of student-centred learning in Chapter 3. Rogers and Freiberg (1994) emphasise that 'trust' underpins these key conditions, which they suggest in reality permeates all mutually beneficial relationships. It is akin to a 'psychological contract' between the practice supervisor and learner, or between unwell person and carer, or colleagues and friends. The two parties also have to be willing to spend time together to maintain this relationship and to work towards the achievement of practice objectives, for instance. Although the learner has to actively seek out relevant learning opportunities, the practice supervisor also needs to take actions that support the learner's learning, by for example familiarising themselves adequately with the student's educational programme. For research on how practice supervisors and learners develop trust in each other, see Hauer et al. (2015) noted under the Further Optional Reading section of this chapter.

EFFECTIVE SUPERVISOR–LEARNER COMMUNICATION

The skills and techniques of effective communication are some of the most important tools the practitioner undertaking the practice supervisor role has to utilise. The healthcare professional should already be a skilled communicator in healthcare settings through initial educational preparation, and therefore it is important to establish which other communication techniques they need to develop in order to extend their skill base. Effective communication skills are essential within all teaching and learning situations.

Various modes of communication are available to the practice supervisor to choose from, including:

- written, for example handwritten, typed, emailed, faxed, printed, as a text message
- oral (spoken), for example face-to-face, one-to-one, in groups, by telephone
- non-verbal, for example body posture, eye contact, tone of voice.

Oral (spoken) communication is always accompanied by non-verbal messages, vocal and non-vocal. In fact, non-verbal hues (or cues) are more powerful than verbal messages. Furthermore, Argyle (1994) suggests that non-verbal signals of a friendly attitude (as opposed to an unfriendly attitude) are:

- *proximity*: closer, leaning forward if seated
- *orientation*: more direct, but side-to-side for some situations
- *gaze*: more gaze for each other, and mutual gaze

- *facial expression*: more smiling
- *gestures*: head nods, lively movements
- *posture*: open arms stretched towards each other rather than arms on hips or folded
- *touch*: more touch in an appropriate manner
- *tone of voice*: higher pitch, upward contour, pure tone
- *verbal contents*: more self-disclosure.

After reflecting on a former framework for non-verbal communication referred to as SOLER (which stands for: 'sit squarely'; 'open posture'; 'lean towards the other'; 'eye contact'; 'relax'), Stickley (2011) suggests that the framework (or model) can be enhanced by using the acronym SURETY (which stands for 'sit at an angle'; 'uncross legs and arms'; 'relax'; 'eye contact'; 'touch'; 'your intuition'). This latter model incorporates the function of touch as a means of non-verbal communication and intuition. Normal communication processes, however, are often presented as the information processing theory in the context of cognitive learning theory, which is discussed in Chapter 2.

GENERIC AND SPECIALIST COMMUNICATION SKILLS

Increasingly widely utilised is the SBAR (situation – background – assessment – recommendation) framework or technique for effective communication in various clinical situations, from patient handover to during crises. From a literature review of SBAR as a tool for communicating patient care information, Stewart and Hand (2017) conclude that it creates a common professional language for healthcare communication and improves efficiency, efficacy and accuracy of communication, and consequently patient safety.

In addition to general communication skills, the practice supervisor is likely to benefit from developing specialist communication skills to manage more complex learner issues. Scammell (1990) suggests a communication continuum that spans generic communication at one end to specialist communication at the other, with the associated specific purposes and specific skills for each component on the continuum. These components and their associated purposes and skills are as follows:

• Primary communications	*Purpose*: initial contacts with others; brief encounters *Skill*: simple interpersonal or social skills, e.g. ability to listen, etc.
• Secondary communications	*Purpose*: ongoing relationships – verbal, non-verbal, written; informal support groups *Skill*: interpersonal or social skills, knowledge of how groups work, etc.

(Continued)

(Continued)

• Advice giving	*Purpose*: to offer factual information; to teach, instruct, supervise *Skill*: when to give advice, ability to impart knowledge of subject area, etc.
• Primary counselling	*Purpose*: support for friend or work colleague *Skill*: listen non-judgementally, help with problem-solving, etc.
• Secondary counselling	*Purpose*: therapeutic counselling for specific mental health problems *Skill*: advanced accurate empathy, self-disclosure, etc.

Primary and secondary communication occurs between practice supervisor and learner when exchanging information and establishing a working relationship. Beyond this level, the practice supervisor may need to give direct advice to the student, especially when teaching, as well as when advice is requested. This, however, does not go as far as counselling, for which the individual requires more extensive training.

Primary counselling is a specialised communication skill that the practice supervisor needs to develop to deal with difficult practice supervision situations. Secondary counselling will be required for more intense psychological or behavioural issues, which the practice supervisor can deal with by directing the student to appropriate support services, or, if trained, by using a systematic approach such as Heron's (2009) six-category intervention analysis (see the box below).

THE SIX-CATEGORY INTERVENTION ANALYSIS AS A SPECIALISED COMMUNICATION SKILL

Authoritative intervention

- Prescriptive: giving advice
- Informative: imparting information
- Confrontational: directly challenging

Facilitative intervention

- Supportive: understanding and encouraging
- Cathartic: allowing the release of emotions
- Catalytic: encouraging deeper exploration

Heron's (2009) six-category intervention analysis therefore entails six possible actions that the counsellor can choose from. In difficult supervisor–student situations, for every interaction the practice supervisor may decide which of the six categories is most appropriate. For instance, for a student who frequently claims to be feeling unwell, physically or psychologically, the practice supervisor might use the prescriptive category of helping, and advise the student to consult the occupational health department. They might also give further information about where the department is, and the likely outcomes of this situation. In other situations, the practice supervisor might use another one of the categories, for example cathartic, to enable the learner to elaborate in detail how they feel about a patient whom they have looked after but who has passed away rather suddenly, for instance.

Ways in which the practice supervisor can usefully apply Heron's model of intervention towards their students are also discussed in Chapter 7.

CHARACTERISTICS AND ROLES OF EFFECTIVE PRACTICE SUPERVISORS

In addition to effective communication skills and the ability to form effective supervisor–student relationships, various researchers have examined the characteristics and roles of mentors that play crucial parts in enabling the learner's learning during practice placements.

CHARACTERISTICS OF PRACTICE SUPERVISORS

ACTIVITY 1.3   ATTRIBUTES OF AN EFFECTIVE PRACTICE SUPERVISOR

Make a list of what you consider to be the characteristics or personal attributes of a registrant who is effective in their practice supervision role for either undergraduate or postgraduate students. Consider their characteristics from such perspectives as personal qualities, approach/actions and skills.

Henricson et al.'s (2018) identify research supervisors as having to be able to coach, to be well-read and knowledgeable, and to collaborate with the research student as well as research colleagues. Responding to Activity 1.3 must have been straightforward, as all healthcare professionals who have undertaken pre-registration programmes that included practice placements will have encountered practice-based learning supervisors (e.g. practice educators) who support learning. Some supervisors may have been excellent, while there might have been reservations about others. Most of the characteristics identified by groups of post-registration students, which also apply to practice supervisors, are listed in the box below.

CHARACTERISTICS OF THE PERSON WHO IS AN EFFECTIVE PRACTICE SUPERVISOR

- Patient
- Open-minded
- Approachable
- Has a good knowledge base
- Knowledge and competence is up to date
- Has good communication skills, including listening skills
- Provides encouragement
- Is self-motivated
- Shows concern, compassion, empathy
- Has teaching skills
- Provides psychological support
- Counsellor
- Tactful
- Diplomatic, fun and fair
- Willing to supervise students' learning, and continuous assessment
- Versatile, adaptable, flexible
- Allows time and commits self to it
- Confident
- Enthusiastic
- Advisor
- Is honest and trustworthy
- Trusting
- A role model
- Non-judgemental
- Resource facilitator
- Able to build working relationship

From their concept analysis of mentoring, Hodgson and Scanlan (2013) identified the characteristics of effective mentors as: approachable, knowledgeable, honest, friendly, patient, experienced and enthusiastic; willing to spend time with the student; having a strong belief in the student's capability; they challenge, support and encourage a learner, but also expect the learner to be willing to learn; they are career committed, competent and have strong self-identity and initiative. Both above sets of characteristics or personal attributes also apply to the effective practice supervisor.

ROLES OF PRACTICE SUPERVISORS IN ENABLING LEARNING

In addition to personal attributes, other researchers have explored the 'roles' of mentors, which refers to the actions that they take to enable or facilitate learners' learning. Deducing from an earlier substantial study on various aspects of mentoring, Darling (1984) identified 14 roles that enable learning, which also apply to the practice supervisor role. These roles are being a:

- role model
- energiser
- envisioner
- investor
- supporter
- standard-prodder
- teacher–coach
- feedback giver
- eye-opener
- door-opener
- ideas bouncer
- problem solver
- career counsellor
- challenger.

Taking a broader perspective, Hall et al. (2008) explored teacher mentors' perceptions of their role in teacher training in the USA and found that it comprises nine roles and responsibilities for supporting learning of individuals engaged in teacher training, which includes being a coach, a counsellor and a source of advice.

Additionally, Health Education England (HEE) (2015) identifies six values that it sees as being fundamental to the accountability and responsibilities of supervisors of practice-based learning. These values are also essential for healthcare professionals in the new practice supervisor role, and they are:

1. ambassador
2. illuminator and reflector
3. broker of learning
4. professional role model
5. energiser
6. promoter of standards.

ACTIVITY 1.4   ASCERTAINING THE PRACTICE SUPERVISOR'S CHARACTERISTICS POTENTIAL

Consider HEE's (2015) or Darling's (1984) roles of the mentor and identify situations from the past when you were in practice supervisor-type roles, or likely to be in the near future.

- For each value or role, do a self-rating of yourself using the numbers 1 to 4, with 1 indicating development or learning need and 4 indicating skilled.
- Next, focus on one or two of the roles on which you rate yourself as low, and consider why this is (e.g. lack of opportunity), and how you can develop your competence in that role.

The above exercise based on roles was referred to by Darling (1984) as 'Measuring Mentorship Potential'. Other mentorship capability tools, or criteria, have been developed since then for different professions (e.g. by Chan et al., 2017). Most of these tools refer to concepts akin to being a role model for practice in the specific field. As importantly, the practice supervisor has to be a role model of teaching, and in healthcare the practice supervisor has to be a role model in care delivery as well.

Each of these roles can be explored in detail as a concept in its own right, and to illustrate this we will explore below the features of being a role model in the section on 'practice supervisors' actions to support learning', after first considering the role of being a 'challenger and supporter' (both roles were identified by Darling, 1984).

CHALLENGES AND SUPPORT FOR LEARNERS

During their practice placements students are likely to encounter service user care situations that they find challenging, and other situations that they will find much less challenging, especially in the latter part of their pre-registration programme as they acquire various clinical skills. How much of the support role identified by Darling should the practice supervisor exercise towards the student when the latter encounters very challenging situations?

REFLECTION POINT 1.1:   LEARNING SUPERVISION SUPPORT AND CHALLENGE

Consider the practice supervisor's roles as challenger and supporter' and think of patient care situations (or clinical interventions) in your workplace that, say, a second-year student will find highly challenging, and others that will be much less challenging. Often practice supervisors have to comment on the level of initiative that their students have shown. So, think for yourself (or discuss with a peer) what level of support you would provide to your student if the student encounters highly challenging service user care situations.

What is the result if the student consistently encounters situations that are of 'low challenge' to them?

Of course, students have to be supervised all the time, either directly or from a distance. There are various examples of situations that present high or low challenges for learners in practice settings, and the level of support required. Asking a third-year student nurse consistently to perform clinical skills for which they have already been signed as competent would provide a lesser challenge to them, and lesser support might be required. But if the same student has not yet learnt how to provide care in epidural pain control, for instance, or catheterisation, then this would present a higher challenge and the student is likely to need a fair level of support.

Daloz (1989) explored the effects of different levels of challenge and of support, and concluded that high challenge and high support can lead to growth and achievement of aspirations (or vision), while low support and low challenge can result in stasis and apathy. However, high challenge and low support, according to Daloz's findings, leads to 'retreat and burnout' (see Figure 1.2).

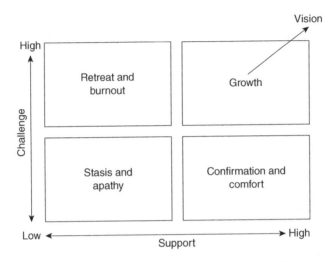

Figure 1.2   Effects of support and challenge on the learner's development

Source: Daloz, 1989

PRACTICE SUPERVISORS' ACTIONS TO SUPPORT LEARNING

The roles and responsibilities of the effective practice supervisor can be regularly researched to ascertain the more contemporary nature and perceptions of this function. Carnwell et al. (2007) explored NHS and HEI managers' perceptions of learning support roles. They found that the primary requirement in clinical practice, that is their primary skills, comprise of clinical expertise, teaching clinical skills and student support; and their primary focus is the individual student, that is student supervision. However, they also identified potential for role conflict, particularly if the supervisor has qualified only relatively recently and therefore is still developing their own repertoire of clinical skills.

No doubt a range of components that support learning can be identified. One of the key functions of the practice supervisor is to help the student integrate into the practice setting, which entails managing the practice placement, receiving the student and conducting initial, mid-placement and final interviews, which are

ACTIVITY 1.5   PRACTICE SUPERVISOR ACTIONS THAT SUPPORT LEARNING

In addition to having the characteristics of an effective practice supervisor, think of and make a list of a number of actions that practice supervisors can take to support learning.

supported by the use of learning contracts or learning agreements. 'Acceptance' of the student (Rogers and Freiberg, 1994) signifies that the practice supervisor accepts the student for their current levels of knowledge and competence, which may be either extensive or minimal.

As for managing the placement, designated practice supervisors may have been nominated before the student starts on the placement and would need self-preparation time beforehand to ensure they understand what the role requires of them. Time would also have been set aside for receiving the student and introducing them to the care team.

Seeing the practice placement from a student's viewpoint suggests that they might be experiencing different feelings in anticipation of the placement. They are likely to appreciate any prior information sent to them, which might include any preparatory reading that the student can do. On the first day, they tend to appreciate an introduction to the practice setting, making them feel comfortable about learning, a professional but friendly environment, student involvement and continuity of practice supervisor. These perspectives are consistent with 'empathic understanding', which is a key condition of effective working relationships identified by Rogers and Freiberg (1994).

Furthermore, the NMC (2018c) and the National Nursing Research Unit (King's College London, 2014) have identified the need for protected time (referred to as 'supported learning time' by the NMC, 2018c: 9), but this has consistently proved difficult to access (e.g. RCN, 2016: 11).

THE PRACTICE SUPERVISOR AS THE ROLE MODEL

Various research studies indicate that practice-based supervisors of learning should be role models for their students (for example, Darling, 1984; Jack et al., 2017).

REFLECTION POINT 1.2:   A ROLE MODEL

Consider the terms 'model' and 'modelling'. Next, consider what a role model is. Consider also why healthcare professionals need to be role models, who else for, and what it is about a person that makes him or her a role model.

In response to Reflection Point 1.2, you might have felt that healthcare professionals who are role models are those who provide holistic, and safe and effective, care and clinical interventions, and to the highest standard. They should, however, also be role models as organisers of care, as evidence-based practitioners and as teachers, albeit within the parameters of their post.

As with most nascent and tentative concepts, a concept analysis or a STEP (social, technological, economic and political) analysis can enable further clarification of the concept, and a systematic understanding of various facets and components of the concept. Alternatively, a SWOT (strengths, weaknesses, opportunities and threats) analysis can be undertaken. Such an analysis can help the individual decide whether any problem-solving, avoidance or developmental actions need to be taken.

ACTIVITY 1.6 STEP ANALYSIS OF ROLE MODEL

Using the headings 'social', 'technological', 'economic' and 'political', conduct a STEP analysis of 'the practice supervisor as a role model'.

Being a role model is a feature of Bandura's (1997) social learning theory, which stipulates that substantial learning occurs as a result of observation of appropriate professionals, which is appropriate for healthcare students as they learn substantial clinical intervention skills working with qualified professionals in healthcare settings, which is also consistent with 'work-based learning', which is discussed in Chapter 4.

There can, however, also be bad role models, that is, those whose behaviour reflects how *not* to come over as a healthcare professional. Bad role models can therefore not be seen as a model at all, considering what the word 'model' means. A role model is 'a person regarded by others as a good example to follow' (Brookes and O'Neill, 2017: 810), that is, someone whose practice standards, attitudes and beliefs can be emulated by the observer. Individuals choose their role models, such as someone who is good at time management, at self-organisation or at how they interact with colleagues.

Donaldson and Carter (2005) report on an evaluation of the perceptions of undergraduate students on role modelling within the clinical learning environment. They indicate that students stressed the importance of good role models whose competence they could observe and practise. Constructive feedback was needed on their practice from their role models to develop their competence and build up their confidence, and to convert observed behaviour into their own behaviour and skill set.

Faugier (2005a) suggests that role models are those whom we look up to, emulate and admire as professionals, but in society in general, she suggests, people base their character identities, values and lifestyles on celebrities and characters in television programmes. All teachers in the practice setting (for example, practice supervisors) should therefore be aware of their impact as role models on students' learning of skills and professional attitudes, but there are mixed views about nurses being role models of healthy habits when off duty. However, a certain level of self-awareness of one's public behaviour should keep their credibility as role models intact.

RESEARCH IDENTIFYING POOR LEARNING SUPERVISION IN CARE SETTINGS

A common experience in nursing in the twenty-first century has been that nurses working in many practice settings feel that they are managing their workload with ongoing staffing constraints. Indeed, Phillips et al.'s (2000) research concluded that mentors have been fulfilling this role as one of several other roles they have during any normal span of duty. Despite 'protected time' for facilitating students' practice-based learning having been advocated for approximately two decades, the implementation of this mechanism has remained slow for many, mainly due to multiple demands on their time. More recently, a study at King's College London (2014) found that such issues persist.

Furthermore, practice supervision can become problematic when several supervisors are allocated to one student while they also have responsibility for providing care to one or more service users, and are likely to be dealing with various other work responsibilities. There is a risk that the student's learning experience can consequently become fragmented and superficial, and the student is left with several service user-related queries. The supervisor–student relationship can thereby also be affected negatively. When working within these constraints, knowingly or unknowingly, the practice supervisor could be taking (or omitting) actions that could result in discouraging learning.

ACTIVITY 1.7   HOW THE PRACTICE SUPERVISOR MIGHT DISCOURAGE LEARNING

Think of, and make notes on, a range of actions on the part of practice supervisors that, deliberately or not, may be seen as discouraging or hindering learning.

The following case study presents an example of recent poor supervision of practice-based learning.

CASE STUDY 1.1: POOR SUPERVISION OF PRACTICE-BASED LEARNING

Mel Alexis is a second-year student nurse on a rehabilitation ward. One day she finished her shift early, having told the staff nurse in charge that she had a terrible headache, while in fact she was extremely upset regarding her placement.

That morning she had felt that the staff nurse had spoken to her in a very unprofessional manner, as she does to patients as well. This is what bothered Mel the most. She also challenged the staff nurse over her drug administration that morning. A patient was left her morning medication in a pot on the table but was unable to swallow it as she needed assistance due to her having a weak side and problems with her other hand. As Mel walked past the patient's room, the patient called her and indicated that she had not taken her tablets yet. As Mel was not the nurse who administered the drugs, she called the nurse to the room for her to administer the medication. The nurse said that she did not have time to do this but the tablets were correct for the patient.

Mel agreed to assist in giving the medication but noticed three tablets lying on the table beside the pot. Mel asked the nurse what these tablets were and she was advised they were morning medications as well. Mel doubted this as they were not in the medicine pot and asked the nurse why they were not in the pot, but the latter did not give an answer and instead picked them up and put them into the pot. The nurse then told Mel to assist with the medications and Mel made it clear that she did not feel that the medications were correct, as there seemed to be more tablets than the patient usually took in the morning. The nurse told Mel not to question her drug administration, so Mel felt that she had no choice but to assist the patient in taking the drugs.

This event highlighted Mel's unhappiness with this ward. She had started feeling like this on day one, when she was not introduced to any staff members or shown around. She had had to find things out for herself during her time on this ward and if she asked where something was, the staff said it would be quicker for them to get the item themselves rather than show Mel. As a second-year nurse, she was expecting to do many nursing activities but instead she felt that she was being treated like a support worker. Although Mel loves providing basic nursing care to patients, she expected a lot more out of this placement than she was actually achieving. Mel appreciates that on a rehabilitation ward nursing takes on a different role, but she feels that she has yet to see what this role is.

Mel says she has always wanted to be a nurse and really loves the job, but this ward has now made her question this and it makes her very sad to feel like this.

In response to Activity 1.7, you may have felt that one of the problems that students have experienced in the past is the lack of opportunities to work with their practice learning supervisors. Actions on the part of practice supervisors that can discourage learning which you might have thought of are:

- lack of interest in students and in their learning needs
- lack of knowledge about the student's course
- lack of evidence-based practice or research utilisation
- hierarchical mindset, and a lack of team approach
- not acknowledging the student's previous experience

- negative attitudes
- reluctant to change practice.

There is a possibility that you have yourself witnessed poor supervision of learning, directly or indirectly. Earlier research has identified personality characteristics of practice-based learning supervisors that discourage learning. For instance, Darling's (1985) qualitative study revealed what she termed the characteristics of the 'galaxy of toxic mentors' (see Table 1.1).

Table 1.1   The 'galaxy of toxic mentors' (or practice supervisors)

Types	Features
Avoiders	Practice supervisors who are not available or accessible, also referred to as 'ignorers' or 'non-responders'
Dumpers	Throw people into new roles or situations and let them flounder, or let them 'sink or swim,' often deliberately
Blockers	Actively avoid meeting the learner's needs by refusing requests, by controlling through withholding information, or by blocking the learner's development by over-supervising
Destroyers/Criticisers	Set out to destroy the learner by subtle attacks to undermine confidence, and open and public verbal attacks and arguments, questioning the learner's abilities and deliberately destroying confidence

The types of activities and demeanour identified by Darling in Table 1.1 are referred to by Proctor (2011: 26) as 'oppressive supervisor behaviour'. Based on extensive experience in management and decision-making, Heirs and Farrell (1986) explored the mindsets of individual employees who enable an organisation to progress with its aims, and those of people who block such development. While the focus is on looking for, and developing, 'talents' in junior employees, in reality the mindset of some employees can stifle development of juniors and learners. The researchers grouped the problematic or disabling traits of those who block development as 'three mental poisons', in terms of the functioning of rigid minds, ego minds and Machiavellian minds (see box). Such ways of thinking are not always obvious, nor easily detected, but do affect learning adversely.

RIGID MINDS, EGO MINDS AND MACHIAVELLIAN MINDS

The rigid mind:

- Personal values are set or stereotyped
- Unable to see the positiveness in others' thoughts if they conflict with their own thinking

- Continually blocks the openness of more creative thinking
- Loyal to traditional thinking and rejects novelty
- Appears to lack imagination or creativity
- Stifles use of originality and encourages complacency

The ego mind:

- Sees elements of a problem only in terms of self-interest and self-importance
- Fairly ambitious and has a high opinion of own abilities
- Looks after number one to the exclusion of other considerations
- Pays little attention to what others think and say
- Unsociable and does not contribute to collective thinking
- Will betray colleagues and even the organisation if it serves his or her ends

The Machiavellian mind:

- Quickly sees the range of likely outcomes of any decision
- Manipulates the feelings and ambitions of others to deceive
- Devious and calculating
- Intimidates and engages in politicking
- Perpetuates worry in the organisation and perpetually currying favour with superiors
- Scheming, cunning and suspicious of subordinates

Source: Heirs and Farrell (1986)

Furthermore, Gray and Smith (2000) conducted a study to explore students' experiences of practice placements, and found that whilst effective and good supervision of learning did prevail, the majority of students also experienced learning-inhibiting activities of some healthcare professionals in supervisory roles: lacking in knowledge and expertise, having poor teaching skills, delegating unwanted jobs to students, breaking promises and intimidating the students.

ACTIVITY 1.8   PRACTICE SUPERVISORS WHO DISCOURAGE LEARNING

Discuss with a peer or in a small group why any practice supervisor might behave in the negative ways described by Darling or Gray and Smith. Discuss also if and how such behaviours can be changed.

Darling (1985) makes a number of suggestions on how to deal with 'toxic' mentors. For instance, the student can try to keep the relationship with the practice supervisor balanced by building a support network with other students or registrants within the team and drawing on his or her own personal strengths (for instance, problem-solving skills). However, line managers are often aware of practice supervisors who under-perform, and conversely Heirs and Farrell (1986) suggest that it is the responsibility of the organisation's managers to identify employees who block development and learning. 'Poisonous' thinking endures but can be changed gradually through formal and informal meetings. Decisions about delegation of responsibilities and roles need to be applied selectively and overseen with appropriate intensity or freedom.

At times, practice supervisors may be ineffective because of a lack of detailed knowledge of their student's educational programme (their course), regarding which the PEF should be able to advise. Other action that can be taken when ineffective supervision is detected is to implement co-supervision, which involves two or more practice supervisors jointly supervising the student's learning. Temporary non-allocation of a student to the ineffective practice supervisor is another alternative that might work. Managers can formally or informally ask the practice supervisor how well they feel they are fulfilling their practice supervision role. The line manager may be able to confront the ineffective practice supervisor if poor learning supervision has been observed, or a complaint received. There can be other alternative strategies, but they will be dependent on local circumstances. Ethical aspects of poor supervision of practice learning are discussed in Chapter 7.

APPROACHES, MODELS, FRAMEWORKS FOR EFFECTIVE PRACTICE SUPERVISION

Despite the multiplicity of likely practice supervisor behaviours that could inhibit learning, practice supervision roles constitute a necessary mechanism for supporting learning in healthcare professions. Due to the humane, personal and suffering-prevention nature of healthcare provision, professional education programmes need to be appropriately structured and carefully monitored. Practice supervision of students must also be a structured exercise, as discussed earlier in this chapter. An appropriate combination of directive and facilitative approaches may be adopted, depending on the knowledge and competence that the student displays.

The underlying principles on which practice supervisors base their role vary according to the personal beliefs and approaches of the individual towards the role, and about student learning, and therefore determine their approach to the role and the model of supervision that they utilise.

The differences between the terms *approach*, *model* and *framework* are as follows. 'Approach' to practice supervision is personal to the individual and is based on his or her own life and professional experiences, and personal views and beliefs. It would therefore depend on the practice supervisor's beliefs about nursing, about undergraduate course design, about student and learner populations and their styles of learning.

A 'model', however, can be defined as a research-deduced, and therefore informed, set of interrelated components that enable the activity to be addressed comprehensively. A 'framework' takes this further, whereby the components of the model are utilised as sections or headings for planning and implementing the activity and may even have been empirically tested.

All three perspectives indicate a well thought-out and systematic approach to the student's placement experience to make it optimally effective. Very few frameworks for mentoring in healthcare have been available, and even fewer for supervision of learning. Darling's (1984) roles of the mentor constitute such a model, the NMC's (2008) eight-domain standards for mentoring are another, and HEE's (2015) values are yet another. For supervision of learning, it is important to examine other approaches and models of practice supervision that are available, such as those identified in Table 1.2, including the CLiP model, which is a novel model of nursing and midwifery mentorship. When using the CLiP model, a clinical educator supports and coaches students, acts as a source of expert advice in such circumstances as underachieving students, etc., and is visible to actively contribute to the ward learning environment (Health Education East of England, 2014: 7).

Table 1.2   Approaches and models of practice learning supervision

Collaborative Learning in Practice (CLiP) model	Entails appointing a 'clinical educator' to guide practice-based learning
Apprenticeship or coaching model	The practice supervisor is a skilled crafts person, and the learner learns by following instructions provided by the supervisor
Reflective practitioner model	Based on learning theories, e.g. andragogy, styles of learning and student-centred approaches, the practice supervisor is a critical friend and co-enquirer
Competence-based model	The practice supervisor enables students to learn specific practice objectives, and monitors and records their progress
Team practice supervision	A team of designated practice supervisors oversee one or more students' learning (as recommended by Phillips et al. [2000] for example), which is also applied to team supervision for doctorate students
Contract supervision	Formal supervision of learning that is time- or objectives-restricted for both supervisee and supervisor, e.g. when on practice placement at another institution
Dissertation supervision	For academic supervision of student's dissertation
Personal coaching	A natural, mutual and self-chosen, one-to-one coaching relationship that can usually be terminated by mutual decision

The approaches and models of supervision of learning identified on Table 1.2 can all be adopted or adapted for practice supervision as found most suitable locally. As indicated previously, the practice supervisor role is novel, and as yet there is a dearth of research on the topic area, and therefore a lack of frameworks or models. However, recently, following on from an RCN-commissioned project exploring mentorship models outside the UK, the RCN (2016) identified three non-UK models, and several other different 'approaches' prevailing in the UK. The three non-UK models, which are notably insufficiently researched, as different from the one-to-one model that has prevailed in the UK, are:

> *Real Life Learning Wards* (Amsterdam model): involves team-based mentoring and students are given responsibility for patient care early in the placement.

> *Dedicated Education Units* (USA and Australia): also involves team-mentoring, but with extra focus on creating a positive learning environment.

> *Clinical Facilitation Model* (Australia): the facilitator assesses the student, but their learning is facilitated by other registered nurses and by student 'buddying'.

In these models, there is more than one student per supervisor of learning. The RCN (2016: 18–19) acknowledges these models and identifies other relatively tentative variations of them, such as coaching, associate mentors and peer-mentoring, lead mentor, etc. In their systematic review of practice education, Jayasekara et al. (2018) found that dedicated education units and 'collaborative clinical placement' models result in enhanced engagement by students and constitute more effective learning environments. In the former model the supervisor receives additional payment for the role, and the latter incorporates joint university–healthcare organisation appointments.

There are also other forms of supervision of practice-based learning, which include shadowing, inter-professional supervision, e-supervision, etc. which are concepts and activities that are transferable, and suggest flexibility as alternative forms of practice supervision. Electronic or e-supervision can be implemented successfully, whereupon the supervisor and the student communicate entirely via their computers and similar devices. Of course, internet-based mentoring (e-mentoring) is not a new concept as its feasibility has been demonstrated for some time, including by Whiting and de Janasz (2004).

With e-supervision, Bear and Jones (2016) researched factors that influence satisfaction with an internet-based practitioner–student learning relationship in which the business studies student participates in choosing their supervisor, and found that satisfaction with the supervisory relationship correlates with trust in the practice supervisor. Consequently, students view their practice supervisor as a role model, and there is a clear understanding of the objectives of the supervision during practice placement (internship).

Long-arm or distant supervision is yet another form of learning supervision that tends to prevail primarily in certain areas of primary and social care where the practice supervisor would not generally be based at the same healthcare site as the student, and yet all criteria and activities constituting effective practice supervision are fulfilled.

ACTIVITY 1.9   APPLICATION OF APPROACHES
AND MODELS OF PRACTICE SUPERVISION

In your own experience of practice learning supervision activities, which of the approaches, models or frameworks referred to in the above sections apply to learning professional skills in your own practice setting, and why? Which ones suit you most? Make some notes.

The apprenticeship model, which is akin to coaching, applies more to the training of support workers, in that an apprentice often learns skills and crafts at the level of task performance, along with the necessary associated practical knowledge, unlike the holistic psycho-bio-social approach taken by nurses and midwives. Johnson (2017) endeavoured to constitute an apprenticeship model of learning supervision based on Bandura's (1997) model of development of self-efficacy, but concluded that the latter covers an insufficient range of concepts for effective supervision of learning for healthcare students.

The reflective practitioner approach is one that is frequently favoured within health profession circles, whereby practice supervisors take a less directive approach to their practice-based teaching. The competence model might also apply, but the reader needs to be aware of varying definitions of the term 'competence'. Some definitions see competence as the ability to perform a skill in accordance with agreed procedures and incorporate practical knowledge, while others see it as including theoretical knowledge as well.

Most of the models and approaches presented in Table 1.2 are not frameworks for practice supervision, although they can constitute systematic, comprehensive and often self-styled ways of supporting practice learning. They are also relatively recent concepts that await further empirical exploration or testing. Furthermore, there are also instances when students and practice supervisors could mutually select each other for their respective roles for facilitation, guidance, assistance and support with student learning. The notion that students can select their practice supervisor also has currency in some situations, such as if one of the members of the learning supervision team's job changes at short notice, or when the student is asked to select a supervisor from the practice supervision team.

Peer-supervision (or peer-teaching) is another emerging model of learning supervision, and Gilmour et al. (2007), for example, report on a highly successful peer-teaching programme in which second-year student nurses oversee first-year students' learning as they embark on their pre-registration university courses. Increasingly, the value of peer-learning supervision is being recognised and the concept implemented (e.g. RCN, 2016: 11, 18).

However, we need to be aware of previously noted shortcomings of peer-teaching and peer-learning in professional practice (peer-teaching also being a component of the CLiP model of practice learning) whence we were advised to guard against the likelihood of senior students passing on poor practice to junior students, and possibly an incorrect knowledge base. Johnson (2017: 17) suggests that one of the risks of peer-teaching is that past mistakes are likely to be repeated even after qualifying, when the individual is no longer closely supervised and consequently the quality of care compromised.

Furthermore, in evaluation of peer-teaching during practice placement, some students have indicated that time spent teaching junior students is time sacrificed that could have been used for their own practice learning working with their own supervisor. Clearly peer-teaching by senior students needs to be encouraged, but it needs to be carefully structured so that these students who are on the verge of becoming RNs do not lose out from lack of access to their practice supervisors, nor from incidental learning. Additionally, any innovation or change in practice needs to be considered in the context of 'management of change', for the implementation to be effective (see Chapter 5 of this book for discussion on management of change).

'Communities of practice' (also discussed in Chapters 2 and 4 of this book) is yet another form of peer supervision. Moreover, increasingly, as inter-professional working and inter-professional learning is being systematically operationalised, the concept of inter-professional learning supervision is also gaining in popularity and credibility. Lait et al. (2011), for instance, document the findings of an evaluative research on the then inter-professional mentoring model, indicating that:

- students learned about the roles of other professions and how to work together to provide patient-centred care
- inter-professional learning can be 'threaded' through all clinical placements rather than being offered only once on the three-year pre-registration programme, or once a year.

Lait et al. (2011: 213) also point out that the activities that students engage in vary in complexity, and that 'provider commitment' is important. Furthermore, although inter-professional learning has been researched substantially, evidence of inter-professional supervision is lacking. Following their small-scale study of inter-professional supervision, Yang et al. (2017) warn against the limitations of the activity. They found that, on occasion, students were supervised by supervisors from other health professions who had not had formal preparation for the role which resulted in student dissatisfaction with the required practice learning; at times inter-professional supervisors were chosen due to shortage of supervisors in their own profession; etc.

Moreover, in a study of students' experiences and staff perceptions of the implementation of placement development teams, Williamson (2009) reports that students indicate a need for more direct, personal and organisational support, and better communication between university and placement areas. Additionally, research also suggests that the effectiveness of the learning supervision role also depends on the level of the healthcare professional's motivation and interest in students' learning (for example, Hallin and Danielson, 2009).

Having delved into and analysed key facets of practice learning supervision, the final section of this chapter concludes the concept and role by suggesting a model and framework for practice supervision based on previous research on the topic area.

FRAMEWORKS FOR PRACTICE SUPERVISION, AND CONTENT OF SUPERVISOR PREPARATION PROGRAMME

As noted earlier in this chapter, in addition to supervision of students' learning in care settings during practice placements, supervision also has a range of other applications in health and social care. Saltiel (2017), for example, highlights supervision of social workers in relation to child protection work, whereupon supervision of qualified social workers incorporates learning that consequently enhances care provision for service users, and thereby reduces child deaths.

Saltiel's research also acknowledges the 'complex skills' that experienced supervisors utilise, and which novice supervisors 'struggle to acquire' (p. 533) in the current under-resourced work environment, and recommends a supportive learning environment for newly qualified social workers. The point highlighted in these findings is the recognition that recently qualified care professionals may not reach high standards in their work if they are not provided with educational, developmental and emotional support, because otherwise they rely only on their managers' instructions and their pre-qualifying education.

Returning to pre-qualifying healthcare students then, it is reasonable to suggest that if qualified care professionals have a need for supervision of learning, then health and social care students need this mechanism even more so. So, what is supervision in the context of pre-registration students' learning? In addition to Nancarrow et al.'s (2014) observation that most definitions of supervision incorporate working relationships, and support, etc., Kilminster et al. (2007) define supervision as: 'The provision of guidance and feedback on matters of personal, professional and educational development in the context of a trainee's experience of providing safe and appropriate patient care.' Moreover, as noted earlier, Johnson (2017: 6) suggests that supervision is relationship-based facilitation of learning, that also heeds ethical and legal parameters. All explanations of supervision, explicitly or by implication, indicate that its focus is on learning professional intervention skills, and that it is founded on development of a trusting relationship that should be initiated by the supervisor, although in healthcare students are explicitly advised to proactively initiate interaction with their supervisor-to-be.

Additionally, Kilminster et al. (2007) note that the features of effective supervision, which essentially comprise a framework, incorporate:

1. Supervision is aligned to the practice setting's and the care organisation's clinical guidelines, as well as being based on the student's HEI practice competencies.
2. Direct supervision – learner and supervisor working together and observing each other.
3. Frequent constructive feedback is provided to supervisees.
4. Supervision is structured, with regular timetabled meetings.
5. The supervisory relationship is developed in conjunction with written learning agreements, and takes into account the assessment components, and maybe appraisal for healthcare apprentices.
6. Supervised learning includes elements of management of care, teaching and research, with structured reflective discussions, in addition to learning care interventions.
7. The supervision process should be informed by a '360-degree perspective', which therefore includes patient feedback, inter-professional supervision, together with reviewing written work by students, and records of supervision.

For pre-registration nursing and midwifery students, the NMC has succinctly stated the roles, responsibilities and educational preparation of practice supervisors. For preparation of practice supervisors, Falender (2014) has previously suggested that competency-based supervision of learning does not refer only to the supervisee developing and achieving practice competencies, but also to the supervisor being provided with competency-based education for the role. This implies an educational preparation for supervisors of learning that is 'fit for purpose', and Falender indicates that there is growing consensus that competency-based preparation of supervisors should include addressing:

•   formation of strong supervisory alliance
•   development of supervisory/learning contract
•   supporting the student with self-assessment
•   providing constructive and positive feedback
•   identification and repair of strains in the alliance
•   complying with legal and ethical aspects of supervision
•   evaluating service user outcomes
•   managing supervisees who are not progressing as expected etc.

The arguments presented above clearly suggest that the content of the practice supervisor preparation programmes needs to be comprehensive so that they can benefit learners and supervisors, as well as ultimately care service users. However, as suggested earlier in this chapter, practice learning supervisors' readiness for the role needs to be ascertained beforehand, and they need to be motivated to fulfil this role.

So, the relatively rich literature on supervision ultimately always tends to incorporate learning, and describes the features of effective supervision and the principles of supervision, which essentially comprise 'good practice' of the activity.

ACTIVITY 1.10 GOOD PRACTICE IN SUPERVISION OF LEARNING

Along the lines of the title of this activity, as well as your own experience of supervision of practice-based learning, take just a few minutes to identify the actions that supervisors of learning in your health or social care profession would take that constitute good practice.

In supervision of learning in care professions, identifying all actions that comprise good practice would result in a lengthy list of considerations and activities, and in addition to the features of effective supervision identified above, they include:

- Ensuring full endeavour to establish a firm working supervisory relationship at the very first formal meeting.
- Incorporating agreed level of direct supervision with nominated supervisors, which entails learner and supervisor working together in service user care situations.
- The supervision process should be enriched by input from multi-professional team members, which should be in written form and include mention of the learner's learning activities and any assigned work.
- Being clear about the initiators of the supervision, assuming it is part of a programme of learning, and inform the initiators of any concerns when they occur.
- Protect supervisor–student interaction time preferably without interruptions, but definitely with privacy.
- Ensure confidentiality, and abide by all other relevant codes of practice set by professional regulators (e.g. HCPC's).
- Ensure non-verbal messages match verbal statements.
- ... (add your own).

Make a note of your own perspectives on good practice activities as you feel appropriate. The supervision features and activities identified above can consequently be grouped under headings of a framework for effective practice supervision related to your specific profession. Kilminster et al.'s (2007) framework comprises an example of effective supervision.

Finnerty and Collington (2013) researched how a model of supervision can be applied to supervising midwifery students' learning and found the model to be beneficial, mainly because it is consistent with coaching, which in turn entails role modelling, reverse role modelling and experiential learning. However, one model of supervision that has stood the test of time for some years now is Proctor's (2011) model of supervision, which comprises addressing the normative, formative and supportive aspects of supervision, as well as restorative.

In concluding the above-discussed tentative models, frameworks and good practice of supervision of practice learning, it is feasible to deduce the content of practice supervision preparation programmes. Falender's (2014) suggestions that are presented in bullet-form above comprise a very good starting point for the content of an effective practice supervision preparation programme if it is complemented by addressing the NMC's (2018a) clauses under 'Effective practice learning' and 'Supervision of students' in *Standards for Student Supervision and Assessment*.

ADAPTING PROCTOR'S SUPERVISION ALLIANCE MODEL INTO A FRAMEWORK FOR SUPERVISION OF PRACTICE EDUCATION

Although intended initially for peer-support-type clinical supervision, Proctor's model of supervision can be adapted effectively to practice supervision in nursing and midwifery and similar roles in other care professions for the achievement of required outcomes. In a little more detail, the model comprises:

- *Formative supervision*: refers to the educational aspect of the placement; etc.
- *Normative supervision*: refers to adherence to clinical guidelines and procedures that have been approved by the organisation; comply with the profession's code of practice, etc.
- *Supportive supervision*: refers to allowing students time to learn and practise newly learnt clinical skills, etc.
- *Restorative supervision*: reviewing student progress with practice objectives; re-establishing placement requirements following sickness or other breaks, under-achievement, etc.

NHS England (2017a) highly recommends the adaptation of Proctor's model to 'clinical midwifery supervision' for RMs. However, the model can also be reconstituted into a framework for effective practice supervision of pre-qualifying healthcare students, as suggested in the box below.

APPLYING A FRAMEWORK OF PRACTICE SUPERVISION

Normative supervision

- Adhering to clinical guidelines and procedures that have been approved by the employer
- Abiding by the profession's code of practice, and exercising ethical competence towards service users, colleagues and peers
- Evidence-based practice and changing practice

- Establishing working relationships
- Negotiating and agreeing on a learning contract for the whole placement
- Enabling supervisee to value the practice placement and the supervision mechanism
- Awareness of quality of care
- Supervisor's leadership

Formative supervision

- Identifying supervisees' practice objectives that must be achieved
- Facilitation of learning for acquisition of knowledge and skills
- Optimising incidental learning opportunities, and relevant spoke visits
- Instituting reflective practice
- Improving care intervention skills resulting in improved care for service users
- Evaluating practice learning provision
- Formative assessment and contributing to students' summative assessment (discussed in Chapter 6 of this book)

Supportive supervision

- Supervisor's positive attitude and skill in the relationship
- Allowing supervisee time to learn and practise care intervention skills
- Acceptance of the student, and mutual respect
- Providing support, and direct help in challenging situations
- Motivating student to learn through feedback on progress with their practice objectives
- Creating a climate for learning in the care setting

Restorative supervision

- Managing under-achieving students
- Mid-placement interview, or more frequent monitoring of progress
- Supportive teaching skills/facilitation of learning
- Using empathy
- Re-establishing placement requirements following sickness or other breaks
- Trust and rapport
- Supervisor's advice to the student
- Developing self-confidence and resilience

The examples identified under the adaptation of Proctor's framework in the box above provide a comprehensive backdrop for constituting a framework of your own for a practice supervisor preparation programme, which is done by taking into account the specific requirements of your own professional specialism. This can be done by populating Template 1.1. Furthermore, the Template can then comprise a self-assessment tool for practice supervisor competence by grading competence level on each item between 1 to 5, 1 being for non-competent to 5 for highly competent.

Template 1.1   A framework of practice supervision for supervisor self-assessment

Practice Supervisor's Name: .... *Date of self-assessment:*	
Components	**Competence level**
Normative supervision • .... • .... • .... • .... •	
Formative supervision • .... • .... • .... • .... •	
Supportive supervision • .... • .... • .... • .... •	
Restorative supervision • .... • .... • .... • .... •	

Incidentally, the examples identified in the box above also address the main component of the previous NMC's (2008) standards for mentorship, but naturally also much more.

A further perspective on supervision of learning for qualified healthcare professionals is provided by NHS England (2017a), which endorses Proctor's (2011: 25) indication that the restorative function should be addressed first, because until the supervisee can relax, and is free of anxiety and stress, they might not be receptive to formative and normative developments. Examples of key components of the restorative function include:

- addressing the emotional needs of staff.
- supporting the development of resilience.
- creating space for reflective conversation, supportive challenge and open and honest feedback.
- contemplating different perspectives.
- processing difficult emotions experienced by healthcare professionals through a supportive, confidential relationship.

However, it is argued that in terms of supervision of learning for pre-registration students, the formative and normative functions take priority, but are underpinned by the supportive function to fully enable the student's progress towards achievement of the agreed placement objectives.

CHAPTER SUMMARY

This chapter has focused on practice supervision for enabling healthcare students to develop safe and effective clinical intervention skills, which is based mostly on research and other literature on supervision and mentorship, and has therefore addressed:

- Relevant perspectives on the practice supervisor role, and definitions of and distinctions between the practice supervisor and various other learning facilitation roles, such as preceptors, clinical educators, assessors, supervisors, practice education facilitators, link lecturers and personal tutors. All these roles are established with the aim of facilitating healthcare learners' acquisition of care intervention skills, knowledge and appropriate attitudes.
- A number of reasons for requiring practice supervisors to support learning for healthcare students on preparatory education programmes during practice placements, and the necessary characteristics of practice supervisors.
- Effective practice supervision, which encompasses effective working relationships; relevant supervisor–learner communication, which includes generic and specialist communication skills.
- Research findings on detrimental effects of poor, inefficient or adverse practice supervision, and ways of addressing these when they occur.
- The use of different approaches, models and frameworks for practice supervision and mentoring, good practice in practice supervision, and then a framework for effective supervision of practice-based learning.

FURTHER OPTIONAL READING

1. For an exploration of research and different perspectives on coaching in a wide range of settings in the UK and abroad and discussion on inherent issues, see:

- Garvey, B., Stokes, P. and Megginson, D. (2017) *Coaching and Mentoring: Theory and Practice*, 3rd edn. London: Sage.

2. For an example of application of coaching in healthcare, see:

- Finnerty, G. and Collington, V. (2013) 'Practical coaching by mentors: Student midwives' perceptions', *Nurse Education in Practice*, 13(6): 573–577

3. For research on how practice supervisors and learners develop trust in each
   other, see:

   • Hauer, K.E., Oza, S.K., Kogan, J.R., Stankiewicz, C.A., Stenfors-Hayes, T., Cate, O.T.,
     Batt, J. and O'Sullivan, P.S. (2015) 'How clinical supervisors develop trust in their
     trainees: A qualitative study', *Medical Education*, 49(8): 783–795.

4. Look out for developments in supervision of learning for other professional
   roles, such as student nursing associates, apprentices, etc.

To access further resources related to this chapter, visit **https://study.sagepub.com/
gopee4e** where a range of learning and teaching materials are provided.

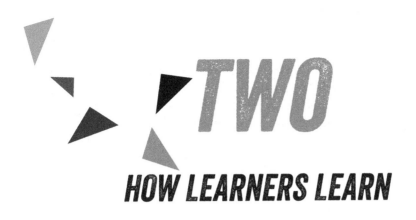

HOW LEARNERS LEARN

INTRODUCTION

As patient care interventions are the main part of healthcare professionals' work, an appropriate proportion of their pre-registration education courses are dedicated to students learning clinical and psychosocial care skills in the work setting. In a nursing pre-registration course, for instance, which amounts to a total of 4600 hours of learning in three years, the NMC (2018e, 2010a) requires a minimum of 50 per cent of this learning time to take place in practice settings (of which a small number of hours of practice learning can be facilitated by 'simulation' in skills laboratories and in other education settings). Learning in practice settings therefore occupies a pivotal role in pre-registration education. Indeed, learning is an ongoing requirement for all healthcare professionals throughout their careers.

Fundamental to the achievement of learning objectives is facilitation of student learning and teaching students the required skills, values and knowledge. Consequently, this chapter and Chapter 3 are based on facilitation of students' learning. The NMC (2018a: 6) indicates that practice supervisors' roles include enabling 'students to learn and safely achieve proficiency and autonomy in their professional role'. Furthermore, the NMC's (2015a) and HCPC's (2016) codes of practice indicate that registrants must support their students' learning, and also share their skills, knowledge and experience with their colleagues for the benefit of healthcare service users. Moreover, the previous NMC's (2008) standards for mentors identified 'facilitation of learning' as one of the eight essential skill areas for supporting learning in healthcare settings, which incorporated ascertaining the student's stage of learning to select appropriate learning opportunities for them, enabling students to integrate learning from practice and academic settings, and reflection.

The NMC (2018a) doesn't provide extensive detail of the practice supervisor role in facilitation of learning, but does provide guidance. Chapter 2 consequently draws on research on the multiple theories of learning, and focuses on ways in which healthcare learners learn the competence and knowledge required for providing care that is 'person-centred, safe and compassionate' (NMC, 2018b: 7) and effective. Ways in which practice supervisors can facilitate learning are examined in Chapter 3, and how practice settings can also be effective learning environments in Chapter 4.

CHAPTER OBJECTIVES

1. Identify the specific knowledge and competencies that healthcare students learn during their pre-registration education programmes, including different types of knowledge and professional skills.
2. Identify various reasons for learning by different individuals, and the nature of professional competence.
3. Analyse prevailing major views and perspectives on learning, teaching and education.
4. Understand and critically analyse key theories of learning and indicate how they can be applied to learning in practice settings.
5. Comprehend the different styles and approaches to learning and ways in which practice supervisors can adapt their approaches to teaching to match students' individual learning styles and approaches.

WHAT DO HEALTHCARE LEARNERS LEARN, AND WHY?

The first section of this chapter begins by identifying the specific knowledge and competencies that learners in healthcare professions learn, in particular during their initial preparatory programmes.

HEALTHCARE COMPETENCIES

For nurse education programmes, in *Standards for Pre-registration Nursing Education* the NMC (2010a) identifies the knowledge and skills that students have to acquire in order to gain the Registered Nurse (RN) qualification. These standards have been implemented since 2011, being preceded by the one published in 2004, and superseded by the NMC (2018b) standards of proficiencies.

The NMC (2010a) standards comprise those that all HEIs currently offering pre-registration nurse education programmes have to incorporate in their pre-registration nursing courses. In its 'competency framework', the NMC (2010a) identifies: first, 'generic competencies' that student nurses in all four 'fields' of practice (previously referred to as 'branches') must achieve during their education programme. The four fields are: (1) adult nursing; (2) mental health nursing; (3) learning disabilities nursing; and (4) children's nursing.

Second, the standards identify a set of field-specific competencies. Both generic and field-specific competencies are grouped under the following four domains:

- professional values
- communication and interpersonal skills
- nursing practice and decision-making
- leadership, management and teamworking.

As can be expected, the NMC provides comprehensive details of all areas of competence that students must achieve to be able to have their name entered into the NMC's register as a 'registrant' in the particular field of practice. Under 'Platform 4 – *Providing and evaluating care*' of the NMC's (2018b: 17) SOP, the related outcome is: 'The proficiencies identified below will equip the newly registered nurse with the underpinning knowledge and skills required for their role in providing and evaluating person-centred care'. A few examples of SOP under this platform and outcome are reproduced in the box below.

EXAMPLES OF SOP UNDER 'PLATFORM 4 – PROVIDING AND EVALUATING CARE'

4.3 Demonstrate the knowledge, communication and relationship management skills required to provide people, families and carers with accurate information that meets their needs before, during and after a range of interventions.

4.6 Demonstrate the knowledge, skills and ability to act as a role model for others in providing evidence-based nursing care to meet people's needs related to nutrition, hydration and bladder and bowel health.

4.7 Demonstrate the knowledge, skills and ability to act as a role model for others in providing evidence-based, person-centred nursing care to meet people's needs related to mobility, hygiene, oral care, wound care and skin integrity.

4.12 Demonstrate the ability to manage commonly encountered devices and confidently carry out related nursing procedures to meet people's needs for evidence-based, person-centered care.

4.18 Demonstrate the ability to co-ordinate and undertake the processes and procedures involved in routine planning and management of safe discharge home or transfer of people between care settings.

Source: NMC (2018b: 17–18)

The standards of proficiency are then translated into specific practice competencies locally that students will need to achieve during practice placements. The overall NMC's (2018b) SOP for pre-registration nursing education identifies course outcomes that are structured under seven 'Platforms' (instead of the 2010 four domains), which are:

1) Being an accountable professional
2) Promoting health and preventing ill health
3) Assessing needs and planning care
4) Providing and evaluating care (see examples in the box above)
5) Leading and managing nursing care and working in teams
6) Improving safety and quality of care
7) Coordinating care

For midwifery students, in *Standards for Pre-registration Midwifery Education*, the NMC (2009) identifies the 'Standards of proficiency' (SOP) that students have to achieve to register with the NMC as 'Registered Midwife' (RM). These standards documents are available free from the NMC. Standards of proficiency for the preparation programmes of the AHPs managed by the HCPC have also been identified in appropriate HCPC publications for each allied health and social care profession that it regulates. The General Medical Council (GMC) and other healthcare regulators publish their own corresponding standards.

These standards will have been translated into specific practice competencies locally that students will need to have become competent in during practice placements. No doubt it should prove useful for all practice supervisors to have a paper copy or electronic copy of the whole standards for pre-qualifying education (e.g. NMC, 2010a, 2018b) document handy to refer to as and when required. Standards for nursing associates have been published by HEE (2017a), which will be superseded by the NMC's (2018d) standards; and for nurse apprenticeships by Institute for Apprenticeships (2016a), which is currently based on the NMC (2010a) standards for pre-registration nurse education.

In addition to the regulatory bodies' standards, each healthcare profession's professional body, for example the Royal College of Nursing and the British Medical Association, tend to publish further guidance to facilitate implementation of the regulatory body's standards in professional preparation programmes.

Furthermore, every two to three years, one or more major organisational inquiry on nurse education publishes its findings and makes recommendations. Because of recent reports, mainly in the media, of poor nursing care, the RCN commissioned one such inquiry with the remit to explore the nature of 'excellent preregistration nursing education in the UK' and how it should be delivered. The recommendations of the inquiry, known as the Willis Report (Royal College of Nursing, 2012: 6), include:

Nursing education should foster professionalism which includes embedding patient safety as its top priority, and respects the dignity and values of service users and their carers.

Professionalism, according to the NMC's (2017b: 3) *Enabling Professionalism in Nursing and Midwifery Practice* publication 'is characterised by the autonomous evidence-based decision making by members of an occupation who share the same values and education ... Professional nurses and midwives demonstrate and embrace accountability for their actions.'

Safety and dignity of service users are key concepts in the Willis Report (RCN, 2012) recommendations, and clearly such recommendations directly indicate elements that pre-registration education should cover and that student nurses must learn – see also the section in Chapter 9 of this book under the heading 'Students raising concerns'. The DH's (2013) *Education Outcomes Framework for Healthcare Workforce* is another prominent publication that is being instituted to influence the content of pre-registration programmes. The framework is a parallel document to the *NHS Outcomes Framework 2016 to 2017* (DH, 2016a) that was developed as a component of the Health and Social Care Act 2012 (DH, 2012a).

The Act has meant a radical change in the management of healthcare delivery in England ever since its implementation in April 2013. In relation to the education and training of the healthcare workforce in England, the Act includes the establishment of Health Education England (HEE) (DH, 2016b) and Local Education and Training Boards (LETB) for the overseeing and operationalisation of funding, respectively. The Act also included other policy changes, such as the establishment of clinical commissioning groups (CCG) for commissioning care and treatment and the strengthening of public health activities through instituting *Public Health England*.

ESSENTIAL SKILLS CLUSTERS AND COMPASSIONATE CARE

The NMC undertakes a number of public and professional consultations periodically to arrive at new content of pre-registration nurse education programmes that aim to meet current healthcare needs. Following one of these consultations it was decided to include 'essential skills clusters' (ESCs) within these programmes. These skills later became fully integrated into both nursing and midwifery pre-registration programmes.

Included in ESCs is compassionate care, which was further strengthened by more guidance jointly issued by the Chief Nursing Officer for England (CNO) and the Director of Nursing at the Department of Health as they identified the 6 Cs of Nursing (Department of Health, 2012b). The 6 Cs stand for: care, compassion, competence, communication, courage and commitment. The guidance has been further enhanced by a framework for high-quality care in the publication entitled *Leading Change, Adding Value – A Framework for Nursing, Midwifery and Care Staff* (NHS England, 2016).

Compassion and the related concepts therefore naturally also form part of pre-registration curricula, and of practice competencies that practice supervisors enable students to achieve during practice placements. 'Compassion' is also examined in Chapter 5.

In nurse education, from 2018 the ESCs are being completely replaced by an extensive range of healthcare skills which are grouped under two headings:

- Communication and relationship management skills – which under four sections include communication skills for assessing, planning, providing and managing best practice, evidence-based nursing care; for working with people in professional teams, etc.
- Nursing procedures – under eleven sections, for example procedures for assessing people's needs for person-centered care.

THE STUDENT'S LEARNING NEEDS: KNOWLEDGE AND COMPETENCE

In addition to the placement competencies that students are required to learn, as adult learners (Knowles, 2015) students are also likely to have their own aims and thoughts on specific healthcare knowledge and competence that they would wish to acquire during particular practice placements. This should be encouraged and explicitly supported, as appropriate.

Students acquire knowledge in, say, human physiology, pharmacology and treatment methods, which is consistent with the generic and field competencies under the four domains identified by the NMC (2010a), and later under the NMC's (2018b) seven 'platforms'. The terms *competence* and *competency* are often used in relation to the skills that healthcare students learn. Different types of knowledge are discussed shortly but, first, what do the terms 'competence' and 'competency' mean?

DEFINING 'COMPETENCE'

There are conflicting definitions of the terms 'competence' and 'competency' in the literature.

Although the term *competence* is at times used rather glibly, it is a term that has several definitions, as identified by Fernandez et al. (2012), and Garside and Nhemachena (2013), for instance. Benner (2001) sees being competent as being at the midway point in the 'novice to expert' stages of the skill-acquisition continuum. This is the point when the learner is deemed able to perform the skill safely and effectively unsupervised, but further learning is required to become 'proficient' or 'expert'.

Benner (2001) suggests that the term competence has different interpretations related to skilled performance, and it is described by its intent, function and meanings (as in competency statement). Policy and research documents therefore indicate that the terms *competence* and *competent* apply to the person, that is, to the professional's overall knowledge, skills and attitudes and their 'fitness to practise'. The term *competency*, however, applies to specific clinical skills, which in nursing also include the associated knowledge and attitude components.

TYPES OF KNOWLEDGE ASSOCIATED WITH PROFESSIONAL SKILLS

The knowledge base required for clinical competence can be grouped or classified in different ways. Schon (1995) notes that healthcare professionals have an accumulated repertoire of knowledge, with mastery over its applications. Benner (2001) identifies practical knowledge and theoretical knowledge, as well as tacit knowledge. She suggests that novices – that is, healthcare professionals who are new to healthcare – are more inclined to use rules and guidelines, such as practical knowledge, while 'expert' healthcare practitioners also use their intuition.

Different types of knowledge that professionals use can also be viewed from Carper's (1978) 'patterns of knowing' perspective. They are:

- *empirical knowledge*: knowledge derived from research and scientific experiments, which therefore can be measured, tested and corroborated
- *ethical knowledge*: knowledge based on morals and philosophy, but which is usually difficult to test
- *aesthetic knowledge*: knowledge based on sensitivity or intuition, such as in the 'art of nursing'
- *personal knowledge*: knowledge of one's self and how it influences one's professional practice.

Each of these 'patterns' of knowledge is seen as equally important for healthcare practice and for developing further knowledge. Therefore, in relation to physiotherapy and knowledge regarding hip replacement, for instance, empirical knowledge relates to the research evidence for hip replacement operations, the patient experiencing less chronic pain and a better quality of life afterwards. Ethical knowledge could refer to whether, say, if an 80-year-old widow consents to such an operation, it would still be right to subject her to such a potentially traumatic experience.

Aesthetic knowledge refers to the expertise, extensive experience and intuition of the physiotherapist to enable the patient to mobilise fully after the operation. Personal knowledge refers to the physiotherapist knowing himself or herself as a person, their preferences and values, and the effect that these might have on their professional practice.

The practice supervisor's role towards the physiotherapy student would be to enable the student to acquire skills and practical knowledge, but includes having a good insight into the student's level of scientific, ethical and personal knowledge.

In a study exploring whether nurses use knowledge from research findings to inform decision-making, Thompson et al. (2002) found that although colleagues are the more immediate source of information on which to base decisions, they are also a source of research (or data-based empirical) knowledge and useful networks. However, although various decisions made by clinical managers are based on empirical knowledge, other decisions are often influenced by previous experience and intuition.

MAJOR VIEWS AND PERSPECTIVES ON LEARNING, TEACHING AND EDUCATION

WHAT IS LEARNING?

How individuals learn has been researched and defined over a number of years. So, what is learning? How do you define 'learning'? Generally, dictionaries provide a broad explanation of the term. For instance, to learn is to 'gain knowledge of something or acquire a skill' and 'gain knowledge or skill by experience or by practice' (Brookes and O'Neill, 2017: 525). More specific definitions have come from philosophers and educational psychologists. The latter generally agree that learning is a process that leads to modification in behaviour or the acquisition of new abilities or responses, and which is additional to natural development, growth or maturation.

Accordingly, Gagné et al. (2005: 3) define learning as a process that leads to a change in a learner's disposition and capabilities that can be reflected in behaviour. This is a near universally accepted definition of learning that suggests that learning something changes the person as a person and adds to the things they are able to do (mentally or physically). After learning, the new disposition or capability persists over a substantial period of time.

Similarly, Curzon and Tummons (2013: 11) define learning as 'the apparent modification of a person's behaviour through his or her activities and experiences, so that his or her knowledge, skills and attitudes, including modes of adjustment, towards their environment, are changed, more or less permanently'.

These definitions tend to concur that:

- learning is reflected in changes in behaviour, physicality and attitudes
- learning occurs in day-to-day life experiences, in addition to planned formal education
- learning a psychomotor skill is permanent in nature in that the individual subsequently has the capacity to perform the skilled act at a future point in time.

Specialist skills may 'decay' (e.g. become outdated) mainly due to such factors as changes in medical devices, social values and so on. Learning in healthcare professions is about learning competence and knowledge, the nature of which was discussed earlier. In healthcare professions, learning is a lifelong process of skill and knowledge acquisition, updating them through planned participation in focused reading and structured programmes of study.

PERSPECTIVES ON LEARNING

Learning experiences are influenced by where the learner 'is coming from', as each person perceives new experiences in a different way, depending on how the new experience relates to the individual's past. However, two opposing views about formal learning are suggested by Ramsden (2003), who identifies learning as either: (a) a quantitative accretion of knowledge, i.e. facts and procedures; or (b) a change in the way in which people interpret and understand the world around them.

However, according to Socrates (2000 years ago), education is not merely transferring knowledge of facts and procedures from 'teacher' to 'pupil'. Rather, it is 'an adventure, an activity of the mind, a pursuit demanding reflection, analysis and investigation, a social activity undertaken by equals freely associated to engage in dialogue' (Jeffs, 2003: 28).

Radical distinctions are also made by Freire (1996), who argues that there are two contrasting perspectives on education and learning, which he identifies as the 'banking' concept of education versus 'problem posing'. On the one hand, the banking concept is the traditional mode of learning and involves the teacher helping a student fill their minds with knowledge, which is later 'cashed out' relatively unchanged, for example in examinations. On the other hand, the problem-posing approach to education is education through dialogue, in which the facilitator and students meet and exchange ideas and experiences through critical discussions and debate. Neither the facilitator nor the students necessarily have the 'right' answer as there is room for 'multiple realities'.

Another perspective is provided by Peters (1966, 1973) regarding the differentiation between training and education. What distinctions would you draw between education and training, between nurse education and nurse training, for example? Peters (1966) notes that training means knowledge and skill development devised to bring about some specific end. However, the aims of education, he notes, are that:

- something of value is being passed on and learned
- the individual comes to care about the learning involved, to develop understanding, and to achieve
- what is being learned must have a place in a coherent pattern of life, that is, relevance among other things in life.

Therefore, education 'implies that something worthwhile is being, or has been, intentionally transmitted in a morally acceptable manner ... The educated person is one whose life has been transformed by the deepening and widening of his understanding and sensitivity. To be educated is not to arrive at a destination; it is to travel with a different view' (Peters, 1973: 122).

These perspectives on learning correspond with the concepts of teacher-centred learning and student-centred learning, which are discussed in Chapter 3. So how do the definitions and these views on learning and education apply to, or compare with, approaches taken in healthcare profession education curricula?

ACTIVITY 2.1   DIFFERENT PERSPECTIVES ON NURSE EDUCATION

Discuss with a course or work-based peer your thoughts on how far Ramsden's (2003), Freire's (1996) and Peters' (1966, 1973) perspectives on learning apply to nursing, midwifery or to AHP professional education. Is there an equally well-researched perspective on learning that is more contemporary?

In nurse education, the difference between education and training is that the word 'training' is usually associated with developing the ability to take an approved set of actions to perform a certain clinical task. This is thought of as a convergent process of learning to complete a task competently. Education, however, is seen as a divergent process that in addition to initially learning the step-by-step actions, the healthcare professional is constantly reflecting on each action in the context of their deep knowledge-base background, principles, values, ethics and effect on the recipient individual.

Education does not stop at a predetermined point of attainment, but progresses further in the development of critical ability and, consequently, the individual remains open to new impressions, principles and perspectives. Education facilitators should therefore provide an environment where students feel sufficiently supported to decide on areas and depth of learning, as long as the core curriculum aims are achieved.

WHERE DO HEALTHCARE LEARNERS LEARN?

Naturally, learning does not occur only in university classrooms through lectures, workshops and books, but also in work-based settings, during healthcare service user contact. Learning also occurs in skill laboratories and in the ward, teaching room or office. Furthermore, learning occurs in the trust's postgraduate or in-service training departments. In the practice setting, learning can be informal and by structured teaching sessions.

Additionally, learning occurs in the student common room, in informal social meetings and even 'in car parks, in corridors, over tea as well as through unnoticed patterns of behaviour and interaction in the classroom itself' (Field, 1999: 12). This notion that learning can occur from friends and peers and in a whole range of settings is referred to as 'social capital' (Gopee, 2002a). A corresponding notion is 'human capital', which refers to the self-investment of time and effort by individuals through learning at university or in public libraries, as well as at home and in the non-traditional places suggested by Field (1999). Learning occurs everywhere, including, for example, in therapeutics. Learning contributes to progress, and notions such as the 'learning society' and 'learning organisation' (in that most companies have training and customer services departments) have evolved.

Lately, other effective ways of 'social' learning have been recognised, such as 'communities of practice' and 'action learning sets' – the first being more informal and the latter more formal, but both are equally effective. Communities of practice refer to groups of people sharing a passion for something of interest, which they want to know more and more about or do, and learn by interacting regularly, as identified by Wenger (2000) and Webber (2017). The learning that ensues is not necessarily intentional, but is achieved by sharing information with each other, and building relationships that enable learning from each other (e.g. Morley, 2016) and by engaging within the community of practice.

The feasibility and benefits of students learning from each other is increasingly being recognised, as also noted, for example, by Nygren and Carlson (2017). Additionally, students studying for a specific subject have an overall common interest, but smaller groups of students may develop a 'passion' for specific sub-topics and meet informally to learn more and more about the sub-topic. The same may apply to health and social care professionals in relation to their specialist area (e.g. Leggat et al., 2014). Action learning sets are more formal classroom- or meeting-room-based discussions on pre-identified curricular topics, as confirmed by research (e.g. Currie et al., 2012; Walia and Marks-Maran, 2014).

THEORIES UNDERPINNING LEARNING

There are a number of theories of learning that can underpin professional education programmes. Exploration of these theories has taken place over several decades. It has swung between theories of learning, models of learning, principles of learning and styles of learning, with theories and styles of learning being the more popular concepts in the twenty-first century.

There are at least ten schools of thought, theories or models of learning, which have all created different definitions and incorporate a variety of concepts, but most of them have evolved from the three more robust learning theories, namely:

- behaviourist learning theories
- cognitive learning theories
- humanistic learning theories.

BEHAVIOURIST LEARNING THEORIES

Most learning theories belong to the field of psychology, which in the earlier part of the twentieth century used to be about introspection, that is, how mental processes are structured. However, gradually there was a move away from this paradigm (see, for example, Nolen Hoeksema et al., 2014) and it was suggested that psychology should be a science, and psychological theories should be based on observable and quantifiable data, that is, those manifested in changes in behaviour. Initially, psychologists worked with animals to observe behaviour changes, and later worked with people.

Behaviourist learning theories refer to learning through response to particular stimuli, resulting in classical conditioning or operant conditioning. Classical conditioning refers to changes in behaviour through stimulus–response, whereby desirable responses to particular stimuli, that is, newly learned behaviours are rewarded. Operant conditioning is a subsequent development by Skinner (1971) and others, whereby approximations of desired behaviour are rewarded and thereby the target behaviour develops gradually. Being rewarded for new learning is also known as 'positive reinforcement', and can be external, in the form of verbal affirmations from the teacher (or close relatives) such as 'well done', or material rewards, or they can be internal through self-satisfaction, for example.

Behaviourist learning theory can be applied in healthcare professionals' education programmes. For instance, operant conditioning can be effectively applied when students with weak academic backgrounds could achieve high levels in academia if earlier attempts are positively reinforced. Overall, healthcare learners are positively reinforced both by feeling a sense of achievement on being able to perform new healthcare skills, and by their practice supervisors acknowledging or recognising their newly developed competence.

Another example is that gaining praise for becoming competent at a particular clinical skill, or part-skills towards the desired competent performance, can positively motivate the student and make them want to learn new skills. Thus, praiseworthy performance or approximations of competent practice or of part-skills by healthcare learners are rewarded or positively reinforced.

Social learning theory builds on these early behaviourist theories whereby the individual observes competent behaviour or skill performance by professionals, learns the behaviour and reproduces it, and if the attempt is positively reinforced then that behaviour or skill is likely to be adopted. It refers to the behaviour, attitudes and values of teachers or other role models that may be copied by learners (Bandura, 1996, 1997) and thus learned in social situations, as discussed in Chapter 1. Sub-theories and inherent concepts of learning can be grouped in different ways by different authors, but such classification is mostly only an academic exercise. However, such groupings can disentangle the multifarious theories of learning, and therefore a tentative summary of sub-theories of learning and some inherent concepts emanating from the three main theories are presented in Table 2.1.

Table 2.1 Learning theories, sub-theories and some inherent concepts

Learning theories	Sub-theories	Some inherent concepts
Behaviourist learning theories	Bandura's social learning theory	Reinforcement for learning Operant conditioning Role model
Cognitive learning theories	Gestalt theory of learning; Piaget's stages of intellectual/cognitive development	Insightful learning Discovery learning Constructivism The 'aha!' phenomenon Experiential learning Reflective practice Ripples model of learning
	Ausubel et al.'s assimilation theory	Information processing 'Flipping' method Situated learning
Humanistic learning theories	Alan Rogers' characteristics of adult education and andragogy	Andragogy or adult learning Self-directed learning Learning contracts Peer learning
	Carl Rogers' student-centred approach to learning	Student-centred teaching Experiential learning Problem-based learning Social capital
	Maslow's hierarchy of human needs	Learning for self-actualisation and growth
	Kohlberg's moral development (Sanders, 2018)	Stages of moral development

COGNITIVE LEARNING THEORIES

As just indicated, behaviourist learning theories initially constituted an attempt to make psychology more scientific and empirical. More recently, various education sectors, including nurse education, have incorporated aspects of behaviourist theories and social learning theory into professional education programmes (for example through systematic feedback to students on their knowledge and competence, and through consciousness of being a role model for learners).

Subsequent work by Piaget (1962), Ausubel et al. (1978) and others led to the evolution of cognitive learning theories, which take the view that learning is an internal purposive action involving thinking, perception, information processing and memory. Cognitive learning theories include:

- Gestalt theory of learning – entailing insightful learning, the 'aha' phenomenon
- Ausubel et al.'s assimilation theory – which incorporates information processing
- experiential learning – learning through engaging in practical activities, followed by reflection.

Cognitive learning theories were initially based on animal experiments by Kohler (1925), but all three above-mentioned theories can be applied to healthcare professional education programmes. They include learning by insight (or insightful learning) which overlaps with Gestalt learning theory, which in turn refers to seeing the whole picture, and insight is gained through the 'aha' phenomenon and the sudden realisation of a solution to a problem, or how various parts fit into a pattern, for instance the 'penny-dropping' experience.

Gestalt theory of learning (e.g. Koffka, 1935) can be applied to professional education programmes by structuring learning so that learners are given problem situations to resolve (such as in problem-based learning), and through group discussions, analysing ideas and trial and error, whereby particular insights are gained. Thus, group discussions as well as project work, self-directed learning and peer learning can enable this process. Implementation of problem situations that can be used in teaching include, for instance, asking a small group of students to resolve a snapshot of a clinical situation such as helping a patient with partial paralysis move from a bed to a chair safely.

To a notable extent, Bruner's (1960) discovery learning theory refers to insightful learning. It involves situations that are devised in such a way that the learner can discover principles and underlying techniques for themselves. It also involves the use of past experience and existing knowledge to form new insights. For instance, a student who witnesses a patient with asthma gain relief from distressed breathing by using their inhaler can gain further insight into the specific functions of bronchioles and alveoli in oxygen transfer previously encountered in books or lectures.

Ausubel et al.'s (1978) assimilation theory is based on the view that most meaningful cognitive learning takes place as a result of interaction between the knowledge (cognitive structures) that the individual already possesses, and new information that the individual encounters. Thus, the single most important factor influencing learning is the knowledge that the learner already has. This forms the basis for the transfer of learning, in that, for instance, once the learner comprehends the principles of asepsis in hospital settings, the knowledge can be adapted in community care settings.

Thus, Ausubel et al.'s (1978) assimilation theory refers to activating the relevant knowledge the student already has so as to assimilate new knowledge into their existing mental structures. This also increases retention, and is therefore also relevant for adult learners, as they already have substantial knowledge prior to starting on an academic course.

For new information to be 'received and assimilated' or subsumed into an anchoring structure or schema, Ausubel and his colleagues suggest giving the learner prior reading or the opportunity to engage in particular activities in preparation for the teaching session (referred to as 'advanced organisers', and more recently as 'flipping'). The advanced organiser creates an anchoring structure for the new knowledge, like a scaffolding of ideas on which to build what the student needs to know. For instance, prior to a practice placement with a physiotherapist, the learner could be advised to revise or learn about the microstructure of muscles, in readiness for learning how they are strengthened through exercises by a patient who has had a broken leg operated on.

Cognitive learning theory therefore involves learning by participation, and continually taking into consideration the person's previous knowledge and competence, such as clinical skills already learnt by the student on previous placements, and university skills laboratories. Cognitive learning is supported through learning by adaptation of technological devices, or digital technologies through the use of customised apps, and is fully endorsed by the NMC (2018b: 20, 28).

Experiential learning refers to learning by doing, albeit supervised, rather than by merely being informed by others about a particular topic. It is achieved by building simulation activities in teaching–learning sessions, for instance, as advocated by Kolb (2014), among others. Experiential learning is therefore a component of reflective learning.

REFLECTION POINT 2.2:   LEARNING FROM EXPERIENCE

Consider the question: Do we learn from all experiences we come across in our day-to-day activities?

In response to Reflection Point 2.2, you might have felt we can't be learning all the time, that is, all of our 16 waking hours each day, every day of the year. On researching how much we learn from all the situations that we encounter each day, minute by minute, Jarvis (2010) found that there are several situations in life that are non-learning situations, while we do learn from other situations but in different ways. Jarvis identified ten types of learning encounters, as briefly summarised in the box below. The list does not include self-directed learning, nor styles of learning, as they are concepts of learning in their own right.

TEN TYPES OF LEARNING ENCOUNTERS

Non-learning	When we encounter a situation that we have dealt with before, we respond to it in the same way as before (also referred to as presumption)
Non-consideration	When we are presented with a new learning situation but we do not take it up, which may be because we are too busy for example, or the topic area is too complex
Rejection	When we consciously or deliberately reject a learning opportunity, maybe because we have had negative experiences related to that situation in the past, or sense information overload
Ambivalence	Conflict between our thinking and our emotions can leave us undecided about whether to pursue a line of learning
Incidental learning	Also referred to as *pre-conscious knowledge learning*, we sometimes learn without realising we have; we also learn through our bodily senses, e.g. by the scent or look of something
Memorisation	Learning facts and recalling them without much thinking being involved, either by brief memorisation or for longer-term use
Emotional learning	When we think about what we are learning which gradually becomes a part of our feelings and attitude
Action learning	Learning from participation in skilled activities, but may include learning by 'trial and error'
Discovery learning	When we find a solution to a problem or by conducting experiments
Reflective learning	Also referred to as contemplation, learning by deliberately reflecting on a situation straight after the event

Jarvis' types of learning acknowledge the reality that there are particular situations that do not lend themselves to much learning for each individual, that is, non-learning experiences. Learning by memorisation is also referred to as non-reflective learning and includes rote learning, and also temporary learning such as a telephone number for one-off use.

However, reflective learning focuses on the important part that experience and deliberate contemplation plays in the learning process. Reflective learning refers to the learning that occurs as a result of systematic reflection on situations encountered. Consider the following reflective recording in the portfolio of a student social worker Sheila.

CASE STUDY 2.1:   SHEILA'S PORTFOLIO RECORDING

I visited Mr J while his care coordinator, who is also my practice supervisor, was on annual leave. At this time Mr J expressed concern about his care coordinator and questioned her supportive abilities. My initial reaction was to explain that different practitioners would use different approaches, and advised him to raise the issue with the care coordinator. In a further conversation by telephone, Mr J reiterated the issue but in a more agitated manner and asked me to speak to the care coordinator. His care coordinator suggested that we visit Mr J to question him about what he actually wanted from the service and what type of support he felt she should offer. She felt Mr J didn't always engage with services (he frequently missed appointments), and that his drug-addiction problem was the issue he most needed to address, but which she did not specialise in. Mr J was receiving services from the drug team but, again, he didn't always attend his appointments. However, it was clear Mr J felt he needed more support. As a result, we discussed a referral to an agency which provided outreach support specifically for people with a history of offending and drug/alcohol abuse problems. Mr J was keen to accept this support.

I deduced from managing Mr J's situation that the negotiated line of care and treatment can be more effective than prescribed routes because it is consistent with person-centred practice that treats the service user as an individual with his own thoughts and preferences.

Reflective recordings from clinical situations provide an essential learning vehicle for students. The above case study demonstrates the purpose of reflection, which is learning from the situation or 'incident', despite being only a brief account. Kolb (2014), for instance, suggests that learning can be conceived of as a four-stage learning cycle that involves identifying the immediate concrete experience or an incident as the basis for observation and reflection. Out of this arise new concepts for hypothesis and theory building. Implications of these are considered in new situations and then theory is confirmed, adjusted or advanced.

This form of learning is widely used in general and professional education programmes. Individuals are encouraged to learn from situations or 'critical incidents' that they encounter, to analyse them in the context of published literature and to record them systematically in their portfolios. These can comprise assessed work components of their programme of study.

The rationale for reflective practice in healthcare is that it is also a means of constructing or generating knowledge from particular incidents. The origins of reflection on incidents go back to times when, for instance, techniques for dealing with aggressive behaviour in mental health nursing were minimal. When clinical staff met after such incidents to discuss the situation, they started realising that if cues and signs of potential violence were identified in the individual patient before the disruptive incident actually occurred, they could take certain actions to prevent it from happening in the first place. This was formalised and seen as a therapeutic means that could be used, step by step, to prevent the disruptive incident, and also gain a better understanding of the service user's thinking. This also constituted constructing knowledge from clinical practice. The lack of knowledge and theory development from day-to-day experiences in practice settings was a weakness identified by Phillips et al.'s (2000) study of learning in practice settings.

Similar 'concrete experiences' have led to changes in clinical practice, such as use of the triage system in Accident and Emergency departments and ensuring that normal saline solution is at room temperature or above prior to using it for wound cleansing. Several of these examples are noted in Chapter 5.

Kolb's (2014) learning cycle comprises four stages in the learning process, from the initial concrete experience or incident, through to exploring the experience retrospectively so that it leads to new learning, generalising from the new learning, to applying new learning to similar new situations. The original Kolb's cycle is presented as a closed circle with the fourth stage (applying new learning) leading to the first (the initial concrete experience). However, it is likely that the new learning may not be fully effective when applied to new situations that are similar, or even identical, to the initial concrete experience or incident, and therefore it becomes another new experience or incident to learn from.

Consequently, the experiential learning cycle can be presented more meaningfully as a spiral that shows that applying new learning to similar situations must be undertaken with an open mind, as further learning might ensue in the light of new evidence and evolving social changes, as well as possibly research (see Figure 2.1).

Adapting (i.e. making small changes) to published models and frameworks in one's teaching and learning is not uncommon, and can in fact be recommended as they are applied to specific groups of people or activities. This is also because Kolb's model of learning has its critics. For example, Bergsteiner et al. (2010) thoroughly examined Kolb's learning cycle and argue that the graphics of the model are flawed and suggest changes. Rogers and Horrocks (2010) argue that since learning from new experiences requires 'critical reflection', all learning cycles need to be adapted in the search for new principles before new conclusions are reached.

Nonetheless, teachers and students can alternatively utilise other models of reflection, such as the one by Boud et al. (2005), Gibbs (1988) or others that are generally available in the published literature. Boud et al.'s model of reflective practice involves identifying the concrete experience, observation and reflections, attending to feelings, re-evaluating the experience and new learning.

For instance, when the student encounters a new experience during the practice placement, they observe the experience as a critical incident and later they recall the incident, and describe it, reflect on it and explore it in the context of existing

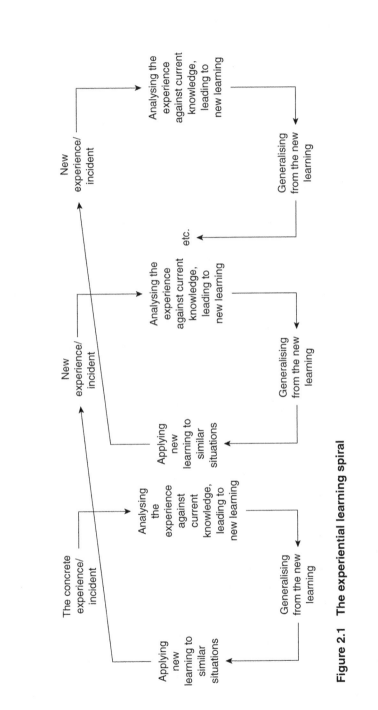

Figure 2.1 The experiential learning spiral

knowledge within professional and other relevant literature. As a result of this, they develop and generate further insight by identifying and redefining the problem in a climate of mutual support (at university reflection-on-action workshops, for instance). They can share their newfound knowledge in as much detail as appropriate, even make a presentation, as it might have teaching implications for future practice. However, to benefit from this concept, the scheduling of the learning process should ensure that time is made available following practice placements for reflection, consolidation and evaluation.

CONSTRUCTIVISM

Also gaining in popularity is a further development from the three groups of cognitive learning theories, one that is referred to as 'constructivism'. As a concept that was earlier pioneered by Berger and Luckmann (1967) as the social construction of reality, constructivism previously signified how individuals construct new thoughts, images, concepts and theories from structured and incidental experiences, that are 'scaffolded' onto the individual's existing current and past knowledge. An evolving ensuing term is 'constructionism', which refers to specific instances of creation of knowledge from life experiences and encounters with learning situations.

Currently, as a learning theory, constructivism is founded on the premise that, by reflecting on our experiences, each one of us constructs our own unique understanding of learning encounters, and in the quest for meaning we construct our own images and models of reality. Thereby the student does not accept verbatim all knowledge presented to them, but assimilates it in the context of their prior knowledge and their current social surroundings. Research findings on constructivism as a basis for effective learning include those of a study by Duane and Satre (2014) that supports the uses of this theory.

Furthermore, Choe et al. (2014) conducted a study examining the effect of two constructivist teaching strategies, namely action learning and 'cross-examination debate', and concluded that both strategies enable active interaction among students which can enhance their adaptability in practice settings and self-knowledge. Problem-based learning is another teaching strategy that can incorporate the principles of constructivism.

HUMANISTIC LEARNING THEORIES

A third group of theories that have been developed with regard to how learning occurs are humanistic learning theories, which include:

- Alan Rogers' characteristics of adult education and andragogy
- Carl Rogers' student-centred approach to learning
- Maslow's learning as self-actualisation.

Humanistic learning theorists claim that preceding theories omit aspects of human existence such as feelings, attitudes and values, and thereby overlook the more holistic perspective that incorporates attitudinal components of learning. They suggest that learning should be concerned with personal human growth. Students can therefore learn concepts, theories, models and propositions (i.e., 'propositional knowledge') from books and other learning resources, and spend more classroom time on experiential learning activities, which include thinking processes that also incorporate exploration of values, attitudes and feelings.

ADULTS AS STUDENTS ON HEALTHCARE PROFESSION COURSES

In the context of the more holistic and humanistic approaches to learning, adult learning is another concept in its own right.

REFLECTION POINT 2.3:   ADULT LEARNERS

Consider the question: Should ways of teaching adults be different from ways of teaching school children or college students? That is, what is different about adult students in contrast to school or college pupils? Think of reasons for your answer.

Both Knowles (2015) and Rogers and Horrocks (2010) suggest various ways in which teaching adults, or adult education, is different from teaching children. A prominent underpinning assumption about the preferred way of learning by adult learners is that they are competent at self-directed learning. Teaching adults includes teaching university students on generic or professional courses. Some of the differences suggested by nurses on post-registration courses are identified in Table 2.2.

Table 2.2   Differences in the ways in which adults and children learn

How children learn	How adults learn
• Children have a shorter attention span, and therefore a variety of learning activities is needed, including starter activities. • Teaching children is pedagogy, e.g. telling them. • Children are more open to new ideas. • There is a need to reinforce information over time.	• Adults are (usually) self-motivated to learn. • Adults may have relevant (or faulty) professional and life experiences. • Open discussion is more feasible in adult groups. • Lesson content can be adjusted based on ongoing evaluation of learning needs.

Source: Gopee (2000)

However, in both instances, the learner–teacher relationship is important and needs to be based on mutual trust. Different teachers may have their own repertoire of different teaching styles and techniques when teaching adult students. Rogers and Horrocks (2010) conclude by identifying the characteristics of adult students or learners as individuals who:

- define themselves and have a self-image as adult students
- are in the middle of a process of growth, not at the start of the process
- bring with them a package of experience and values
- come to learning with intentions
- bring with them expectations about the learning process
- have competing interests
- already have their own set of patterns of learning.

REFLECTION POINT 2.4:   ADULT EDUCATION IN HEALTHCARE COURSES

How far is the adult learning approach relevant or applicable to nursing and other AHP education?

Rogers and Horrocks' characteristics of adult learners suggest that adult students' learning can be facilitated more effectively within an ethos of self-directed learning. Practice supervisors can build self-directed learning into practice placement programmes for learners by allocating time for exploring further relevant clinical experiences or consulting relevant learning resources.

ANDRAGOGY AND SELF-DIRECTED LEARNING

Andragogy is an approach to teaching and learning aimed at enabling individuals to become aware that they should be the originators of their own thinking. Accordingly, although substantial knowledge and skill acquisition begin on qualifying (for example, becoming a registered nurse), it is up to the individual professional to determine the necessary areas of learning for themselves. This learning could be instigated by ward-based experiences and the self-direction developed should become career-long.

In a qualitative study of lecturers' and students' perceptions of self-directed learning (SDL) and factors that facilitate or impede them, Lunyk-Child et al. (2001) found that students who engage in self-directed learning undergo a transformation that begins with negative feelings (i.e. confusion, frustration and dissatisfaction), but ends with confidence and skills for lifelong learning. Based on a qualitative study in which Embo et al. (2014) tested the usefulness of the 'Midwifery Assessment and Feedback Instrument' (MAFI), which already functions as a framework for facilitating SDL, they concluded that MAFI does promote SDL in practice settings, except it needs to be supported by a feedback culture for enhanced effectiveness.

However, another side to SDL is highlighted by Hughes (1999), who indicates that this approach is not necessarily 'emancipatory' as it can be a 'repressive instrument' in that it can marginalise the benefits of collective and cooperative learning, that is, learning in groups in classrooms. Hughes suggests that governments can use SDL to argue that less central funding would be required to educate self-directed students.

Nonetheless, Phillips et al. (2015) used the 'Self-directed Learning Readiness Scale' to ascertain student nurses' readiness for SDL and found that first-year students show less readiness for SDL than more senior students. However, they also found readiness for SDL by those with a previous first degree to be higher than those with a postgraduate qualification.

Additionally, Du Toit-Brits and Van Zyl (2017) concluded their research on SDL by identifying the characteristics of effective self-directed learners, which include: self-determination to learn, assertiveness, self-discipline, being organised, perseverance, high degree of self-motivation, inquisitiveness, and being goal oriented, that facilitators of learning should help learners develop or strengthen in themselves.

REFLECTION POINT 2.5:   CHARACTERISTICS OF SELF-DIRECTED LEARNERS

Consider the characteristics of self-directed learners identified by Du Toit-Brits and Van Zyl and reflect for yourself whether you already have these characteristics. Do you find these characteristics desirable in an effective learner?

Knowles (2015) suggests that learning facilitators need to develop specific competencies to accommodate effective SDL. In light of these issues, and reservations related to andragogy and the benefits, as well as Rogers and Horrocks' (2010) general characteristics of adult learners, it can be concluded that in healthcare:

- Adult education constitutes collaborative activities between teachers and learners (and can include use of a learning agreement).
- Teaching should build on learners' professional experiences.
- Learners should participate in identifying learning needs, setting objectives and evaluating learning.
- The level of effective application of theory to clinical practice must always be identified.
- The role of the teacher is that of a facilitator.
- The outcome of the teaching and learning encounter should be to enable the individual to develop into a responsible autonomous practitioner.

The implications of the above examination of SDL for practice supervisors is that it cannot be assumed that, even as adults, students are necessarily competent or willing to be self-directed learners, and therefore several may need guidance on which areas of knowledge and skills they should pursue to enhance their learning during practice placements.

STUDENT-CENTRED TEACHING

Carl Rogers (1983) is well known for suggesting that teaching may be an overrated activity, as it is learning that should be in focus. For this to happen, he advocated the use of empathic understanding, genuineness and being non-judgemental in learning situations. These activities are helping skills that Rogers successfully trans-ferred from therapeutic counselling situations to student-learning situations (Rogers and Freiberg, 1994). The teacher thus becomes the facilitator of student-centred learning, as is also advocated by Freire (1996) and Knowles (2015). The facilitator achieves this by creating the appropriate environment for learning and identifying resources, and therefore empowering students to become responsible, to develop self-awareness and to think of alternatives. Student-centred teaching is discussed in some detail in Chapter 3.

LEARNING AND SELF-ACTUALISATION

Maslow's (1987) theory of a hierarchy of human needs suggests that our highest-level need, which is also often lower priority, is our need for self-actualisation. Our physiological needs are highest priority, followed by safety needs, the need for belongingness and love, our self-esteem needs and finally the need for self-actualisation. It could be argued that the goal of education is to assist indi-viduals to achieve self-actualisation, to help the person to become the best that they are able to become with the resources that are accessible. Maslow observed that there are a number of characteristics of self-actualising individuals, which include:

- demonstrate acceptance of self and others
- are problem-centred
- demonstrate democratic character
- have a philosophical, non-hostile sense of humour
- show creativeness
- seem to transcend any culture.

Teachers might argue that they apply the above-mentioned theories of learning as appropriate, with particular groups or with individual learners. However, from adult educators' professional perspectives, andragogy also requires consideration of whether the adult student is merely biologically adult or merely of legally adult age, or is also a psychologically and socially responsible adult.

Furthermore, Race (2014: xii–xiii) reviewed the main prevailing theories of learning and observed that most theories are worded in academic technical language used by educational psychologists that the majority of readers find cumbersome and not easy to comprehend. He therefore constituted his theory of learning using much simpler words, which he termed the 'ripples on a pond' model of learning, which in turn identifies fundamental factors underpinning successful learning, namely:

- wanting to learn
- taking ownership of the need to learn
- learning by doing
- learning through feedback
- making sense of what is being learned
- verbalising or speaking – to deepen learning
- making informed judgements – assessing.

The ripples model of learning is a more recent further development of experiential learning and is therefore rooted in 'learning by doing'. Race argues that the seven factors underpinning learning occur in sequence, with each stage interacting with those next to it, much like a pebble falling into a pond and creating ripples, with each stage moving in backward and forward directions. It is presented as concentric circles. It is interesting to note that the first three 'ripples' tend to represent learners' motivation and the actions that they take to learn, both being components that have featured for decades as crucial for effective learning.

Race's ripples model of learning can be implemented in educating healthcare profession students by ensuring that each factor is achieved, such as enabling students to become motivated to learn, creating the medium for 'learning by doing', by giving feedback and creating opportunities for students to teach others.

HOW ELSE DO WE LEARN HEALTHCARE SKILLS?

In addition to different theories of learning, learning is also influenced by the different styles and approaches to learning adopted by individuals. The distinctions between theories and styles can be explained as follows.

A theory tends to imply cause and effect, that is, if we do x, then y should happen. For instance, if the Smiths send their child to an independent school, then they will have a better chance of securing a student place in a reputable university. According to the dictionary (Brookes and O'Neill, 2017: 970), a theory is a 'set of ideas based on evidence and careful reasoning, which offers an explanation of how something works, or why something happens, but has not been completely proved'.

Alternatively, Lindberg et al. (1998: 62) define a theory as 'a group of concepts, definitions, and statements that presents an organised view of phenomena … with the intent of describing, explaining, or controlling these phenomena'. A learning theory, the humanistic theory for instance, is an organised view of a group of concepts that should result in a better understanding of how we learn and more effective learning.

In contrast to a learning theory, a learning style refers to the unique way in which the particular individual tends to, or prefers to, respond to learning situations so that they acquire the targeted skill or knowledge. For example, do they accept new learning instantly, or do they prefer to reflect on it before accepting it fully? Do they question first whether the learning has practical applications, or do they first accept new concepts at theoretical levels? Alternatively, approaches to learning tend to depend on the level of individual commitment to particular episodes of learning, as discussed shortly in this chapter.

MAJOR LEARNING STYLES

The foregoing paragraph on learning styles was largely linked to learning theories and concepts, and partly to learning clinical skills.

REFLECTION POINT 2.6: WHAT IS YOUR LEARNING STYLE?

We are all unique as learners. How does each of us prefer to learn? What is your preferred learning style, for learning in practice settings and for learning in classroom settings? Which style does not suit you?

Learning styles (or learning preferences) have been researched over a number of years, and Honey and Mumford's (2000) classification (or framework) of styles of learning is one that has been most widely published. You might have responded to Reflection Point 2.6 by identifying that you prefer to learn by attending a course or lecture, that is, in formal teaching situations. Others may prefer to learn by:

- watching others and seeing the end-product first
- trial and error, generally through experience
- reading and other forms of personal study such as distance learning
- discussion with others.

Another well-accepted proponent of learning styles is Kolb (2014), who identifies four styles of learning manifested by students, namely the converger, the diverger, the assimilator and the accommodator. Honey and Mumford (2000) suggest that individual learners vary between whether they are activists, reflectors, theorists or pragmatists. Jarvis (2010: 86) suggests yet another learning style that comprises focusers, scanners, impulsivity and reflectivity. The main learning styles inherent within frameworks like those just mentioned are summarised in the box below.

POPULAR LEARNING STYLES

Converger vs Diverger	Convergers are individuals who tend to use abstract thinking, progress to active experimentation and generate a single correct solution; divergers tend to start from concrete experiences, generate ideas then speculate on broader perspectives.
Impulsivity vs Reflectivity (similar to Accommodator vs Assimilator)	Using the 'impulsive' style means the individual tends to respond first, at times spontaneously (is accommodating) and reflect later; those who use reflectivity tend to reflect first (assimilate) and respond subsequently.
Activists vs Reflectors	Individuals who are activists tend to involve themselves fully in new experiences; reflectors ponder on experiences from different perspectives, thoroughly analysing them before participating in the experience in practice.
Theorists vs Pragmatists	Theorists are individuals who start from observations and develop or synthesise them into theories; pragmatists tend to consider the practical application of novel encounters first and theorise afterwards.
Focuser vs Scanner	Focusers are individuals who examine the whole problem and develop solutions from them; scanners tend to solve one aspect of the problem at a time and assume that it is the correct one unless it is disproved.
Holistic vs Serialistic	Individuals using the holistic approach tend to prefer to see a phenomenon as a whole; while serialists prefer to identify its components and their roles as part of the whole phenomenon.
Visual, Aural, Read–write or Kinaesthetic	Using the acronym VARK, this model distinguishes between students who like to be shown the correct way of performing a task (visual), prefer to be instructed (aural), etc.

Styles of learning are explained in full detail in the relevant literature. For instance, the style 'Impulsivity vs Reflectivity' implies that some individuals respond to new learning stimuli first and reflect later, while other individuals reflect first and respond afterwards. Although the latter might be intellectually sounder, the former has its uses in certain situations, especially by those who are in a position to use intuitive knowledge.

ACTIVITY 2.2   LEARNING STYLE
SELF-ASSESSMENT

Locate the 16-item VARK questionnaire on the internet (e.g. see http://vark-learn.com/the-vark-questionnaire/) and print a copy. Subsequently, perform a self-assessment and look at the results to identify which learning style you tend to veer towards.

Activity 2.2 shows version 7.1 of the VARK questionnaire, but VARK version 7.8 is also visible online. To enable utilisation of styles of learning, Honey and Mumford (2000) designed a Learning Style Questionnaire (LSQ) that is also widely used. The LSQ constitutes a self-assessment tool that indicates which style is generally utilised by the individual completing it. The main uses of knowledge derived from the LSQ are:

- increased awareness of learning activities that are congruent with the individual's learning style
- a better choice of activities leading to more effective and economical learning
- identification of areas in which an individual's less effective learning processes can be improved
- development of ways in which specific learning skills can be improved, for example reflective learning.

A number of questionnaires and inventories on learning styles are available in education literature and through the internet (e.g. VARK Learn Limited, 2017), but research on learning styles almost always indicates that students do not choose and use only one fixed style of learning as they use different styles or a combination of styles.

Anderson (2016: 59) also advocates adapting teaching styles to accommodate students' learning styles, but also suggests that learners should be 'stretched beyond their comfort zones' so that they are able to adapt to different learning settings and opportunities. However, logically, in teaching in academic or practice settings, whenever teaching more than one student, it is difficult to adapt to every student's learning style.

On examining the application of learning styles in pre-registration midwifery education, Power and Farmer (2017) agree that identifying particular styles of learning for each student may have only limited practical value as it is educationally limiting in that it suggests narrowing down approaches to teaching. In their longi-tudinal study on student nurses' learning styles Fleming et al. (2011) conclude that students do not use only one 'dominant learning style', and therefore educators should endeavour to maximise students' learning potential by utilising a range of teaching and learning methods. In their exploration of two highly popular models of teaching, Ng (2014: 484) also concludes that lesson plans for teaching practical skills should use a blend of activities that stimulate visual, aural, verbal as well as kinaesthetic senses to enhance learning effectiveness because the majority of students possess 'multimodal' learning styles.

However, despite the difficulty adapting to each student's learning style when teaching groups of students in universities or practice settings, it is when practice supervisors work on a one-to-one basis with the student during practice placements that identifying learning styles could well enable the practice supervisor to adapt their teaching to the student's style of learning more fully. A potential problem is that, for example with the learning style 'Impulsivity vs Reflectivity', a learner who leans towards impulsivity may be a fluent or quick learner, or a 'surface' learner (discussed shortly in this chapter), which is akin to superficial learning. The learner who tends to use the reflectivity style may either be a 'deep' learner, or one who takes time and can be indecisive.

Furthermore, on examining the literature on learning styles, An and Carr (2017) identified a number of issues such as lack of research linking learning style to achievement, lack of frameworks for learning styles, etc. An and Carr recommend considering individuals' behavioural or personality differences such as fluency in learning, the learner's attitude to the topic area, or their temperament, and adopt a wide range of teaching styles so that learners can understand their learning weaknesses and can thereafter decide whether to work on their weaknesses and rectify them.

ADAPTING TO STUDENTS' STYLES OF LEARNING

As implied in Reflection Point 2.6, the individual's learning can also vary, depending on whether the individual has to learn clinical skills or professional theories and concepts. Despite different research findings, it is arguable that, where feasible, the practice supervisor should endeavour to assess their student's learning style and approach to see if they can adapt to them in order to make their teaching more effective. This could make the achievement of practice objectives easier and more efficient.

An example of the adaptation of the 'Theorists vs Pragmatists' style of learning is as follows. For instance, if the practice supervisor finds that a particular student has leanings towards the pragmatist style for any particular component of learning – that is, they immediately want to know how the learning applies to actual patient care situations – then the practice supervisor can first focus on the practical application of the learning and subsequently move on to the underpinning theories. The practical knowledge can follow immediately afterwards and the theoretical knowledge later. Another student may wish to acquire all necessary theoretical knowledge before engaging in its practical application.

APPLYING THE 'PRAGMATIST STYLE' TO LEARNING DRUG CALCULATION

Another example of the application of learning styles can be with regard to students acquiring drug calculation skills. Competent drug calculation is naturally a crucial nursing or midwifery skill, as too much or too little medication can either harm the patient or delay their recovery (which the 'theorist' would need to know before learning the skill). But some students struggle to become competent at drug calculation, which is a problem that has been highlighted for over a decade. A literature search in just one journal (*Nurse Education Today*) presented over 100 articles on the topic area, and recently there has been a proliferation of books (and even e-learning packages) on drug calculation. Many universities also have a mathematics support department to help students who need to refresh their calculation skills.

Coincidentally, practice supervisors are in a suitable position to help their students or supervisees learn these skills, as instead of being a classroom-based potentially dry topic, during practice placements drug calculation directly applies to each individual service user in their care. During drug administration, the practice supervisor could seize the opportunity to ascertain his or her student's drug calculation skills. Subsequently, if appropriate, for the learner who is more of a pragmatist than a theorist (or leans towards the 'visual' style), the practice supervisor can show the learner step by step how patient X's medication dose is calculated, preferably long before they learn to administer the medication. It is a competency that simply has to be mastered (e.g. NMC, 2009, 2010a, 2017c).

To conclude this examination of learning styles, there are also individuals who do not adhere to a specific learning style, as noted by Fleming et al. (2011) for instance, and the individual may even consciously change their learning style according to the situation. Learners could develop their ability in all styles of learning and change or adapt them as new knowledge and skills are encountered, which might depend on how novel the experience is to the individual. Style may also change through new experiences and at different stages of maturation. Furthermore, practice supervisors usually already make their facilitation of learning even more efficient by the use of learning contracts.

USING LEARNING CONTRACTS

Learning contracts are very much a feature of adult education (or andragogy, as discussed earlier in this chapter) and involve negotiated learning between teacher and student. As the word *contract* implies, a learning contract is a written and signed agreement between teacher (practice supervisor in this case) and learner resulting in the latter's active involvement in decisions over practice objectives and other components of learning. Therefore, it is often a feature of practice placement learning whereby the practice supervisor and student agree on specific practice objectives and on each party's responsibility in the achievement of the objectives.

The use of learning contracts is advocated by Knowles (2015) in the context of adult learners needing to exercise more self-direction in their learning. The agreed set of objectives in the learning contract includes those of the course curriculum for practice learning, and those of the student and the practice supervisor. Therefore, the learning contract affords the student some control and responsibility over their learning, motivates them to engage with the placement experience and to learn. It is also a medium for identifying the student's pace of learning, to explore the means of theory and practice integration, and can be supported by ascertaining the student's preferred learning style.

However, the requirements and objectives set by the course curriculum have to be met. A learning contract section or template may already have been included in the student's placement competencies booklet. Basically, the practice supervisor and student discuss and agree on specific practice learning objectives for the student, how the learning will take place and precisely how they will know that the objectives have been achieved. These are usually written down by the student and, when agreed, both practice supervisor and student sign and date the contract. Learning pathways based on patient journeys can be incorporated as a strategy for achieving particular objectives. An example of a learning contract is presented in Template 2.1.

Crucial components of the learning contract are also the specific resources (human and material) that are required to enable the student to achieve the agreed objectives and also the specific dates by which each objective will have been achieved. An alternative to a learning contract is a 'learning agreement' (RCN, 2017a; University of St Andrews, 2017), which has similar features but might not include the signatures of those involved, nor rigid 'achieve-by' dates.

REFLECTION POINT 2.7:   THE LEARNING CONTRACT

What would logically happen after both parties have signed the learning contract? Do you feel that it should be constantly reviewed to monitor the student's progress with its content, or only reviewed on the 'target date'?

Learning contracts may be seen by some as a chore. Others may prefer to write something, treating it as a mere formality. But the benefits of learning contracts have been reported by Boitel and Fromm (2014), for example, who identify a learning contract as a vehicle for integration of theory and practice in the practice setting for social work students. They suggest that the learning contract requires the student to think about the relationships among the classroom-taught application of learning, the practice placement experiences, and the competencies that need to be achieved, and does so with efficacy.

Template 2.1 A learning contract

Name of student:

Placement:

Cohort:

Practice supervisor's name:

Learning needs	Objectives	Resource and strategies	Target date	Evidence
What do I want to learn? – Topic area	What do I want to have achieved at the end of this learning? – Specific objectives	How will I learn, and who will support me? – Learning strategies	Date of achieving the objectives	How will I know I have achieved my intended learning?
1. Assessment of a new patient	Able to assess the health and social care needs of newly admitted/referred patient/ service user	Practice supervisor, social worker	30–11–2018	Practice supervisor reviews and agrees with my assessment and care plan
2. Teach patients	Able to teach a type 2 diabetic patient how to control their dietary intake	Practice supervisor, dietician. Consult diet sheets, guidelines. Read up on type 2 diabetes	30–11–2018	Practice supervisor observes my teaching and signs me as competent in this skill
3. ……….	...			

Pre-contract

Signature of student: Date:

Practice supervisor's signature: Date:

Name of link lecturer/practice education facilitator: Name of personal tutor:

Comments on achievement of contract objectives

Signature of student: Date:

Practice supervisor's signature: Date:

An important step involved in constructing a learning contract is the practice supervisor facilitating self-assessment of clinical skills and knowledge by the student and identifying prerequisite learning. Naturally, when a contract has been drawn up, then on the 'achieve-by' date there will be a need to ascertain whether the activities identified in the contract were undertaken and the objectives achieved. The review time will of course have been determined at the beginning when the content was being discussed and documented.

The practice supervisor will have developed knowledge and understanding of the use of learning contracts as part of the practice supervisor preparation programme, along with how they can deliver these functions in the context of other roles that they have to fulfil.

Rogers and Freiberg (1994) indicate that learning contracts endow the student with some freedom to learn aspects that they wish to learn and pursue areas that they find particularly interesting. A learning contract is also a medium for resolving any doubt that there may be about specific purposes of the learning experience. It clarifies the activities that the student would engage in and provides motivation and reinforcement through the achievement of objectives.

For learning contracts to be effective, they need to be skilfully constructed. Guidelines for constructing them are provided by educational researchers such as Knowles (2015), and an example of a well-constructed learning contract is presented in Template 2.1 above.

LEARNERS' APPROACHES TO LEARNING

Evolving from different theories and styles, research has also identified different approaches to learning. Marton et al.'s (1997) research on approaches to learning identified individuals who take a deep approach to learning, those who take a surface approach and those who take the strategic approach. Students tend to use one of these three approaches. The defining features of each approach are presented in the box.

DEEP, SURFACE AND STRATEGIC APPROACHES TO LEARNING

Deep approach	• Relates ideas to previous knowledge and experience • Looks for patterns and underlying principles • Checks evidence and relates it to conclusions • Examines logic and argument cautiously and critically • Engages with full interest with the course content

(Continued)

(Continued)

Surface approach	• Studies without reflecting on purpose and strategy • Treats the course as unrelated bits of knowledge (discrete elements) • Memorises facts and procedures in relation to assessments • Finds difficulty in making sense of new ideas presented • Feels undue pressure and worry about coursework
Strategic approach	• Puts consistent effort into studying • Ensures conditions and materials for studying are appropriate • Manages or organises time and effort to greatest effect • Is alert to assessment requirements and criteria, and pays attention to cues about marking schemes • Gears work to the perceived preferences of lecturers

Whether a student takes the deep or surface approach to learning (Marton et al., 1997) might also depend on the stage of development of the subject area. Social sciences and arts may warrant a deep approach, while parts of science subjects such as biology and law might only require surface approaches, at least at earlier stages because they often constitute factual, single-answer knowledge. Newer and less factual subjects might also warrant a deep approach.

Approaches to learning also relate to the quality of the learning undertaken. Ramsden (2003) reports that if someone treated learning as an external imposition and concentrated on memorising facts, then that person was taking a surface approach to learning, and this would result in poor knowledge and understanding of the subject. Alternatively, 'if they intended to understand, and interacted vigorously with the content of the text (a deep approach), they stood a better chance of getting the author's message and being able to remember the supporting facts' (2003: 19). As for adapting to the student's approach to learning, the practice supervisor would prefer the student to take a deep approach but, during very busy times, strategic and surface approaches might temporarily be relevant.

PRINCIPLES OF LEARNING

Based on the views, theories, styles and approaches to learning discussed in this chapter, there are certain generally agreed principles of learning that can be concluded from them, which can make learning more effective from the standpoint of both facilitators and learners. Partly derived from Gagné et al.'s (2005) and Knowles' (2015) research, these principles are:

- Whatever a student learns, they must actively learn it themselves – no one can learn it for them.
- Each student learns at their own chosen pace, as this varies depending on their particular circumstances, mental abilities and various other factors.
- A student learns more when each step is immediately reinforced or corrected.
- Full, rather than partial, mastery of each step makes the total more meaningful.
- When given responsibility for their own learning, the student can become more highly motivated and likely to learn and retain more.
- The teacher as manager of learning should assume that McGregor's (1987) theory Y prevails, that is, learners are self-motivated to learn, and they seek out learning opportunities for themselves (theory X implies learners have to be directed or coerced to learn).
- Students who come to education expecting to be passively fed information and knowledge should be eased into andragogical principles of learning and teaching soon after.

CHAPTER SUMMARY

This chapter has focused predominantly on the 'what' and 'how' of learning professional knowledge and competence, and has therefore explored:

- What healthcare learners learn, and why, in the context of the student's learning needs and the different types of knowledge associated with professional skills.
- The definitions of competence and healthcare competencies, and issues related to them.
- Major views and perspectives on learning, teaching and education, which include what learning is, and where and how individual healthcare learners learn.
- Theories underpinning learning, in particular behaviourist learning theories (including Bandura's social learning theory), cognitive learning theories and humanistic learning theories, such as andragogy and self-directed learning, student-centred approach to learning and learning as self-actualisation.
- How learners learn healthcare skills, which included an examination of major styles of learning, and approaches to learning, such as deep, surface and strategic learning, and how the practice supervisor can adapt their teaching activities to students' individual styles and approaches; use of learning contracts.

FURTHER OPTIONAL READING

1. For a detailed discussion on 'vicarious learning' in relation to social learning theory, see:

   - Roberts, D. (2010) 'Vicarious learning: A review of the literature', *Nurse Education in Practice*, 10(1): 13–16.

2. For a systematic review of research on simulated learning, see:

   - Cant, R.P. and Cooper, S.J. (2017) 'The value of simulation-based learning in pre-licensure nurse education: A state-of-the-art review and meta-analysis', *Nurse Education in Practice*, 27(November): 45–62.

To access further resources related to this chapter, visit **https://study.sagepub.com/gopee4e** where a range of learning and teaching materials are provided.

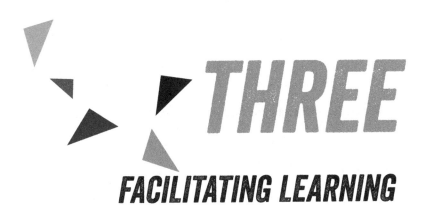

THREE

FACILITATING LEARNING

INTRODUCTION

Having explored in Chapter 1 the meaning of practice supervision and similar roles, why we need these roles, and how they are performed, and then in Chapter 2 the different major perspectives on learning, along with learning theories, styles and approaches, this chapter focuses on the practice-based facilitation of learning or teaching duties of practice supervisors.

The chapter therefore considers the various professional groups of learners whose learning healthcare professionals facilitate; whether to teach or facilitate learning; systematic ways of facilitating learners' acquisition of practice skills and knowledge; as well as some of the main issues related to facilitation of learning in practice settings.

CHAPTER OBJECTIVES

1. Identify a wide range of students and learners whose learning qualified healthcare professionals facilitate.
2. Differentiate between teaching and facilitation of learning, and the different contemporary perceptions of, and approaches to, teaching and learning.
3. Evaluate a number of ways in which practice supervisors can enable healthcare students to acquire health and social care skills, the steps involved in effective planning for skills teaching, along with the underpinning knowledge base.

(Continued)

(Continued)

4. Demonstrate knowledge of structured and systematic methods of teaching that can be implemented by practice supervisors to enable students and learners to acquire health profession skills and knowledge; and of some of the issues related to facilitation of learning.
5. Evaluate various methods of teaching and the teaching aids that can be selected for effective teaching for all categories of learners, including students with special educational needs and disability.

WHOSE LEARNING DO HEALTHCARE PROFESSIONALS FACILITATE, AND WHY?

ACTIVITY 3.1   WHO DO HEALTHCARE PROFESSIONALS TEACH?

To start exploring facilitation of learning, first make a list of all the groups of people who nurses and other healthcare professionals teach, mainly in healthcare settings. Having done this, add the exact healthcare topic areas that they are likely to teach to the different groups of individuals.

The healthcare professional's role includes a substantial teaching component and you might therefore have felt that Activity 3.1 was rather simplistic. However, it does reflect the reality of the extent of teaching that RNs, RMs and AHPs do, and in response to the activity you might have mentioned:

- Nurses teach student nurses (first, second and third year), healthcare support workers on national vocational qualification courses, student nursing associates, students on nurse apprenticeship programmes, patients/service users, patients' relatives/carers, and junior doctors.
- Midwives teach women/service users, for example new mothers and fathers, how to look after a new baby.
- The practice nurse teaches primary (and secondary) level ill-health prevention, for example how to quit smoking, lose weight, expectant mothers regarding their diet and relaxation for those with high blood pressure.
- SCPHNs teach mothers with different needs, such as single teenage mothers or those in different age groups.

AHPs and doctors have a teaching role towards healthcare service users and might also teach other healthcare staff.

WHY DO HEALTHCARE PROFESSIONALS NEED TO KNOW HOW TO FACILITATE LEARNING?

On a day-to-day basis, the healthcare professional's role focuses largely on attending to healthcare service users' health problems. Teaching activities generally tend to be more sporadic and are engaged in at opportune moments, in addition to timetabled work-based teaching of target learners. Nonetheless, there are several reasons why healthcare professionals teach and facilitate learning. First, in addition to teaching colleagues and juniors being a job requirement for most healthcare professionals by virtue of their contract of employment, teaching also constitutes one of the four essential components of healthcare professionals' groups of duties (HCPC, 2016: 3), the other three being clinical practice, management of care, and research. Six categories of healthcare professional roles are also identified by Gopee and Galloway (2017: Chapter 1) as:

- care interventions (i.e. direct patient care activities)
- the organisation and management of care
- training and educating colleagues and students
- teaching and promoting health and well-being
- using research and evidence-based practice
- leadership.

Correspondingly, the *NHS KSF* (DH, 2004: 57) notes under 'personal and people development' that healthcare professionals have to contribute to 'the development of others during ongoing work activities [by] structured approaches ... informal and ad hoc methods' and demonstrate and share skills and knowledge (see also NHS Employers, 2010).

Similarly, teaching usually forms part of healthcare professionals' codes of practice, which stipulate that they must be willing to share skills and experience. For instance, the NMC's (2015a: Clause 9) and HCPC's (2016: Clauses 2.5 and 2.6) codes of practice specify that registrants 'must' share their skills, knowledge and experience for the benefit of their colleagues and service users, and also support their students' learning. This form of teaching includes teaching new skills to colleagues (RNs/RMs), for example the use of new medical devices such as a new glucometer, how to conduct a patient assessment using a new form, applying a new wound care ingredient, using national early warning system (NEWS).

Developing teaching skills is also an integral component of healthcare professionals' pre-registration education programmes as identified by the NMC (2018b: 30), which under the heading '*Communication and relationship management skills*' for example states: 'Demonstrate effective supervision, teaching and performance appraisal', and provide 'clear instructions and explanations when supervising, teaching or appraising others'. Under 'Platform 5 – *Leading and managing nursing care and working in teams*' (NMC 2018b: 20), clause 5.8 reads 'support and supervise students in the delivery of nursing care ... and documenting their performance'.

Furthermore, sometime after registration with the regulatory body, specialist RNs and other healthcare professionals are at times required, or invited, to do small-group teaching on specific aspects of their specialist areas within the healthcare trust or classroom teaching on specialist university-based courses. Moreover, research by Campbell and Evans (2016) confirmed that managers have a central role as facilitators of workplace learning, particularly so if they adopt a coaching approach and act as role models for teaching and learning.

Additionally, healthcare professionals might also seek out opportunities to teach merely to advance the teaching or presentation skills that they have previously acquired to varying degrees. They could thereby also start to develop public speaking skills. For more experienced practice supervisors, teaching provides them with an opportunity to apply the principles of teaching and learning, and experiment with new teaching techniques. Furthermore, practice supervisors have to teach because of variable levels of success in joint education–trust roles such as lecturer–practitioners and the clinical teaching role of nurse lecturers.

FACILITATING LEARNING OR TEACHING?

At times we hear the statement, 'John (or Jane) is an excellent (or a born) teacher', but, as with most skills, teaching can be regarded as an 'art' and a 'science'. This means that although someone may appear to have a natural knack for teaching, it is also a skill that can be learned, using scientifically deduced theories. Teaching courses such as the *Diploma in Education and Training* (Education and Training Foundation, 2018) offered at colleges of further education and the 'Postgraduate Certificate in Education' courses are specifically designed for this purpose.

After several years of teaching experience, eventually the skill becomes so well developed and refined that it appears akin to an artistic talent. However, thinking about some of the concepts discussed in Chapter 2, such as self-directed learning and reflective learning, consider the question: Should practice supervisors teach students and juniors, or facilitate their learning? Both concepts are suggested for contemporary practice supervision activities.

APPROACHES TO TEACHING AND LEARNING

Dictionaries tend to define teaching as 'to tell or show someone how to do something' and 'to give instructions (or lessons) to students' (Brookes and O'Neill, 2017: 959). Such definitions tend to signify teaching as one-way traffic, that is, the teacher controls the content, volume of content and the sequencing of the content. They also reflect one of the earlier approaches to teaching. However, various other approaches to teaching and learning have evolved over the years, so much so that Joyce et al. (2009) indicate that there are more than 22 models of teaching, some of which are well researched whilst others still need rigorous testing.

An underlying trend that figures clearly in all these approaches and models of teaching is the transition from the rather derogatory term 'teacher-centred' teaching to 'student-centred' teaching. Three stages of evolution of approaches to teaching can be identified, which are as follows:

1. In the earlier stage, teaching was seen as the teacher imparting selected and pre-determined knowledge and skills to students as he or she is the expert in that subject area. In such approaches, students in turn are passive recipients of the instruction, but this results in students feeling inhibited from exploring alternative views.
2. In a gradual change in attitude towards teaching and learning, teaching was viewed as enabling active learning, an approach in which teachers structure learning activities for students so that the latter actively engage with the subject matter and explore specific topic areas in the curriculum or syllabus. Thus, the teacher leads students to conclusions by enquiry and questioning.
3. In the third and current stage, teaching is viewed as 'facilitating learning', whereby teachers work in partnership with students and jointly determine their learning needs in the overall context of the curriculum and the means by which those learning needs will be met. The teacher creates the conditions for learning and does not control all learning outcomes, thus allowing the student a substantial degree of choice in what to learn.

These three stages of development in ways of teaching therefore reflect an evolving trend from the earlier one implying a teacher-centred approach to the latter as much more student-centred, and therefore progressing from teaching to facilitation of learning. Thereby the approach to student learning shifts from a focus on teaching and the teacher, to learning by the student. The approach chosen of course depends on several factors such as the particular student group's motivation to learn, the teacher's own beliefs about teaching and learning, and the subject matter, or a deliberate combination of these as the teacher feels appropriate.

The three teaching approaches can also be categorised as didactic, Socratic or facilitative, respectively. Contemporarily, Ramsden (2003) refers to these approaches as theories 1, 2 and 3. However, Biggs and Tang (2011: 16–20) interpret these three approaches as three 'levels of thinking about teaching' and note that at stage (or level) one, if the student does not 'absorb' the knowledge and skills imparted to them, because they either have not got the ability or the motivation to do so, then the teaching is unlikely to be as effective.

In the level (or stage) two approach, in addition to the ability to impart knowledge and skills, the teacher needs additional skills such as that required to structure learning activities and to negotiate student learning so as to ensure the curriculum's learning outcomes are met. Yet further skills are required at the third and current level of thinking about teaching, which is facilitation of learning, as this is based on the student's own learning needs and is about enabling students to engage with their learning more actively. The earlier approaches were also reflected in the method of assessment used by educators, which had negative effects on students' learning and achievement.

The trend in moving away from teacher-centred approaches to student-centred approaches was suggested several years ago by Bruner (1960), for instance, who advocated 'discovery learning' theory, indicating that this approach can make learning more effective as it is an active process that is stimulated through student curiosity. The teacher therefore devises situations, poses problems or questions, and creates the medium for the student to discover the structures and principles underlying the situation or topic area. This approach feeds into the currently advocated methods such as problem-based learning, which is an instructional method in which students work in small groups or individually to gain knowledge from simulated problem situations and acquire problem-solving skills at the same time.

Practice supervisors can use these approaches in their learning facilitation roles. Problem-based learning can be implemented in the form of self-directed learning in clinical practice, in, for example, management of a staff conflict situation, management of a new illness or syndrome and the use of limited learning resources. The teacher, however, must ensure that the learning is directly linked to achieving learning outcomes or competencies identified in the module or the course.

Current definitions of teaching take these evolving learning philosophies into account. For example, according to Curzon and Tummons (2013: 20), teaching is 'a system of activities intended to allow learning to happen, comprising the deliberate and methodical creation and control of those conditions in which learning does occur'. The definition thus does not reflect teacher-centred one-way information-giving.

TEACHER-CENTRED OR LEARNER-CENTRED APPROACHES

Teacher-centred teaching approaches clearly imply that the teacher directs the content and parameters of the teaching session. This may have advantages in being economical, in that with their deep knowledge of the subject the teacher can maximise the allocated time by selecting and focusing on the most significant areas of the topic.

Drawing on the theories underlying patient or service user-centred therapy for people with psychological problems, Rogers (1983) formulated the student-centred approach to learning, which formed a major defining shift in approaches to teaching and learning. Rogers suggested that:

- Human beings have a natural potentiality for learning.
- Much significant learning is acquired through doing.
- Learning is facilitated when the student participates responsibly in the learning process.
- The most socially useful learning in the modern world is the learning of the process of learning, a continuing openness to experience and incorporation into oneself of the process of change.

ACTIVITY 3.2   TEACHER-CENTRED OR STUDENT-CENTRED TEACHING

To follow up on the aforementioned approaches to teaching, identify a number of factors that you consider to be the strengths and weaknesses of teacher-centred and student-centred teaching methods in healthcare professional education programmes.

Jarvis (2010) notes that using teacher-centred methods of teaching reinforces hierarchical social relationships between teachers and learners (or practice supervisors and students), and thereby replicates models of authority in which the teacher might be seeking to control and mould individuals to fit into social systems. Rogers (1983) suggested earlier that such approaches cause learners to become dependent on teachers and thereby obstruct growth and development. The possible weaknesses of teacher-centred methods or strategies include the following:

- They assume that students usually lack discipline and are irresponsible.
- They disregard experience as a resource for learning.
- The orientation to learning is subject-centred rather than building on the individual student's existing knowledge.
- The motivation to learn is external, for example by passing coursework.
- They can suppress the individual's creative powers.
- Student's opinions and questions tend to be largely overlooked.

Consequently, pivotal to effective facilitation of learning is the relationship between individual learners and the facilitator. Rogers sees the teacher as a facilitator of learning, a provider of resources for learning and someone who shares feelings as well as knowledge with learners. The prerequisites for being an effective facilitator of learning are awareness of self and being oneself in the teaching situation, through (as mentioned in Chapter 1 in relation to building an effective working relationship):

- *Genuineness* – The facilitator demonstrates full honesty and willingness to declare their strengths and the areas in which they are lacking, where appropriate. They remain a real person and are not sucked into the image of a distant and authority-vested teacher.
- *Trust and acceptance* – The facilitator must be able to gain and retain the student's trust, and vice versa, and overtly accept any limitations that students might have.
- *Empathic understanding* – The facilitator consistently endeavours to see situations from the learner's viewpoint.

Rogers contrasts the kind of learning that is concerned solely with cognitive functioning, for example acquiring knowledge, with that involving the whole person. The learning naturally needs to be guided by the approved curriculum for the course the student is on to be able to obtain the relevant award (i.e., qualification). Rogers suggests that it is possible for the teacher to build into a programme this freedom to learn. This can be done by using students' own experiences and problems so that relevance is more obvious, and by identifying relevant resources – both material and human – for their students. The goal of education is therefore to enable the student to become a fully functioning person as a whole (Rogers and Freiberg, 1994).

In healthcare learning, the student-centred approach is reflected in andragogy, but the latter needs to be tailored to the individual student's responses to it. Facilitation of learning is also consistent with the andragogical approach to teaching and learning, as advocated by Knowles (2015) (and discussed in Chapter 2) and with 'learning by insight', that is, 'a perception of a whole group of relationships ... a suddenly occurring re-organisation' of one's thoughts (Curzon and Tummons, 2013: 62). A concept analysis of facilitation of learning by Cross (1996) revealed that the:

- prerequisites of being a facilitator are the facilitator's qualities of realness, that is, caring and empathy, access to learning situations and the motivation of students and social influences
- defining attributes of facilitation are a process of enabling change, a climate of learning which includes mutual trust, acceptance and respect, and the nature of interaction being student-centred, negotiated and collaborative
- consequences of facilitation are reciprocal change and feedback, and increased independence.

On exploring the effectiveness of supervisors as facilitators of 'informal learning' in the workplace, Macneil (2001) recommends that more concerted effort is required to facilitate informal learning, through providing for continuous learning based on unanticipated eventualities in work settings. This idea is reinforced by Amy (2008: 212) whose research concluded that learning can be 'institutionalised' in organisations (e.g. healthcare trusts) through facilitative leadership.

CASE STUDY 3.1:   FACILITATING JANE'S PRACTICE-BASED LEARNING

Consider the following case study. Jane is a 34-year-old ex-schoolteacher who is now a first-year midwifery student. Jane is a graduate, who, after initial teacher training, soon found the job easy but had no wish to take on management responsibilities. The job was soon becoming too routine when she realised that in fact she had always wanted to be a midwife instead. Jane is also raising her own family and has remained an active member of the Parents and Teachers Association.

Consider the ways in which Jane's practice supervisor, Julie, can take a learner-centred approach to learning facilitation during the practice placement. Make some notes taking into account Jane's previous vocation.

Practice supervisors can consider ascertaining and adapting their facilitation of learning role to the learner's previous knowledge of health and their preferred styles and approaches to learning, as noted in Chapter 2. Jane's age, responsibility and discipline as a qualified teacher and a mother can be taken into account when taking a learner-centred approach to placement learning. A self-directed approach to learning in collaboration with Jane, with guided study if required, can be warranted to make learning more meaningful and complete for her.

Despite these benefits of the student-centred approach to teaching, there could also be drawbacks, some of which are identified in the box.

ARGUMENTS FOR, AND CRITICISMS OF, THE LEARNER-CENTRED OR PERSON-CENTRED APPROACH TO TEACHING

Arguments for:	Criticisms:
• Motivates, as aims and objectives are clear and relevant. • Learning is meaningful. • Encourages divergent and critical thinking through dialogue. • Allows autonomy and creativity.	• Can be time-consuming if emphasis is on the nature of learning, rather than how much of the curriculum is covered. Rogers (1983) was aware of this and suggested that there should be freedom within a system of constraints. • Structure and guidelines may suffer. • Timetables and deadlines might not get adhered to. • Assumption that everyone engages in self-directed learning.

Despite likely weaknesses, the student-centred approach to facilitation of learning is preferred as it entails more active involvement in learning. This is also consistent with Biggs and Tang's (2011: 63) assertion in relation to the senses and remembering, in that in general learners learn 80 per cent of what they do as learning activities, 50 per cent of all they see and hear, but only 10 per cent of all they hear.

In experiential learning, as a way of adapting learning theories to methods of teaching, students need to be given opportunities for 'doing', that is, applying or using the knowledge or skill. For example, most healthcare courses include the topic 'moving and handling patients'. This is an apt example that lends itself to experiential learning, in that having been exposed to the knowledge base (for example, principles of moving and handling), students can then learn by doing. This can occur in university skills laboratories under close supervision of the facilitator. Students can be given problem situations to solve, which could enable them to make the topic their own and internalise it.

A concluding suggestion on facilitation of learning is that, in the context of the current-day vehement push towards efficiency, practice supervisors and their learners need to seize learning opportunities as they arise, which is also referred to as opportunistic learning or teachable moments.

FACILITATING LEARNERS' ACQUISITION OF CLINICAL SKILLS

Healthcare professions are skill-based vocations, which means that pre-registration education leads to individuals becoming competent at performing specific clinical interventions to improve patients' or service users' health. Competence was defined and discussed in Chapter 2. Alternatively, a skill signifies having expertise in an activity that has been developed as the result of training under the supervision of an expert or is self-taught, that enables the individual to perform the particular task adeptly, and also flexibly. The skill requires mind and muscle coordination and effective movement that ends with the desired result. The features of a skilled activity include dexterity, the ability to respond quickly, and the capacity to share attention among a number of more or less simultaneous requirements, which are also features of clinical skills exercised in contemporary healthcare settings.

LEARNING MOTOR SKILLS

Progression with learning and mastering clinical skills can be placed along a continuum that identifies early attempts at learning a skill to becoming proficient. A widely used framework for categorising levels of psychomotor skill development and testing in healthcare courses is that suggested by Steinaker and Bell (1979) in a taxonomy of experiential learning. The term *taxonomy* broadly refers here to levels of learning, that is, learning from lower levels to higher levels. In Steinaker and Bell's model, skill development progresses from the lower-level exposure, through participation, identification and internalisation to dissemination.

Experiential learning refers to learning that involves going through the experience of actually doing or engaging in the skill. Competency or skill development through the different levels occurs over the three-year course. Steinaker and Bell's five levels of learning and the likely interpretation (or criteria) related to a clinical skill are presented in the box below.

TAXONOMY LEVELS AND CRITERIA

Levels	Criteria
Exposure	Have some knowledge of concepts, terms and methods used in clinical practice Show willingness to participate
Participation	Interact well with patients/service users Carry out activities under supervision Explain activities when questioned
Identification	Apply theory to practice Demonstrate awareness of situations Interpret information correctly Act on one's own without having to be prompted
Internalisation	Consistently apply theory to practice in a range of settings Compare and contrast different approaches to practices Determine implications of practices Solve problems by analysis and evaluation Show willingness to share experiences
Dissemination	Use opportunities to teach service users and families Share experiences with peers and others Accurately write and verbalise information about teaching and management issues

Consider a mental health student who has to demonstrate a certain level of proficiency in helping or counselling skills by the end of their third year of professional education:

Exposure – refers to the student observing the practice supervisor helping or counselling appropriate service users and becoming aware of the preconditions and specific helping skills being used by the practice supervisor.

Participation – refers to when, under supervision, the student attempts to use selected helping skills, e.g. low-level self-disclosure.

Identification – is when the student starts to feel competent at some of the helping skills and this is acknowledged by their practice supervisor.

Internalisation – can be difficult to achieve within the constraints of the pre-registration course, as this implies that the learner is so proficient at these skills that they see them as part of themselves as a person.

Dissemination – refers to being so knowledgeable and competent in a skill that the person can have specific and valid opinions about the skill, can explain them and even teach them, which is difficult to achieve in a pre-registration course.

To teach competencies at the appropriate level entails careful planning that determines the teacher's approach, student behaviour and assessment techniques. Another well-established model of learning a clinical skill is Benner's (2001) stages of skill acquisition, which is based on a framework initially deduced from how trainee pilots learn their vocations and eventually become experts in flying aeroplanes. These stages are novice, advanced beginner, competent, proficient and expert, in this sequence, and they relate to longer-term activities on expertise development as they progress from initial cruder attempts to more refined performance with a substantial associated knowledge base.

Fitts and Posner (1973) earlier on identified three phases of learning most skills – the cognitive phase, associative phase and autonomous phase:

Cognitive phase – concerned with the learning of the procedure, but the more complex the skill, the longer the learning will take.

Associative phase – engaging in skilled performance of part-skills or in whole practical skills, and interfering responses are eliminated.

Autonomous phase – in the long term, the skill becomes automatic and can be performed without the student thinking much about it.

The three phases are not completely distinct, as they overlap, with one phase leading to the next.

TEACHING PSYCHOMOTOR SKILLS

A major component of the practice supervisor's role is to teach clinical skills. Various aspects need to be considered in relation to this. On and off, PEFs have complained that the previous mentor courses haven't adequately equipped course attenders with teaching skills, a major limitation noted by Jayasekara et al. (2018) as well.

ACTIVITY 3.3   SKILL ACQUISITION AND MAINTENANCE

Think of, and list, all factors that the practice supervisor as a teacher needs to consider, and all preparations that they need to make to teach a particular clinical skill in the practice setting. Then list all the factors that might affect enabling efficient acquisition of the psychomotor skill in the practice setting. Finally, list all the factors that might affect maintenance and performance of the clinical skill at the same or higher standard in practice settings.

There are several factors that need to be considered when preparing to teach a clinical skill. Those required for teaching blood glucose monitoring, for instance, include:

- which patient?
- condition requiring it
- equipment needed
- approved procedure for taking a blood sample
- gain patient's consent
- factors affecting reading of results
- ensuring there's enough blood on the test strip
- safety aspects
- own knowledge
- the student's knowledge base – practical and theoretical
- reading result – up/down/normal
- record the result, and take any necessary action
- opportunities to practise
- frequency of measurement
- testing the equipment and cleaning it after use
- evaluate, observe, supervise
- what if?
- time allocated
- record learner's competence.

A list of factors that need to be considered for a particular clinical activity like the one above is rarely fully prescriptive as there are other variables that need to be taken into account in relation to the individual health service user's health problems or needs, and the equipment and other resources that are available.

Teaching a clinical skill requires first of all a skills analysis. Generally, the trust's procedure for the clinical action constitutes a very good basis for structuring a lesson plan for the skill. The practice supervisor can also consider how the task is performed or executed, step by step, by those who are recognised as competent at the particular clinical action. These are discussed shortly. Such a detailed analysis of the clinical skill constitutes its performance or assessment criteria, which is discussed in Chapter 6. In the box below a set of principles of teaching a skill or competency is presented that stands the test of time (adapted from Curzon and Tummons, 2013). These are generally fully used when teaching a skill in the HEI's skills laboratory but can be easily adapted by the practice supervisor when teaching in the practice setting.

The principles presented in the box constitute a firm foundation for developing a skill-teaching session. Achievement of competence at one level ought to be accepted as a necessary preparation for moving to higher level of skill. The learner should be able to progress from competent to proficient performance, etc. Drawing on this, and on healthcare professionals' perceptions of factors that need to be considered when preparing to teach a psychomotor skill, the teacher should also consider taking the following actions before the actual skill-teaching session:

PRINCIPLES OF TEACHING A SKILL OR COMPETENCY

1. *Initially demonstrate the skill in its entirety as a fully integrated set and cycle of operations.* The demonstration needs to be accompanied by a clear step-by-step commentary, and it must be a demonstration of mastery of the skill. The correct movements that go to make up the skill must be in evidence from the outset.
2. *Break the skill down into its component and subordinate activities.* Each action must be demonstrated, explained and analysed. The relation of separate activities to one another and their integration into a hierarchy of sequences that make up the skill must be stressed.
3. *Skill acquisition lessons require supervised, reinforced and carefully spaced practice by students.* It is only by experiencing and repeating the essential movements that the learner can discover the kinaesthetic cues of successful performance.
4. *Continuous, swift and accurate feedback must be provided for the learner.* Delayed feedback on performance makes the feedback less effective.
5. *Assess part-skills or the whole skill regularly and in work-related realistic conditions.* Evidence should also be sought on the ability of the student to transfer the acquired skill to related situations.

Source: Adapted from Curzon and Tummons (2013)

- Practise the skill yourself, using the relevant procedures and equipment.
- Ensure that, as the teacher, your practice is up to date and evidence-based.
- Have all equipment and materials ready.
- Arrange for your learner(s) to hear and see the skill demonstration.
- State the aim of the session.
- Show the finished product if possible.
- Ask the student/patient to verbalise the action.
- Arrange for the student/patient to practise the skill.

DOMAINS OF LEARNING AND LEVELS OF SKILL ACQUISITION

Precisely which areas of knowledge and competence do healthcare students learn on their pre-registration courses? Well, students learn a comprehensive range of knowledge base and competencies that are required for healthcare interventions. Each intervention comprises three domains of activity: psychomotor (skill), cognitive (knowledge) and affective (attitude) (for example, Bloom, 1956; NMC, 2018b – includes values, compassion, empathy).

The psychomotor domain refers to motor, muscular and coordination skills; the cognitive domain refers to the use of knowledge and information; and the affective domain refers to attitudes, emotions and values. The three domains equating broadly with skills, knowledge and attitudes, also equate largely with doing, thinking and feeling, respectively. The three domains are integrated essential components of each competency and not necessarily distinct and separate activities. All health-care interventions incorporate these three domains and therefore learning the clinical skill must also incorporate all three components.

The sequence of events that both teacher and learner should engage in during skill acquisition is summarised in Table 3.1. It captures the principles of teaching and facilitation of learning of a psychomotor skill or competency that incorporates the cognitive and affective domains. The five components of the affective domain to be achieved by the learner are: *receiving*, *responding*, *valuing*, *organising* and *characterising* (Krathwohl et al., 1999).

Table 3.1   Skills teaching sequence

Psychomotor domain	Cognitive domain	Affective domain
Awareness that learner lacks the skill or is deficient in it	Establish learner's existing knowledge base underpinning the skill	Receiving – i.e., ensuring learner realises that it will be beneficial to learn the skill
Ensure the learner is motivated to learn the skill	Permit learner to be active in seeking related knowledge	Responding – learner is willing, and takes action to learn the skill
Analysis of the step-by-step procedure/components of the skill	Having clear objectives in learning the skill, and seeking out possible sources of learning	Responding – learner appreciates the step-by-step procedure and the materials required at every step
Prepare equipment, etc., to teach the skill	Assembling appropriate equipment/devices and materials	
Demonstrate the skill at normal speed	Enable learner to observe and assimilate all details of the procedure	

(Continued)

Table 3.1 (Continued)

Psychomotor domain	Cognitive domain	Affective domain
Discuss each step just performed; re-demonstrate part-skills as required ↓	State rationale for each action; emphasise important points; discuss safety points; encourage learner to ask questions	Valuing – the rationales for each step taken; learner is willing to participate in performing the skill or part-skill
Allow learner to perform whole skill/part-skills ↓	Select components to work on, and actually 'doing' the skill, i.e. experiencing it	Organising – mental rehearsal of each skill component, with rationales; asking questions when unsure
Allow learner to perform the skill under supervision ↓	Observe in silence, and with confidence in the learner	
Praise and review ↓	Give feedback on performance. Reward progress. Correct any mistake.	Organising – reinforcement and sense of achievement, confidence
Allow to apply/repeat the skill under supervision ↓	Using the learning in real situations. Assess progress and knowledge of rationales	Characterising – accepting the procedure is the correct way of performing the skill

After practising the skill on several occasions, a summative assessment of competence will be performed by the practice assessor and, if the learner is deemed competent, he or she is usually permitted to practise the skill without direct supervision. One of the key purposes of Table 3.1 is to highlight how the cognitive and affective domains of learning are integral components of learning any clinical intervention.

As a general guide, 25 per cent of the lesson time should be used to demonstrate the skill, 15 per cent in verbal explanation and 60 per cent for guided practice. So, for effective acquisition of the skill or competency, it is important to consider the requirements for effective teaching. Other factors that shape effective and efficient acquisition of the skill include:

- the complexity of the skill
- individual differences in speed of learning, or background
- its transferability to real-life settings
- teaching situation – environment, light, space, room temperature
- the quality of instruction
- knowledge of progress
- availability of practice opportunities
- availability of necessary equipment – checking it beforehand, describing it
- getting feedback on skill performance

- a positive approach
- a running commentary if appropriate
- a true-to-life setting
- allowing time for discussion
- time for practice – with positive reinforcement.

An example of a 'lesson plan' (examined closely shortly) for teaching a clinical skill to a learner is presented in the following template, with a few dotted lines for completion depending on the learner group who is being taught. It provides details of the sequence of activities involved in teaching skills effectively, by providing an example of a lesson plan for teaching a clinical skill, which in this instance is manual measurement of blood pressure (MMBP). Very briefly, this comprises five steps: introduce the skill > demonstrate the skill > explain key actions taken > demonstrate and give rationale for each action > practice by the learner(s).

The template may need adapting according to whether the skill being taught is in a skills laboratory (in university or in the healthcare trust), and to the number of students being taught (which can be from 1 to 30), availability of extra lecturers to supervise each learner practising the skill, the complexity of the skill, whether each student has to be summatively assessed during the session, etc.

Template 3.1 represents an effective step-by-step lesson plan for teaching any clinical skill. Alternatively, see Gagné et al.'s (2005) *Principles of Instructional Design* for comprehensive detailed analysis of skills teaching. Moreover, at times authors (e.g. Ng, 2014) cite the use of Peyton's (1998) 4-step model of teaching a clinical skill which constitutes: (1) demonstration of the skill; (2) deconstruction, i.e. identifying each distinct step of the skill; (3) explanation of reasons for each step; and (4) performance of the skill by the learners. However, oversimplifying a task in this way can mask the complexity of the whole task; and also not stating clearly the objectives of the lesson, or not ascertaining the learners' existing knowledge, can result in ineffective or erroneous skills learning.

The types of knowledge associated with skills teaching is practical knowledge (i.e., 'knowing how') and theoretical knowledge (i.e., more in-depth 'knowing that'). Healthcare courses involve acquisition of both types of knowledge, and students are assessed on them at different academic levels, as detailed shortly in this chapter. Also see https://study.sagepub.com/gopee4e for an example of a lesson plan for teaching a component of knowledge or healthcare theory.

FACILITATING KNOWLEDGE ACQUISITION

Despite the current paradigm shift away from teaching to facilitation of learning, formal teaching also has its place in professional preparatory programmes. Many clinical skills and knowledge components are best imparted to learners through teaching. There will be times when the practice supervisor will have to conduct short structured teaching sessions, probably in a room in the practice setting that

Template 3.1 Steps in lesson planning for teaching manual blood pressure measurement

Date:	Cohort:	Number of students: ....

Title of the course & module: ....

Subject of lesson (clinical skill being taught): Manual measurement of blood pressure

Lesson aims: ....

Lesson objectives:
1. ....
2. ....

Duration of the lesson: 1 hour 50 mins		Classroom:	
Time (minutes)	Lesson content	Teaching method	Teaching aids
2	State and explain lesson topic and **objectives**	Verbal exposition (VE)	ppt slide
5	Ascertain students' existing **knowledge** of MMBP, and rationales	Questions & answers (Q&A)	--
5	Explain the clinical skill, and the **rationales** for performing them, including recapitulation of related anatomy and physiology	Q&A	ppt slides
5	**Demonstrate** MMBP at normal speed	Demonstration	Equipment & student volunteer
10	**Explanation**/overview of rationale for each step	VE	
15	**Demonstrate** the skill at slow pace, explaining/ascertaining rationales for each step	Demonstration	Equipment & another student volunteer
30	Supervise students handling equipment and **practising** MMBP on each other	Supervision	Sets of equipment
3	**Recapitulation**, and invite and respond to any question	VE & Q&A	--
3	Indicate location of paper or electronic copies of clinical **guidelines** or procedure for performing MMBP	VE	ppt slide
20	Intensive **practice** of MMBP by each student	Practice	Sets of equipment
10	**Test** each student (if required), or evaluation of session	Test/evaluation	MCQ/gapped handout papers
2	**Evaluation** of session and announce title of next clinical skill session	VE	Time-table slide

ppt = PowerPoint; MMBP = manual measurement of blood pressure; Q&A = questioning students and responding to their answers; Equipment = includes sphygmomanometer and stethoscope; ...

can be used for this purpose. These sessions can be quite short or last an hour or more, delivered to a small group of learners or colleagues. Therefore, a good insight into how to structure and deliver a teaching session is a useful component of the practice supervisor's armoury of capabilities.

Effective teaching requires careful and thorough planning. The lesson needs to be fully structured, with flexibility built in, depending on whether it is being delivered to a large group or to smaller group workshops.

PLANNING A STRUCTURED TEACHING SESSION

Logical sequencing of a structured teaching session constitutes lesson planning, an example of which is presented in the box below.

STEPS IN LESSON PLANNING

1. Identify the topic of the lesson.
2. Research the subject.
3. Consider the students in relation to their previous knowledge.
4. Write down the aims and objectives.
5. Jot down as many points as possible in keeping with the objectives; then select, prune, sequence and structure these points.
6. Select the appropriate teaching methods.
7. Screen the activities against the objectives.
8. Write the lesson (include teaching aids).
9. Prepare aids, equipment and classroom.
10. Give the lesson.
11. Evaluate the lesson.

Each step presented in the box requires specific attention in its own right. For instance, the third step requires the teacher to consider the students in relation to the knowledge they already have, as well as any prior reading that was required or suggested before the teaching session. This accords with the use of appropriate learning theories such as Ausubel et al.'s (1978) assimilation theory (discussed in Chapter 2). It is also consistent with Bruner's (1960) notion of linking new learning to previous knowledge.

As to the sequencing of lesson content and teaching methods (steps 5 and 6 in the box above), the Herbartian (Encyclopaedia Britannica, 2018) rules (or approach) for lesson presentation has stood the test of time and is also referred to as 'traditional rule'. It involves proceeding from:

The known to the unknown – link new concepts to what is already known by the learner (e.g. water to blood, water pipes to blood vessels).

The concrete to the abstract – demonstrate a link between visible or tangible materials with invisible concepts (e.g. aspirates or infusion to acidity vs alkalinity).

Observation to reasoning – from how things are done to why.

The simple to the complex – simple explanations to more complex areas; increasing level of complexity (e.g. diffusion in a jar to movement of oxygen and CO_2 between alveoli and alveolar capillaries; intra- and extra-cellular movement of potassium).

The particular to the general – use specific examples to illustrate general theories (e.g. giving information reduces anxiety, people generally have a need to know what is happening).

The whole view, to the parts, then return to the whole view – the subject matter as an entity, analysis of component parts, return to the overall view.

Step 6 in the box above suggests selecting the appropriate teaching methods. A range of teaching methods is available to the teacher (see the box below). The teaching method(s) selected for the session must be based on principles of teaching and on learning theories. The appropriateness of the method depends on the teacher's level of knowledge of theories and principles and their values, research and verbal skills, facilitative skills and on the aims of the lesson, for instance.

MOST FREQUENTLY USED TEACHING METHODS

- Lectures
- Buzz groups/work in sub-groups
- Seminars
- Skills demonstration
- Guided study and self-directed learning
- Role plays
- Problem-solving games/exercises/workshops
- Case study/patient-centred discussions
- Simulation
- Video recording of student presentations
- Tutorial – individual/small group
- Ideas free flow exercises (previously known as brainstorming), e.g. concept-mapping
- Questions and answers
- Formal lessons
- E-learning and distance learning (or blended)
- Using apps and 'usable learning objects'
- Group discussion
- Team teaching

Each of these methods has its advantages and disadvantages that are examined later in this chapter. The eighth step in the box above titled 'Steps in lesson planning' is to 'write the lesson' and includes identifying the teaching aids to be used. An example of a lesson plan is presented in the Template above for teaching a clinical skill.

In relation to steps 8 and 9 in the box titled 'Steps in lesson planning', or the use of an appropriate range of teaching aids such as whiteboard/flipchart or PowerPoint slides, some of these will be explained briefly and their advantages and disadvantages will also be explored later in this chapter.

In planning the lesson, the teacher needs to consider likely constraints such as class size (for instance, is it 10 students or 200 students?), the number of pages of handouts if any are given and the accessibility of articles that will be recommended as further reading. The teacher's aim in a lesson is to motivate, stimulate and communicate, to hold the class's attention and to achieve the defined objectives, and therefore further essential considerations by the presenter are:

1. The lesson must be appropriately pitched.
2. The teaching objectives must be realistic and clear.
3. Exposition must be ordered, simple and clear.
4. Development must be logical and sequential (flows coherently).
5. Presentation must be based on the essential 'social character' of the lesson (e.g. laboratory work or lecture).
6. Presentation must involve a variety of media.
7. Presentation must be carefully adjusted in the light of fluctuations in class attention.
8. Appropriate body language should be used.

Furthermore, a well-constituted presentation requires a clearly defined structure, the elements of which will normally include:

- an introduction, main part and conclusion
- a logical sequence within each of the three parts
- regular sign-posting – this is what we have covered so far, this is what we will explore next, and these are what we will address afterwards
- key learning points or main headings
- built-in monitoring and review – checking that the main learning points are being understood.

Appropriate communication and delivery skills are crucial. The presenter's role is also to engage with the audience, to challenge, to enthuse, to support, to motivate and to clarify. The next step is to give the lesson based on the lesson plan, and to evaluate it at the end of the lesson. The evaluation of the lesson can include use of an evaluation form, or the students can be asked to write three things that they liked or found most useful about the session, aspects that can be seen as weaknesses, and suggestions for improvement (see Chapter 9 for more on evaluation).

LEVELS OF THEORY ACQUISITION

The objective of many a teaching session is to impart knowledge and understanding of the designated topic area and, depending on various factors, it can cover application, analysis and synthesis. These concepts are largely enshrined in the cognitive domain of Bloom's (1956) taxonomy of learning, which follows six hierarchical levels. The first or lower level of learning is the acquisition of knowledge, followed by the higher levels – comprehension, application, analysis, synthesis and evaluation, as illustrated here:

1. *Knowledge* – refers to knowledge of topic area and content.
2. *Comprehension* – refers to knowledge, and comprehension or understanding of why things work the way they do.
3. *Application* – refers to knowledge and comprehension, and application of knowledge and understanding to general and specific settings.
4. *Analysis* – refers to knowledge, comprehension, application, and analysis of all components of knowledge and application; and alternative perspectives.
5. *Synthesis* – refers to knowledge, comprehension, application, analysis, and synthesis of components to arrive at solutions to problems.
6. *Evaluation* – refers to knowledge, comprehension, application, analysis, synthesis and evaluation (research, etc., on the topic).

Knowledge is the most basic level of learning, in which the student shows recall of specific facts, classifications, categories and sequences or methods in the topic area. It is a significant component of student assessment, as when the student has to demonstrate knowledge of human biology or of research methods. *Comprehension* refers to understanding and interpretation of the topic area, and can be shown by the student explaining theories and reasoning in their own words. It answers the question 'why' certain things happen, or certain actions are taken, and the possible implications and consequences of these. *Application* occurs when the student applies knowledge and understanding to 'real-life' situations such as patient care.

Analysis entails the ability to break down theories and concepts into their component parts and explain the relationships between elements and the whole. It considers strengths and weaknesses, and separates the important aspects of information from the less important ones. *Synthesis* requires the individual to recombine various components of the topic area into a newly reconstructed whole. The student thereby utilises creativity in producing something unique, for example a plan, a design or a proposal. *Evaluation* implies the ability to make judgements regarding the value of material learned.

A simple and brief example of levels of learning related to 'the heart and blood pressure' is presented here to illustrate how cognitive levels of learning (Bloom, 1956) apply to learning in healthcare:

- *Knowledge* – knowing the anatomy and physiology of the heart and that pressure is exerted on the blood vessels each time the heart pumps a certain volume of blood through them.
- *Comprehension* – understanding that the reason for the heart beating rhythmically at approximately 60 beats every minute, generating a blood pressure (BP) of approximately 110/70 mm Hg is to ensure that essential ingredients such as glucose and oxygen are transferred to every tissue in the human body, and continuously.
- *Application* – awareness that the above BP reading can change for a variety of reasons, which might include diseased organs, and its significance for patient care.
- *Analysis* – when a person is seen to have high BP, the nurse needs to consider the whole range of reasons for this.
- *Synthesis* – designing, and advising the individual on, a set of actions to take to reduce their BP, and explaining the effects of unstable or high BP based on their own unique aetiology and perceptions of high BP.
- *Evaluation* – ascertaining the value of the above set of actions, the skills and compliance of the patient in relation to them, and any research evidence on which actions are based.

The analysis of the cognitive domain of learning is essential as it involves critical analysis, which as already noted above entails breaking down information, exploring relationships between elements, or organisation and structure of information. Critical analysis involves the use of critical thinking, whereby we:

- examine all the component parts of a situation
- identify what existing knowledge or information we have, related to the situation
- distinguish relevant information from irrelevant
- challenge generalisations, assumptions and rituals
- imagine and explore alternatives and choose appropriate options.

Gopee (2002b) and Gopee and Deane (2013) discuss effective ways in which students can demonstrate critical analysis in their written assignments. Furthermore, Krathwohl (2002) has suggested a refinement of Bloom's (1956) level of knowledge acquisition by suggesting that the sequence be represented as follows:

1. Remember	2. Understand	3. Apply	4. Analyse	5. Evaluate	6. Create

Krathwohl reverses the fifth and sixth levels, and this revised taxonomy is also a useful tool for identifying educational objectives but, as with any new framework, it requires further work in its applicability to education programmes for healthcare professions.

TEACHING METHODS AND TEACHING AIDS

As discussed in the preceding section, skill demonstration is an effective way of teaching how to perform a professional skill. For structured lessons, effective teaching requires choosing and applying the appropriate teaching methods and aids, which are selected based on such factors as class size, aims of session, the students' existing knowledge levels, and so on. The most frequently used teaching methods were identified in the box presented earlier titled 'Most frequently used teaching methods'.

TEACHING METHODS – THEIR ADVANTAGES AND DISADVANTAGES

Lectures remain an efficient teaching method for imparting knowledge and comprehension of a selected section of a subject area. A lecture is economical in that the knowledge can be imparted to hundreds of students by one lecturer during a particular teaching session. In fact, the lecture can be televised live to other lecture theatres in the same or other universities, even in other countries.

However, only a limited level of application and analysis can be achieved, as in very large groups it is difficult to cite examples of application to each student's field of interest. Moreover, it is easier for students to let their minds wander off the subject, which they generally cannot do in smaller groups. Discussions, workshops and group work to explore application, analysis and synthesis of components of the lecture should therefore always follow lectures. Similarly, the advantages and disadvantages of other teaching methods also need to be appreciated.

ACTIVITY 3.4   TEACHING METHODS: ADVANTAGES AND DISADVANTAGES

Taking an analytical approach, the strengths and weaknesses of each of the examples of different teaching methods listed in the box titled 'Most frequently used teaching methods' can be identified. Consider these different teaching methods, and feel free to add others of your own, and identify as many advantages and disadvantages as you can for each of these methods.

You should have been able to identify one or two advantages and disadvantages of each of the aforementioned teaching methods. With *skill demonstration*, for instance, the advantages include visual display of the skill being performed. It reinforces previously acquired knowledge of the skill, activates many senses, enables procedure-directed practice, correlates theory and practice and is economical on time. The disadvantages could be that the learner might be left-/right-handed related to positioning of equipment, the skill might involve movements that are too complex and too much information might be given. As learning and mastering a skill take time, there is also a danger that the learner might be expected to perform the demonstrated skill at similar speed to the skilled demonstrator too soon.

The advantages of using *case studies* or *patient-centred discussions* as a teaching method are that there is active participation by students, they are useful in the application of theory to practice and they present an opportunity for structured problem-solving. This increases understanding of the situation, diagnosing the problem, creating alternative solutions and predicting outcomes or implications. The disadvantages include insufficient patient data and extent of relevance for each student.

PRESENTATION AND TEACHING AIDS

There are several types of presentation aids that the teacher can utilise to vary the session and thereby to retain the audience's attention or to add emphasis to aspects of the session. These aids include:

- flipchart and pens
- whiteboard
- PowerPoint slides
- showing video-cassette or DVD recordings
- plastic models of body parts/objects
- gapped handouts
- simulated materials or liquids
- visualisers.

The purpose of teaching aids is therefore to introduce variety into the teaching process, to extend sensory perception, to extend visual perception, to give meaning to abstractions and to assist in conceptualisation of complicated issues. The choice of visual aids involves consideration of appropriateness to the context or message, their cost-effectiveness, their availability and their suitability for your style of presentation. Each teaching aid requires a good understanding of how it works.

ACTIVITY 3.5   STRENGTHS AND WEAKNESSES
OF DIFFERENT TEACHING AIDS

Consider the strengths and weaknesses of the different teaching aids listed earlier, add other ones that you know of, and discuss with someone who has had some experience of classroom teaching what the strengths and weaknesses of each of these aids might be.

The *PowerPoint presentation* is a highly favoured method of presenting the knowledge base of a topic area to small or large audiences. The advantage is that it is prepared in advance and can be made very lively and colourful with pictures, cartoons and short films for more impact. The likely disadvantage might be that too many words are inserted in each slide, or if the slides are presented at a high speed this may not allow time for the audience to take the content in properly, or the equipment (for example, computers) may fail.

FACILITATING LEARNING FOR STUDENTS WITH
SPECIAL EDUCATIONAL NEEDS AND DISABILITY

In addition to theories and individual styles of learning, facilitators of learning should also heed the special education needs and disability (SEND) of individual students (e.g. Department of Education & Department of Health, 2016). The number of students disclosing that they have a disability is increasing (e.g. Olofsson et al., 2015), including those who are students on healthcare profession courses. Universities have an obligation to comply with legal requirements, such as the Equality Act 2010 (Equality Challenge Unit, 2012), and practice supervisors have to be aware of this obligation towards students with disabilities as well under the Act.

The Quality Assurance Agency (QAA) (2010: 7) prefers to refer to the student with SEND as a 'disabled student' but retains the DDA's (GOV.UK, 2018: 1) definition of disability, which is 'a physical or mental impairment, which has a substantial and long term adverse effect on his or her ability to carry out normal day to day activities'.

The above-mentioned Act also identifies a list of different impairments that constitute a disability, including dyslexia, visual or hearing impairment and mental health conditions. In addition to disabilities, the Equality Act, which came into force on 1 October 2010, encompasses other human characteristics that employers could consciously or inadvertently discriminate against. It identifies nine such 'protected characteristics', namely:

- age
- disability
- gender assignment
- marriage and civil partnership
- pregnancy and maternity
- race

- religion or belief (including lack of belief)
- sex
- sexual orientation.

Furthermore, the above Act indicates that institutions must provide 'reasonable adjustment' facilities to support SEND students with their learning and with their course assignments. Almost all organisations concerned with the education of healthcare profession students, including the RCN (2017b) and the QAA (2010), prepare their own written statement on how they make 'reasonable adjustments' for SEND. The RCN's (2017b: 21–22) guidance on how reasonable adjustments can be made in the practice setting for students with dyslexia is as follows:

- the use of coloured overlays to assist in reading text on white paper
- the use of coloured paper
- additional training and support
- giving verbal rather than written instructions
- allowing plenty of time to read and complete the task
- giving instructions one at a time, slowly and clearly, in a quiet location
- reminding the person of important deadlines and reviewing priorities regularly
- using a wall planner, and creating a 'to do' list
- the use of modified/specialised equipment
- provision of a quiet area to write up notes, or for when specific tasks require intense concentration
- flexible working hours/frequent breaks.

For advice and support on how to make adjustments for students with SEND, practice supervisors can consult various named individuals and departments such as the local university's lecturer(s) who specialises in this topic area, Occupational Health services and students' unions.

Research on the extent to which the needs of students with SEND are met include that by White (2007) and Lavender (2017). White, for instance, conducted a qualitative study to explore how far the education needs of students with dyslexia are met during their prequalifying programme. She found that students experienced particular problems during practice placements, but none of the mentors in the study felt adequately educationally prepared to help students with disabilities. Students with SEND do develop their own coping strategies, and the study recommends that a more concerted effort should be made to support both students and their practice supervisors to make the necessary 'reasonable adjustments'.

Other than in the context of policies related to disabilities, there is also an abundance of literature and research on the topic area. Scullion (2010), for instance, identifies the two most prominent perspectives on disability: the medical model and the social model. The medical model, as the term implies, endeavours to enable people with disabilities to function to their maximum by rectifying the problem as far as they can at the pathophysiological level.

The social model tends to view those with disabilities as those who should not be stereotyped and stigmatised, but adjustments should be made to their social environment to enable them to function to their maximum. Scullion indicates that, as a strategy to challenge discrimination, healthcare professionals should promote and enhance the social model of disability through 'social advocacy'.

Furthermore, Olofsson et al.'s (2015: 346) study found that almost half of students with dyslexia need a longer period of study than other students, and Tee et al.'s (2010) study revealed that disabled students require 20 per cent more contact time with lecturers than non-disabled peers, and they therefore recommend the appointment of a 'student practice learning advisor' for extra support. Additionally, Lavender's (2017) study of modes of learning by paramedic students with dyslexia concluded by reinforcing the need to allow SEND students planned extra time for their learning in practice settings.

CASE STUDY 3.2:   STUDENTS WITH DISABILITIES

Student nurse Vicky informed the pre-registration Course Director by the end of the first week of the start of the course that she has been told previously when she was at college that she might have dyslexia. The Course Director advised the student to attend the Student Welfare Department of the university for an assessment of her particular difficulties, and to determine the adjustments that should enable her to undertake her course activities with more ease. Consequently, Vicky was issued with the following facilities and advice, some of which should help in academic settings, others in the practice setting:

- Provision of notes from the lecturer on coloured paper if possible, or use of coloured overlays
- Use of coloured overlays for reading text on white paper
- A spell checker, or a specialised computer with built-in spell checker, etc.
- Permission to have a person take notes for Vicky at lectures or to use a tape recorder to audio record lectures
- Visual diagrams to explain things
- Allowing additional time when taking written examinations
- Allowing extra time to complete nursing tasks in the practice setting
- Giving instructions one at a time, and allowing to request clarification, or double checking on instructions
- Use of pocket books to write words or instructions to remember during a clinical shift
- Use of check lists
- Allocating a quiet uninterrupted area and additional time to write up nursing patients progress notes

---

Vicky was understandably apprehensive about how quickly she was going to be able to adapt to activities in the practice setting during practice placements, and on the other hand although her practice supervisor has attended sessions on 'students with special educational needs and disability both during practice supervisor preparation and at an update session some months earlier, she hadn't actually anticipated that one of her own students would be dyslexic. At the initial individual interview with the student, when the student mentioned her disability, and also indicated that she had been able to use certain contraptions to cope with university lectures and simulation activities, the practice supervisor remembered that in the course of her normal duties she had to adjust to people with various individual differences, and did not pursue this aspect of the conversation too far at that point in time.

However, by the end of the second shift with the student, the practice supervisor had investigated various ways in which students with special needs or disability could be supported in practice settings, including in a Royal College of Nursing (2017b) document, and noted continuing use of the term 'reasonable adjustments'. Giving the student extra time with clinical activities and extra support was deemed essential by the supervisor, as well as asking Vicky how she normally managed her particular dyslexia problems. By the end of the practice placement, the student had achieved all her practice objectives and passed her first placement.

ISSUES WITH FACILITATION OF LEARNING IN THE PRACTICE SETTING

The practice supervisor's role includes teaching learners on a one-to-one basis, and at times in small groups in the practice setting. In both situations, the practice supervisor needs to have a clear view of various components of the session, for example the content and sequence of the presentation, in order to ensure that the learner gains an orderly, systematic understanding of the topic or clinical skill. However, the problematic situations that might arise when facilitating student learning may present challenges to practice supervisors.

For a variety of reasons, in practice settings it cannot be guaranteed that a planned teaching session will go ahead, although most do go to plan. Urgent need to cover for sickness, emergencies such as cardiac arrest, or the patient not consenting to student involvement, are some of the reasons. However, many care provider settings now have dedicated teaching areas, which can help focus attention on teaching sessions.

Furthermore, there can be confusion in the interpretation of students' 'supernumerary status' during placements, in that the student may claim that they are there only to observe clinical activity, while the practice supervisor believes that they should participate as well as observe. Supernumerary status can be manipulated by some students to the extent that they take excessive time off from practice settings for study time, to the detriment of learning hands-on care and clinical skills, as many practice supervisors claim that healthcare delivery is learned by doing, not by merely knowing about it.

In opportunistic learning, negotiating access to opportunities is a skill in its own right.

CHAPTER SUMMARY

This chapter has focused on the practice supervisor's role in the facilitation of learning, both formal and incidental, and has therefore examined:

- Whose learning healthcare professionals facilitate, and why; the various reasons for teaching; and the definitions and different perceptions of teaching, along with why healthcare professionals need to know how to facilitate learning.
- General perspectives on learning, indicating a move away from teaching to the notion of facilitating learning, with teacher-centred methods and student-centred approaches to teaching and learning, with the latter constituting a shift away from formal teaching to much more learner-centred facilitation of learning.
- Facilitating learning of clinical skills, teaching a psychomotor skill, the domains of learning, levels of psychomotor skills and stages of skill acquisition.
- Facilitating knowledge acquisition, include undertaking planned and structured short teaching sessions, either on a one-to-one level or in small groups of learners or peers.
- The types of knowledge associated with skills, such as practical knowledge and theoretical knowledge, along with levels of theory acquisition, and levels and stages of skill acquisition (taxonomy levels).
- Step-by-step planning of teaching sessions, including utilisation of different methods of teaching and teaching aids, and an analysis of how they can be used effectively.
- Strategies for facilitating learning for students with SEND, and some of the issues that might surface in the facilitation of learning in practice settings.

FURTHER OPTIONAL READING

1. For further discussion on facilitation of learning see:

   - Warburton, T., Houghton, T. and Barry, D. (2016) 'Facilitation of learning: Part 2', *Nursing Standard*, 30(35): 41–48.

2. For updates on the current provision for students with SEND and detailed guidance on how to support learning for students with disabilities, see:

   - Quality Assurance Agency for Higher Education (2010) *Code of Practice for the Assurance of Academic Quality and Standards in Higher Education, Section 3: Disabled Students*. Available at: www.admin.cam.ac.uk/univ/disability//practice/pdf/qaa.pdf (accessed 26 February 2017).

3. For a concept analysis of the concept of facilitation in the context of facilitating the implementation of new evidence into practice, see:

- Harvey, G., Loftus-Hills, A., Rycroft-Malone, J., Titchen, A., Kitson, A., McCormack, B. and Seers, K. (2002) 'Getting evidence into practice: The role and function of facilitation', *Journal of Advanced Nursing*, 37(6): 577–588.

To access further resources related to this chapter, visit **https://study.sagepub.com/gopee4e** where a range of learning and teaching materials are provided.

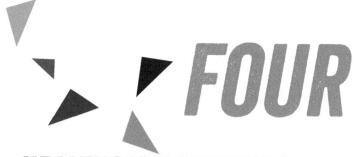

FOUR

HEALTHCARE SETTINGS AS EFFECTIVE LEARNING ENVIRONMENTS

INTRODUCTION

Having explored the concept of supervision of practice learning in Chapter 1, perspectives, theories and styles of learning in Chapter 2, and facilitation of learning in Chapter 3, this chapter focuses on the factors that make healthcare settings effective learning environments for healthcare profession students, as well as for qualified staff. Ensuring that the practice setting has an effective learning environment is an essential responsibility of workplace student placement providers.

In *Standards Framework for Nursing and Midwifery Education* under 'student empowerment', the NMC (2018c) states that HEIs together with their healthcare provider partners must ensure that all students have opportunities to learn from a variety of practice placements in healthcare settings. Under 'Learning culture' it indicates that students must be supported and supervised in practice settings that are 'conducive to safe and effective learning ... and where ... inter-professional learning and team working are embedded' (p5). The setting has a culture that is fair, transparent, and fosters good relations between individuals and diverse groups.

This chapter therefore examines the nature of effective learning environments in practice settings, ways in which healthcare professionals can be involved in creating, maintaining and monitoring such environments, and educational policies, along with the issues related to student practice placements.

CHAPTER OBJECTIVES

1. Clearly identify the various reasons for healthcare students being required to undertake practice placements.

2. Recognise the reasons for ascertaining students' previous clinical experiences before identifying their learning needs, and identify their hopes and expectations with regard to the placement.
3. Identify how a functional learning ethos can be created and maintained in the practice setting, which includes inter-professional learning, implementation of research findings and conducting annual education audits of practice placement settings.
4. Analyse the benefits of, and issues related to, work-based learning and identify ways in which the utilisation of learning pathways can enhance the student's learning.
5. Identify guidelines, policies and standards for clinical learning environments, and how practice settings can become learning organisations.
6. Recognise the likely problematic aspects of practice placements, such as integration of theory and practice, and supernumerary status, and the likely solutions to these.

STUDENTS ON PRACTICE PLACEMENTS

This section of the chapter explores why practice placements are required, and students' perspectives, hopes and expectations in relation to practice objectives and clinical experiences during placements.

THE REQUIREMENT FOR PRACTICE PLACEMENTS

The key reasons for practice settings having to be learning environments for student practice placements are as follows. First, healthcare professions comprise skill- or competency-based activities, and these skills are acquired predominantly in practice settings. Several hundred student nurses, numerous AHP and medical students start their pre-registration or pre-service courses each year, and each student requires practice placements in practice settings to learn patient care skills directly, or to consolidate and extend their learning from university skills laboratories. Most suitable practice settings in the local trusts and the independent sector are used for placements, and the placement of all these students is arranged by the education institution's placement department.

Each practice setting is advised in advance of which students are starting on placement with them and when. Students arrive on placement with a document containing practice competencies that the student must achieve during the placement, which takes into account the specific clinical skills and knowledge that the particular setting can offer.

Pre-service education requirements include those identified in the *European Union Directive 2005/36/EC* [amended by Directive 2013/55/EU] (European Parliament and The Council, 2013: 20; NMC, 2018e) for nursing qualifications, which states that the duration of learning in practice settings must comprise at least one half of the minimum duration of the training (i.e. half of a total of at least 4600 hours' duration of the total education programme). The NMC also indicates that learning environments includes any environment where learning takes place, along with a system of shared values, beliefs and behaviours within these settings. Furthermore, the HCPC (2017a) indicates that practice-based learning must take place in an environment that is safe and supportive for learners and service users (Clause 5.4).

Another reason that practice settings need to be learning environments is the increasingly popular concept of work-based learning (discussed later in this chapter), which clearly recognises the wide occurrence and value of learning in practice settings. However, various research studies have in the past revealed weaknesses of practice settings as learning environments. Consequently, for learning to occur, the practice setting must embody an ethos that nurtures and supports learning, and does not deter it. Poor clinical learning environments as a major factor in student attrition emerged from a study by Crombie et al. (2013) who explored the factors that enhance rates of course completion by student nurses.

STUDENTS' PERSPECTIVES, HOPES AND EXPECTATIONS

A number of practice settings have an established welcome and orientation programme for students starting practice placement with them, and an induction pack with specific clinical objectives for newly qualified healthcare professionals. Nominated practice supervisors are allocated to each student prior to the start of the placement. Both practice supervisors and the student have certain hopes and expectations of each other for the span of the practice placement. So, what does the student anticipate encountering at the start of the placement?

ACTIVITY 4.1   STUDENT EXPECTATIONS FROM THE PLACEMENT

Your work base clearly has a wide range of specific knowledge and competence to offer students during practice placements. From your experience of having students on placement, make some notes on what you feel are the expectations that students might have on starting placement in your practice setting.

On exploring students' expectations of mentorship, a study by Foster et al. (2015) at one UK university concluded that students value teaching, explaining, support and encouragement as some of the key features of a successful practice placement. In addition to students' expectations, the staff in the practice setting naturally also have certain expectations of students. They hope that the student will be punctual, make every effort to integrate with the team and be open-minded about the ways in which care is delivered in the particular practice setting. Practice supervisors usually expect students to seek out learning experiences and opportunities, and ask questions about aspects that they do not understand. The box below lists some of the personal qualities of 'good' learners that were identified by registrants on a previous mentor course.

ATTRIBUTES OF EFFECTIVE PRACTICE-BASED HEALTHCARE LEARNERS

- Keen, enthusiastic and motivated to learn
- Open-minded
- Identifies own learning needs
- Open to feedback and constructive comments
- Is punctual
- Reflects on experiences
- Knows own limitations
- Able to adapt to different practice settings
- Does not have negative thoughts prior to start of placement
- Utilises learning opportunities
- Communicates effectively
- Wants to self-improve
- Reads round the subject area

ADVANCED PREPARATION OF LEARNERS

Universities strongly advise students to contact practice placement settings prior to the placement start date, mainly to introduce themselves, but also to enquire about practicalities such as what time shifts start, a room for changing into uniforms, possibly travel or car-parking facilities, as well as any other information that can be given (for example, contact names). Initiating contact can be pivotal for a smooth and successful placement as, according to Webb and Shakespeare's (2008: 563) research, good learning support depends to a great extent on students themselves initiating and building a relationship with those who are supervising their learning.

However, students find it useful if, prior to the practice placement, they receive a welcome letter from the practice setting, which may even invite the student to come over for an informal pre-placement visit. It is useful if the student can also be advised of any recommended preparatory reading related to the clinical specialism. This action is in line with Ausubel et al.'s (1978) concept of 'advanced organiser', which suggests that learning is likely to occur more effectively if new experiences are linked to prior knowledge.

The value of communication prior to the beginning of the placement is that the student begins to become familiar with the practice setting, gets to know more about the clinical specialism and meets one or more practice supervisors, and staff get to know the student as well. The aim of this would be to ensure that the clinical experiences that students will encounter meet their learning needs and enable the achievement of their practice objectives.

CREATING AND MAINTAINING A LEARNING ETHOS IN THE PRACTICE SETTING

Healthcare students acquire knowledge and competence at universities that are seen as well-established learning environments. This is because they create and maintain environments that are conducive to learning through ensuring a relaxed and pleasant atmosphere in and outside campus buildings, encourage peer-learning and small-group learning by providing spaces where students can discuss their course-related issues and share knowledge in twos, threes or very small groups; they provide cafés and refreshment areas, departments that help students with course-related special issues, etc. For learning in practice settings, the value of work-based learning (WBL) in enabling healthcare practitioners to achieve fitness to practise was referred to briefly in Chapter 1. However, to what extent are practice settings learning environments?

ACTIVITY 4.2 A LEARNING ETHOS IN THE PRACTICE SETTING

Using your current and past experience of factors that are significant in creating an effective learning experience for students during practice placements, make notes on the following: Who are the key people who are role models for learners (undergraduate and postgraduate, other) in practice settings? What are the factors that are important for the creation of a positive learning environment (including research-based factors) for everyone within any particular practice setting?

To be a role model for anyone can be a sobering prospect for most people. In response to who the role models in practice settings are, you would have identified a range of qualified healthcare professionals and probably even some unqualified staff involved in practice-based learning, including:

- everyone acting as a practice supervisor
- ward sisters/charge nurses
- team leaders

- specialist nurses (e.g. pain specialists)
- PEFs
- other RNs on pay bands 5 to 8
- allied healthcare professionals (e.g. physiotherapists, occupational therapists)
- link lecturers
- other students
- senior doctors, mainly consultants
- outreach workers
- clinical managers
- healthcare assistants, for specific skills
- maybe everyone who works in the practice area.

The concept of role models was noted in different contexts in Chapter 1 which includes health and social care professionals being practitioners of best practice in service user care. However, poor care and neglect of patients were reported in the recent Francis (2013) Report at one English NHS Trust. A number of actions were subsequently taken in response to the report, which included:

- enhancement of patient safety
- staffing levels, 'to ensure the right people, with the right skills, are in the right place at the right time' (NHS England National Quality Board [NQB], 2014: 1)
- more openness and transparency, by providing information and acquiring feedback from healthcare service users and their families or friends.

These standards have to be met by the service provider to qualify as a practice placement for health and social care profession students. Similar recommendations were made in the Willis Commission Report (RCN, 2012) as noted in Chapter 2.

PRACTICE SETTINGS AS LEARNING ENVIRONMENTS

In response to Activity 4.2, that is, identifying the factors that are important for the creation of a positive learning environment, you might have noted friendly and knowledgeable staff, positive attitude and allocated time for teaching. Good communication is of course essential, as is the learner feeling that they are part of the team. Team members with up-to-date knowledge of the latest research in their specialism generally make a positive impression. The availability and accessibility of research literature in the working environment, stocked in a learning resources section or in a resource room, also create a positive image.

Furthermore, you might have noted that staff showing some awareness of students' likely learning needs and their stage of knowledge and competence development also create positive impressions. The enthusiasm of team members with responsibility for teaching in practice settings, and the input of PEFs/CHEFs, generate the impetus for learning. Constructive comments on performance of care interventions in an appropriate environment are usually appreciated by learners. A culture in which clinical staff are open to new ideas and share new learning from courses also presents healthy perspectives, as does good staff morale.

Numerous research studies have been conducted on the effectiveness of practice settings as learning environments over the years, and new research in this area continues as the dynamics in practice settings evolve. A study by Newton et al. (2009), for instance, revealed that a supportive social and cultural environment that enables the student to become part of the clinical team is very important. From their study of nursing homes as learning environments, Carlson and Idvall (2014) report with conviction that the 'supervisory relationship' (that is between practice supervisor and student) has the greatest impact on student nurses' learning, and recommend that the work of supervisors of learning in the independent sector should be fully recognised and that they should be supported through collaborative activities (for example, university-led workshops, practice supervisor updates).

More than three decades ago, Fretwell (1980) coined the term 'clinical learning environment' (CLE) as her research concluded that key components of an 'ideal' learning environment include 'anti-hierarchy', effective communication and teamwork between all those involved in the specific practice setting, and the availability of trained nurses to enable learners to meet their learning needs. Fast-forward to today, when the acronym CLE is extended to CLES+T (S signifying supervision, and T signifying additional input from academics and practice-based teachers), and CLEI (I signifies inventory), as will be discussed shortly.

ACTIVITY 4.3   CREATING A LEARNING ETHOS IN THE PRACTICE SETTING

1. Based on the perspectives and ideas discussed above on practice settings being CLEs, make a list of your own of the factors that you consider make a good learning environment in the health or social care practice setting.
2. How far does your own practice setting meet with the recommendations and factors that you have identified?
3. Identify areas in which your practice setting is weak or could benefit from further improvement.

The responses to studies on clinical learning environments could be categorised as factors that promote learning in the practice setting and those that can hinder, a number of which are identified in the box.

Due to a dearth of literature identifying ways in which non-hospital areas such as primary care settings are CLEs, Gopee et al. (2004) make the following recommendations for enhancing these settings as learning environments:

- matching practice supervisor and student in accordance with seniority of practitioner and the student's particular learning needs
- management support to enable designated time to be given for enabling learning, so that students and supervisors of learning feel time spent in this way is valued by their seniors
- raised awareness of the need to integrate theory and practice
- ensuring student practice learning objectives are achievable, for example carrying out dressings might not be available in, say, placement with school nurses
- prior notices of placement and appropriate timing, for example not allocating student to school nursing placement during school holidays
- ongoing professional development for all grades of staff
- more effective communication at all levels, and trust–university–supervisor partnership
- all supervisors of learning (and practice teachers) ensuring that they maintain the relevant NMC standards
- access to clinical supervision for all qualified staff.

FACTORS THAT PROMOTE LEARNING AND THOSE THAT HINDER LEARNING IN THE PRACTICE SETTING

Factors that promote learning	Factors that hinder learning
• Registrants' level of knowledge of their clinical specialism	• Interruptions
• Adequate time to teach	• Over-busy ward area
• Practical demonstration of skills	• Lack of time
• Students feeling that they can take their time to practise the skills	• Staff, patients' and learners' attitudes
• A learning ethos	• Standards of equipment
• Teaching on a one-to-one basis	• Not enough information communicated
• Adequate staffing levels	• Learner–staff ratio too high
• Adequate planning and preparation	• Inadequate staffing levels
• Supporting learning resources and information	• Student uninterested
• Approachable staff	• Disorganised programme of teaching
	• Poor leadership

The need to ensure adequate staffing levels to safeguard patients and provide effective patient care was highlighted in the Francis (2013) Report as noted earlier in this chapter, and subsequently also by the CNO for England (NHS England National Quality Board, 2014: 45), who indicates that all 'nursing, midwifery and care staffing levels, and key quality and outcome measures should be discussed at Trust Board in a public meeting'. For this to happen, the Board has to receive monthly report of 'actual staff available on a shift-by-shift basis versus planned staffing levels' (ibid.). NICE (2014) has also published guidelines on staff capacity and capability with its own perspectives on the issue.

Clearly, staffing levels have been a cause for concern for some years, and without sufficient and capable staff to provide safe and effective care, time might not be available to supervise students' learning. Additionally, the CNO has continually emphasised the need to ensure that a culture of compassionate care prevails, with concomitant staff education in this area (e.g. NHS England, 2016) (discussed in Chapter 5).

Furthermore, according to Campbell and Evans' (2016) qualitative research, managers' beliefs, attitude and roles related to effective facilitation of learning in their workplace have a major influence on the workplace being also a place for learning. A wide range of research studies has been conducted over the years on what contemporarily constitutes an effective CLE, as the character of practice settings evolves with the times. On exploring the experiences of a group of pre-registration mental health nursing students during practice placements, for example, Wood (2005) found that students experience 'conflicting pressures', while their mentors experience difficulty supporting them because of high clinical workload, as also noted by King's College London (2014).

Henderson et al. (2010) explored the organisational culture of practice settings that influence learning, which they discuss under the headings:

- Recognition of learners and learning in the organisation
- Accomplishment, i.e. acquisition of new knowledge and skills
- Affiliation, i.e. feeling part of the organisation, the team in the practice setting
- Influence, i.e. feeling safe to express opinions and suggest ideas.

Later, Henderson et al.'s (2012) research on CLE revealed that students tend to value 'task accomplishment' highly, but although the practice settings valued safe practice, they were 'not readily open to innovation and challenges to routine practices' (ibid.: 299). Thus, with continuing research and recommendations for enhancement of practice settings as CLEs, more positive findings are also reported. Students emphasised, however, that the working relationship with their supervisors of learning was particularly significant in their achievement of their practice objectives.

Based on the above accounts of the subject area, a clinical learning environment can be defined as a practice setting that manifests a psychosocial ethos and culture, with related supportive resources, that fosters mutual learning amongst all healthcare professionals, learners and clientele, and where care and treatment are founded on evidence-based practice. The recommendations from earlier and recent studies regarding aspects that constitute good and effective learning environments form key components of annual educational audit documents.

EDUCATIONAL AUDIT OF PRACTICE PLACEMENT SETTINGS

After Fretwell's (1980) and others' research, later studies on clinical learning environments focused more directly on exploring the factors that can be identified as the necessary criteria in educational audit documents (or tools) that are used for identifying and monitoring the continuing suitability of practice settings for student placement. The criteria for suitability include evidence of a systematic approach to care delivery and holistic care (and the practice setting's philosophy of care). Orton et al. (1993) focused specifically on educational auditing, and asked qualified staff and students the same questions separately in relation to:

1. orientation to the placement
2. theory and practice integration
3. supernumerary status
4. staff attitudes and behaviour
5. mentors
6. progressive assessment.

Thus, having gathered data on the views of key players under the above-mentioned headings, Orton et al. (1993) then designed an educational audit tool with specified criteria that they referred to as 'ward learning climate indicators' to ascertain the practice setting's suitability for student placement. It is an NMC (2017c: 22) requirement that educational audits are continually updated and undertaken at least once every two years for each practice setting where students are placed for learning clinical skills (some require annual educational audit).

More contemporarily, Newton et al. (2010) go a step further by empirically testing the recently advocated 'Clinical Learning Environment Inventory' (CLEI), which comprises 42 criteria grouped under the sections: personalisation, student involvement, task orientation, innovation, and satisfaction and individualisation. They conclude their test by suggesting modifications to the inventory, and by recommending further research to establish the consistency of the modified inventory, which implies that even in 2010 the best educational audit tool had not yet been established. However, later research on CLEI by Shivers et al. (2017) found that overall students are actually satisfied with practice settings that meet all CLEI criteria.

Based on various research on CLE like that cited above, each university, in partnership with the local healthcare trusts, devises its own research-informed educational audit tool. These audit forms contain a range of criteria for determining whether a practice setting is suitable for practice placement of healthcare profession students. Evidence needs to be available to auditors to demonstrate how each criterion is achieved.

The CLEI is designed to measure students' perceptions of the placement practice setting as a learning environment and, in doing so, Brown et al. (2011) found that there are significant differences between the students' perception of their 'actual' CLE and their 'ideal' CLE. However, A. Anderson et al. (2014) report on the implementation of an *Inter-professional Clinical Placement Learning Environment Inventory*, and found it to be a reliable, feasible, easy to complete tool, and preregistration healthcare students felt that the items in the inventory were appropriate for CLE audit tools.

The other prevailing educational audit tool that measures the practice setting as a learning environment from the students' viewpoint is CLES+T, which stands for clinical learning environment, supervision and nurse teacher, consisting of a total of 34 criteria under five sections (Papastavrou et al., 2016).

ACTIVITY 4.4   STRENGTHS AND WEAKNESSES OF YOUR WORK BASE AS A LEARNING ENVIRONMENT

Locate a copy of the current completed educational audit document for your workplace, a copy of which is usually lodged in the practice setting as a paper copy or electronically. If you cannot find the form, ask the ward manager or the PEF where the form can be found.

Then peruse each item or criterion in the document to decide for yourself whether the item has been fully achieved in your practice setting or otherwise. This exercise will be your own professional judgement of areas of strengths and areas where improvements can be made to your practice setting as a learning environment. Discuss your impressions with a peer if you have the opportunity.

Can you do anything about the weaker points? In fact, can you devise a SMART (specific, measurable, achievable, realistic and time-limited) action plan to make tangible improvements to the weaker areas/audit criteria?

Alternatively, view the CLES+T scale in Papastavrou et al. (2016: Table 3), or Mikkonen et al. (2017: Table 3). The scale is designed and worded in such a way that it endeavours to measure the students' perception of the practice setting as a learning environment. Yet another alternative is to use the Inter-professional Clinical Placement Learning Environment Inventory (ICPLEI) in A. Anderson et al. (2014: Appendix). Using either of these two articles, peruse each item in the same way as indicated above for the educational audit document. (Full details of the articles are given in the References list at the end of this book.)

Further research on the CLEI and CLES+T evaluation scales continues. As noted, CLES+T has 34 criteria under five sections, which are: (1) supervisory relationships; (2) pedagogical atmosphere on the ward; (3) the leadership style of ward managers; (4) premises of nursing; and (5) the role of nurse teachers. Warne et al. (2010) conducted a multinational European study using the CLES+T scale of factors that enhance students' learning experience during practice placement and found that student learning 'requires both significant time being spent working with patients and a supportive supervisory relationship' (ibid.: 809).

Furthermore, Gustafsson et al.'s (2015) research concluded that the CLES+T scale is a useful and reliable measure of student nurses' perception of the learning environment within practice placement.

The educational audit document usually includes a section for recording the qualifications of each member of staff, of particular significance being which part of the profession's regulatory body's register they are on, and also whether they hold a practice assessor or similar qualification and have been attending annual update sessions related to practice supervision and assessment. Other post-registration qualifications are also recorded. Template 4.1 shows the content of the section at the front of the audit document that contains key information about the particular practice setting.

Template 4.1 Placement details page of educational audit document

Multi-professional Practice Environment Profile
Placement Details

1) Name of NHS Trust/Healthcare Organisation:
2) Site/Location and Address:
3) Name of Ward/Department/Unit/Team:
4) Placement Area Telephone No.:
5) Name of Manager of the Placement Area:
6) Contact Email address:
7) Type of Service Provision/Speciality:
8) Work/Shift Patterns:
9) Names of Reviewers:
10) Name of Academic Link Lecturer:
11) Name of Practice Facilitator/Practice Educator:
12) What is the maximum number of students that your practice setting normally supports at any one time to date?
13) Please identify the type of students regularly allocated to the placement area to date (child branch, adult branch, midwifery, work experience, ...)
14) What factors influence the number of students you can accept?
15) Name(s) of Academic Institutions Placing Students (University/College of Further Education/ Other, e.g. for work experience):
16) Other:
17) Date of Previous Review:
18) Date of Review:

Naturally, each item in this section of the audit document is important. In addition to the placement details on the first two or three pages of the audit document, it identifies a number of 'standards' that have to be met for the practice setting to qualify as suitable for practice placement of healthcare students. They are often based on national guidelines and can include, for example:

- Care planning documentation reflects appropriate NHS England/NICE guidelines and DH directives.
- Confidentiality is in place to protect patients, staff and student.
- Training records demonstrate all staff have attended mandatory training sessions.

The document also tends to have a section for clinical staff to identify and to list all the formal and informal teaching and learning opportunities that are, or can be, available in the particular practice setting.

ACTIVITY 4.5   FORMAL AND INFORMAL LEARNING OPPORTUNITIES

Identify and make two lists, one of all the formal learning opportunities that are available in your own practice setting, and one of the informal ones. You might find it useful to make the lists in discussion with a colleague in the same practice setting.

For formal learning, you might have mentioned teaching sessions by the clinical nurse specialist, for instance; and for informal learning opportunities, you might have mentioned when you explain to the student why the doctor has changed a patient's medication. There are likely to be various teaching and learning opportunities in your work-base setting. Maybe one of the consultant medical officers holds regular formal teaching sessions for junior doctors, which all healthcare professionals in the particular area are welcome to attend. Maybe pharmaceutical or medical devices company representatives give talks and demonstrations/updates on their products in the practice setting. Further examples of teaching and learning opportunities that tend to be identified when completing educational audit forms are presented in the box.

FORMAL AND INFORMAL LEARNING OPPORTUNITIES

Formal teaching	Informal learning opportunities
• Lectures by senior doctors	• Learning about or from a patient with a new condition
• Patient assessment-related teaching	
• Student interviews – initial, mid-placement and final	• Change in patient's condition discussed at handover
• Teaching while carrying out patient care, i.e. work-based learning	• Asking questions informally
• Setting learning tasks to students	• Reflection-in-action and reflection-on-action
• Practice development nurse's guidance	• Informal chat in the staff room during coffee break
• Teaching by PEFs or by 'cascade trainers'	• Updating procedures and clinical guidelines' folders and learning resources
• In-service/postgraduate training	
• Observing RNs, physiotherapists and other AHPs, or doctors performing clinical interventions	• Access to computer databases and internet

If preferred, the resources for learning available in the practice setting can be grouped as human and non-human resources. Formal learning opportunities, such as teaching sessions and skill demonstrations, require human resources and include inter-professional learning. Non-human resources include printed instructions on how to use equipment, learning about medications, ventilator monitors or 'care programme approach'. Many of the resources needed to deliver patient care can also be used for learning and for achieving clinical and managerial objectives. Other learning resources include a room that can be used for teaching and learning, with internet-enabled computers, whiteboard or flipcharts, for instance. The learning resource files containing project or research reports compiled by individuals in the team, research articles, etc., are also usually available for consultation and learning.

INTER-PROFESSIONAL LEARNING

As for inter-professional learning (IPL) in practice settings, the concept is promoted in various authoritative documents (for example, DH, 2001; NMC, 2018c: 5). Successful education programmes and projects (for example, Goldsmith et al., 2009) are documented and presented at conferences. The Centre for the Advancement of Inter-professional Education, 'CAIPE Inter-professional Education Guidelines 2016 indicate that inter-professional education (IPE) 'occurs when students from various professions learn from and about each other to improve collaboration and the quality of care' (CAIPE, 2016: 5). CAIPE indicates that IPE includes such learning in academic and work-based settings before and after qualifying, and also provides guidelines on a variety of aspects of implementation and evaluation of IPE.

Another definition of IPE is provided by Buring et al. (2009: 59): 'Inter-professional education involves educators and learners from two or more health professions and their foundational disciplines who jointly create and foster a collaborative learning environment.' They indicate that IPE results in improved health service user outcomes and satisfaction, better teamwork, lower error rates, etc.

The basis for IPL is inter-professional working, in that to resolve the individual health service user's health problem (or to avert it), a group of different healthcare professionals such as nurses, doctors, dieticians, physiotherapists and speech and language therapists input their own areas of professional expertise as appropriate. Multi-professional or multidisciplinary working can involve different healthcare professionals attending to the patient, delivering their clinical input and withdrawing. However, these actions can be fragmented and inadequately coordinated and recorded.

Inter-professional working, on the other hand, implies collaboration, and better coordinated patient care with fuller communication, verbal and written, between different healthcare professionals. Inter-professional learning extends the concept to the exchange of knowledge, of understanding and clinical skills, and is a more holistic term. It signifies collaboration to identify patient goals and exercise expanded problem-solving beyond discipline-specific boundaries/work.

IPL also comprises informal and formal learning. Informally, for instance, the nurse explains to the occupational therapist the plan of care for a particular service user and the rationales for each action. In turn, the occupational therapist designs a plan of action and explains the rationales from their perspective. This could also form the basis for work-based learning, which is explored in some detail shortly. Informal IPL refers to all modes of unstructured, incidental or opportunistic teaching and learning between different professional groups, while inter-professional education (IPE) refers specifically to university-designed courses that result in students being awarded diplomas or degrees.

Formal IPL involves attending structured learning programmes, such as courses that are designed for specified healthcare professionals, covering the physical, social and psychological basis for health and illness and the clinical skills that aid recovery. Some courses (or part of them) are designed for shared learning by, say, nursing and medical students (for example, Lockeman et al., 2017; Hood et al., 2014). Others, such as a course on counselling, might be designed for nurses, social workers and specific allied health professionals.

Furthermore, the Academy of Medical Royal Colleges (2017), which is an organisation that represents the majority of healthcare professions in the UK, supports multi-professional team working, indicating that it delivers better outcomes for patients and more effective and satisfying work for clinicians. It adds that multi-professional work requires flexibility in attitude and behaviour and for professionals to value and respect the distinct contribution each professional makes. The academy's position regarding multi-professional work is supported by a subsequent CAIPE statement.

REFLECTION POINT 4.1:   IPL AND IPE

Consider to what extent IPL occurs in your work setting. In those settings where it does occur, is it linked to IPE?

Hean et al. (2006) report on a study that concluded that different AHP student groups tend to see themselves as distinct from other professional groups. This is healthy as it enables them to establish their professional identity prior to exploring commonalities between them. However, when they identified the characteristics that made them different – for example physiotherapy students indicating that they believe that being a team player made them different – other groups also stated having this characteristic. This suggests that many of the characteristics of each AHP group are largely very similar.

Naturally, the areas of clinical expertise of each profession have different focuses. Furthermore, Lockeman et al.'s (2017) research findings suggest that inter-professional education can enhance inter-professional practice and increase understanding of the roles of different professions. However, Foronda et al. (2016)

conducted a review of research on inter-professional communication in healthcare and noted that doctors and nurses have different communication styles which are based on their pre-qualifying education. They identify structural hierarchies, lack of confidence, etc., as issues that hinder effective communication and relationships. They suggest commonality in pre-qualifying education of healthcare professions in patient-related communication, wider use of such constructs as inter-professional handover, etc.

Education programme planners need to be aware of such issues and solutions related to IPE, so that they can make relevant adjustments to their teaching. However, healthcare students benefit from IPL, when for example care and treatment of healthcare service users is planned and delivered inter-professionally through integrated care pathways. These in turn can form the basis for constituting learning pathways for students.

However, we also need to ascertain the learner's perspectives in terms of their motivation and readiness to engage with IPL. McLeod et al. (2018) for example conducted an IPL research to test physiotherapy and adult nursing students' attitude towards IPL using a Readiness for Inter-professional Learning Scale questionnaire and found very positive attitude towards IPL by the majority of students, in addition to greater understanding of other healthcare professionals' roles and acquisition of new skills.

Alternatively, Holt et al. (2010: 264), for instance, report on a project that explored ways of assessing communication, team working and ethical practice, which are three essential competencies for all health professionals at five HEIs and in 16 professional groups in the UK. They took into account the stance of 'professional statutory and regulatory bodies', practice-based and academic staff, and service users and carers on assessment of these skills, and reported that multi-professional assessment is feasible in the endeavour to 'accurately and fairly measure capabilities to help students develop into proficient and effective practitioners' (ibid.: 264).

UTILISING LEARNING PATHWAYS

The student's placement could in many settings beneficially incorporate patient journeys and patient care pathways, which are concepts that have also been identified for some time (e.g. McCarthy et al., 2016). 'Care maps', 'collaborative care pathways', 'multidisciplinary pathways of care', 'clinical pathways' are all terms that are used interchangeably. Once the care pathway for a particular patient has been formulated, it can be included in the student's learning pathway whereby the student can track the patient's journey through healthcare, and thereby gain knowledge of the interventions undertaken and the underpinning rationales for them, in order to enable the patient to recover from their health problem. The student's learning can then be supplemented by pre-arranged lectures and workshops held at the university or within healthcare trusts, and by self-directed study.

The majority of service users' journeys through the health services begin and end in primary care. The Department of Health (2007: 1) defines a patient pathway as:

> the route that a patient will take from their first contact with an NHS member of staff (usually their general practitioner [GP]), through referral, to the completion of their treatment.

Care pathways specifically designed for particular illnesses are well documented in healthcare literature. Examples of this include van Wijngaarden et al. (2006) on thrombolysis in acute ischaemic stroke, and Bowker et al. (2005) on Type 1 diabetes mellitus. Several care pathways are also available on the internet, for example from the National Institute for Health and Care Excellence (NICE) (2017) website.

Research on care pathways includes a quasi-experiment conducted by de Luc (2000), who found that the use of care pathways resulted in increased patient satisfaction and an ability to make staff focus more on the clinical care they were providing. Furthermore, an evaluative study of patient journeys conducted by Baron (2009) found various benefits of this approach, including greater patient involvement in their recovery from illness and more effective interprofessional working.

A student on practice placement could encounter a patient whose relatively straightforward journey through healthcare takes them along the pathway identified in Figure 4.1.

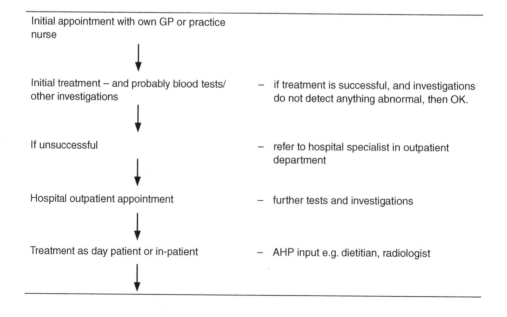

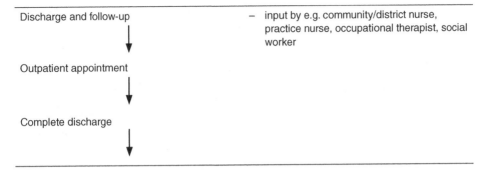

Figure 4.1 A service user's journey through healthcare

The student can follow a service user's care pathway through the healthcare system closely to gain knowledge and understanding of the care and treatment required in particular illnesses. The student's learning pathway through the practice placement would involve exposure to, and engagement with, selected care pathways, supplemented in various ways, for example by practice-based teaching by the PEF, practice supervisor and other healthcare professionals.

HEIs work in collaboration with local trust clinicians to develop and implement learning pathway programmes in healthcare course curricula based on patient journeys, with web-based scenarios for students to investigate. A suitable definition of learning pathways related to healthcare students' learning is difficult to locate. Essentially, a learning pathway constitutes a combination of retrospective and prospective care interventions that are determined by the beginning of the service user: health problem, current state of the problem and how it progresses. Furthermore, as care pathways incorporate involvement of an appropriate combination of nursing or midwifery, medical, social work and AHP staff, learning pathways are increasingly being referred to as 'inter-professional learning pathways'.

The learning pathway for a student on an Emergency Department placement could include the student starting with a day with the ambulance services, following a healthcare service user with a suspected fracture to the X-ray department, spending time working with plaster technicians, and so on. Furthermore, if the same patient or service user also suffers from, say, Type 1 diabetes or displays aggressive or even violent behaviour, these themselves present instances for further learning for the student, the management of which can be explored up to maximum patient recovery.

The effectiveness of learning pathways in making learning more comprehensive was also explored by Anderson (2009: 835), for instance, who conducted a qualitative study, which revealed that the use of learning pathways enabled students to develop 'a greater awareness and understanding of the delivery of healthcare in primary care settings and they expanded their nursing knowledge and skills'. However, Anderson also notes that some students felt that learning pathways fragmented their learning in the base placement area.

The downside of the fragmentation of learning needs to be heeded as the subjects of Anderson's study were final placement student nurses who felt that their priority in this placement was to consolidate their clinical skills. This can clearly also impact on the achievement of standards of proficiency by students during the final practice placement, which is an NMC requirement for them to register their qualification with the NMC. Furthermore, the Centre for Policy on Ageing (2014) indicates that care pathways are designed to provide the best-known standard of care to patients with specific conditions, but they are also contrary to the concept of person-centred care, unless 'variances' to care pathways allow for changes based on the service user's specific health needs.

It is useful to note, however, that the notion of learning pathways is found in at least another two contexts. One of these is the arena of adult education in which individuals who have missed education opportunities during the compulsory education years are enabled to learn through NVQ routes, and so on (for example, McGivney, 2003). The notion of learning pathways also belongs to neurophysiology when new learning can be identified along neuronal paths (for example, Brown et al., 1999). Moreover, Lindquist et al. (2006) conducted a phenomenological study of physiotherapy students' experiences through their pre-registration education programme, and concluded that students dip in and out of four specific professional growth pathways, namely: 'reflecting on practice', 'communicating with others', 'searching for evidence' and 'performing skills'.

Students' learning pathways during practice placement is increasingly a concept that is being favoured widely, with some useful developments that can counteract the weaknesses of learning pathways identified by Anderson (2009). The model is referred to as the 'hub and spokes' model. The hub is the base placement setting to which the student has been allocated and at which their practice supervisors are based, and from there the student can accompany the health service user to whichever department of healthcare or social care personnel he or she has been referred (the spoke).

The 'hub and spokes' model of learning pathways is now widely available to students. Nonetheless, a spoke visit by a student on practice placement cannot be downplayed as 'you might find it interesting', for instance. In fact, to optimise learning from the spoke experience, the student should articulate in writing, usually on relevant pages of the practice competencies document, one or more aims for the spoke visit against the name of the spoke to be visited – see Template 4.2.

Template 4.2   Record of learning from 'spoke' experience

Date of visit to spoke area	Name of spoke	Aim(s) of visiting spoke area	Summary of learning from spoke	Nominated practice supervisor's comments (optional)

After the visit the student needs to write down specific learning acquired from the spoke visit. A number of studies have already been conducted on the hub and spokes model, which include Roxburgh et al.'s (2012) research that in conclusion identified the beneficial effects of using this model of placement learning as a mechanism that promotes deep and more meaningful person-centred learning than the concept of practice placement, which can imply that the student has to spend most or all of the placement time in the placement area itself.

The results of an evaluative study by Thomas and Westwood (2016) of students' experiences of the 'hub and spoke' model of placement allocation identified that the model enhances students' understanding of the whole patient journey which in turn offer students a wide breadth of experience and transferable skills such as communication and adaptability, and also increases a sense of belonging to the hub area. However, when the aims of the spoke experience weren't clearly identified, the experience was problematic.

Yet another study on hub and spokes as a student learning pathway during practice placement conducted by Millar et al. (2017) revealed similar beneficial findings to the above-mentioned study, but also other potential issues such as some spoke areas being in high demand and possibly becoming 'resistant' to students, as well as benefits such as being able to appreciate the patient/service user as an individual, their lifestyle's effect on their health, and thereby also enhance person-centred practice.

In conclusion, recognising the components of patients' journeys or pathways through healthcare can provide healthcare students with fuller insights into the beginnings of an individual's ill-health and the stage-by-stage events that they undergo in the endeavour to resolve their health problems. Under the guidance of their practice supervisors, students can personally witness some of the clinical interventions that occur away from the practice placement setting, which should enrich their learning.

WORK-BASED LEARNING

Learning professional skills in the workplace is also referred to as work-based learning (WBL), except that this term applies to learning in the workplace in all professions, and is equivalent to the term 'practice placement' or 'practice education' in nursing and midwifery and to 'internship' in some university-linked programme such as business studies. Thus, WBL is an overarching term, which has been defined by several people, including Barr (2003) who indicates that WBL is learning that takes place at work, or learning that takes place away from work with the objective of improving performance at work. The definitions of WBL imply that, in addition to apprenticeship-type learning in workplaces, learning is supplemented by some classroom-based lessons or skills-laboratory-based learning.

If WBL is a component of a university-based programme, then it also awards credit points or CATS (credit accumulation and transfer scheme) points, the number depending to a good extent on the duration of the placement, such as whether it is for eight weeks or year-long. An extensive study of WBL by Moore (2010) revealed that managerial support in workplace development is crucial for WBL to be successful as a learning activity.

Marshall (2012) reports on the beneficial effects of a work-based learning module in midwifery, writing that it enables participants to improve multi-professional collaboration and the consequential further development of maternity services within the local Trusts; it is efficient and cost effective to employee and employer and serves to strengthen the link between higher education and the workplace; it also helps to bridge the theory–practice gap, which all in all has the potential to influence directly the development of global midwifery education and maternity services and ultimately benefit mothers, their babies and families.

Lester and Costley (2010: 561) also note that 'the evidence indicates that well-designed work-based learning programmes are both effective and robust'. However, they note too that WBL is often associated with training because employer-led courses lack wider relevance, and are focused on short-term solutions at the expense of quality education. Nevalainen et al. (2018) tend to see WBL as informal incidental learning in work settings, and conclude from their literature review that appropriate workplace culture, physical structures and spaces, as well as inter-personal relations underpin effective WBL.

BECOMING A LEARNING ORGANISATION

Going beyond the concept and practice of practice settings being effective learning environments, is the suggestion that whole healthcare organisations should establish such a culture of learning that they can become learning organisations. The development of a learning culture needs to be a dominant theme in the strategic plans of healthcare organisations, and incorporate a drive to improve the quality of practice by creating the means of integrating learning with practice. Some of the initiatives that support such a change include CPD, reflective practice, clinical supervision and WBL.

A learning organisation is therefore one that facilitates learning for all team members. This concept is part of a trio of notions that include lifelong learning and learning society. It evolved with the development of various non-healthcare organisations such as banks, supermarkets, etc., as learning organisations, on the basis that they all learn from customer feedback and actively engage in ongoing staff training. As for learning societies, de la Harpe and Radloff (2000: 169) note that they comprise a society in which 'every person has the opportunity to be educated to the level of achievement of which they are truly capable'.

In line with the general acceptance that various forms of formal and informal learning occur in the workplace and can be recorded on educational audit documents, and also based on the increasing value derived from inter-professional learning in practice settings, Holland and Lauder (2012) suggest that practice learning should be part of the wider concept of 'communities of (learning in) practice', and that healthcare providers should become 'learning organisations'. The concept of 'communities of practice' has prevailed for some time, and Wenger (2000), for example, explains that they constitute groups of people who share a common passion for something, about which they extend their learning together, some of which may also be incidental, i.e., unintentional.

As for the whole of the healthcare provider, for example an acute NHS Trust, becoming a learning organisation, this can only be healthy in that all its practice settings as well as all departments that are not practice settings have learning and open-mindedness structured within their culture. This ethos is usually well established in UK hospices and university-linked healthcare providers, except that at times senior healthcare managers tend to think of learning organisations only in terms of 'learning from mistakes or incidents' (e.g. Dixon-Woods et al., 2014). Alternatively, Macneil (2001) argues that when supervisors and line managers, who are themselves effective facilitators of learning, tend to encourage and support formal and informal learning whereby the team values learning and benefits from improved team performance.

A learning organisation, according to one of its earliest advocates Peter Senge, comprises several approaches promoting members' learning and development, many of which are informal, and constitute five areas, namely – shared vision, mental model, personal mastery, team learning, and system thinking (Choi et al., 2016). The concept of a learning organisation is consistently becoming a feature of healthcare settings, as lifelong learning is not merely 'keeping up to date', but encompasses a flexible and enquiring approach to the development of a culture of learning as an important part of the work setting. The key features of a learning organisation, which also applies to health and social care providers, are identified by Wilkinson et al. (2004), for example, as one with:

- celebration throughout the organisation of the success of individuals and teams
- absence of complacency, that is always seeking improvement
- tolerance of mistakes and failures, and learning from them
- belief in human potential for creativity and innovation
- recognition of tacit knowledge
- openness and sharing knowledge, and learning across teams
- trusting staff to work towards corporate goals, without close monitoring
- outward looking at competing organisations, and potentially learning from them.

You might wish to check for yourself how far your employing organisation demonstrates the above-mentioned features of a learning organisation, and maybe you will be nicely surprised. See Akhnif et al. (2017) under 'Further Optional Reading' at the end of this chapter for more ways in which the learning organisation idea applies to health services.

GUIDELINES, POLICIES AND STANDARDS
FOR PRACTICE PLACEMENTS

In *Helping Students Get the Best from their Practice Placements*, RCN (2017a) specifies the responsibilities of various stakeholders, that is, those of the student, the HEI, service providers, personal tutors, etc., for ensuring effective learning during placements. The responsibilities of the student encompass those before, during and after the placement. The student's responsibilities before the placement include:

- reading the practice competencies that must be achieved by the end of the placement, and comprehending them
- recognising the purpose of the practice placement experience, that is to learn nursing or midwifery care
- contacting the placement
- acting professionally with regard to punctuality and attitude, and dressing according to the local uniform policy.

During the placement, the student's responsibilities include being proactive in seeking out learning experiences. After the placement, the student has a responsibility to take stock of their achievements, evaluate the placement itself, ensure that all practice placement documentation is completed by due dates and reflect on the experience after completing the placement.

The RCN publication also states that a successful practice placement depends on well-planned learning opportunities and the provision of support and coaching for students. It lists and explains several actions that supervisors of practice-based learning should take to fulfil their responsibility, which include:

- contributing to a supportive learning environment and quality learning outcomes for students
- being approachable, supportive and aware of how students learn best
- having knowledge and information of the student's programme of study and practice assessment tools.

In a subsequent publication that constitutes guidance on facilitating practice-based learning, the RCN (2017b) addresses both ways of helping students maximise their learning during practice placements, including students with special needs or disability, and areas of accountability.

The underlying principles of the DH (2001) guidance document *Placements in Focus* include the need for a dynamic and proactive approach to the organisation, provision and assessment of practice experience. It indicates that HEIs and service providers have to think creatively about how to plan and provide practice placements that meet the needs of the NHS, the wider healthcare sector and developments related to public health. Planning and provision should both take into account and value ideas and suggestions from students and draw on the experience and knowledge of other stakeholders. The guidance is intended to constitute a model of good practice. It focuses on four key aspects of practice placements, namely:

1. providing practice placements
2. practice learning environment
3. student support
4. assessment of practice.

For the practice learning environment, the DH (2001) indicates, for instance, that:

- The practice area should have a stated philosophy of care that is reflected in practice and in the curriculum aims.
- Care provision should be founded on relevant research and evidence-based findings where available.
- Students should gain, where possible, experience as part of a multi-professional team.
- A learning resources area with relevant materials should be available for learning activities in the practice environment.
- Student feedback should be actively sought.

It also identifies how each component will be achieved by different parties, such as placement providers, HEIs and students. Another authoritative body that provides guidelines on placement learning for quality assurance is the QAA (2008, for example). Mulholland et al. (2006) make further recommendations under the *Making Practice-Based Learning Work* project.

ISSUES RELATED TO PRACTICE PLACEMENTS

One of the issues related to pre-registration nursing students has been their supernumerary status (discussed at the end of Chapter 2), accompanied by a relatively small bursary. The latter is a reason for a number of students holding down part-time jobs. This, along with some students having a family to support, may result in their learning being compromised to some extent. Consequently, the student is likely to need extra structured support while on practice placement. Link lecturers can provide this support, which does not necessarily require their physical presence.

A study by Young et al. (2010) evaluated the use of short message service (SMS) texting between university staff and students as an additional means of support for healthcare students (including nursing, radiography and occupational therapy students) during practice placements. They found that texting can improve students' access to additional support when needed during practice placements.

One of the reasons for various guidelines on practice placements being issued by the RCN, the QAA and the DH at the turn of the century is the publication of some research (for example Phillips et al., 2000) identifying various weaknesses in the prevailing practice-based teaching and learning. Another reason is the increase in the number of students due to the shortage of qualified nurses. This means that more learners were to be allocated to fewer RNs. This also coincides with other research findings that some students were being given a pass for practice competencies with scanty evidence of their competence (discussed in Chapter 7), and that some newly qualified RNs were not 'fit for practice', that is, not clinically competent.

Furthermore, the Care Quality Commission (CQC) – which is an organisation that was set up by the government to regularly monitor the quality of care and treatment being provided to healthcare service users by each service provider in England – can also decide whether a practice setting is suitable as a learning environment for students. If deemed unsuitable it has the authority to instruct the particular practice setting to stop having students on placement with them until the weakness identified is rectified.

The CQC's (2017) fundamental standards are for service providers such as hospitals, care homes, GP services, and can be accessed on the CQC's website. These standards are based on five key questions against which service providers will be assessed. The five key questions are (see box below for more details):

- Are they safe?
- Are they effective?
- Are they caring?
- Are they responsive to people's needs
- Are they well-led?

Further details are available from the CQC website (see CQC, 2017 in the References section of this textbook).

THE CARE QUALITY COMMISSION'S FUNDAMENTAL STANDARDS

- Safe – people are protected from abuse and avoidable harm.
- Effective – people's care, treatment and support achieve good outcomes, promote a good quality of life and are based on the best available evidence.
- Caring – staff involve and treat people with compassion, kindness, dignity and respect.
- Responsive – services are organised so that they meet people's needs.
- Well-led – the leadership, management and governance of the organisation assures the delivery of high-quality person-centred care, supports learning and innovation, and promotes an open and fair culture.

Source: Reproduced with permission under the terms of the Open Government Licence

However, the heightened awareness of evidence-based practice means that students are more inquisitive about reasons for each step within clinical interventions. Nevertheless, for various day-to-day reasons, some procedures are not performed exactly as the procedures' manual states and consequently the so-called theory and practice gap at times surfaces. From qualified healthcare professionals' and their managers' viewpoint these still constitute competent practice because procedures are adapted in accordance with resource availability and patient circumstances.

For instance, if the moving and handling procedure or guidelines state that a hoist should be used to help a patient above a certain weight, but a hoist is not immediately available, then the RN could use alternative measures. The reason for this might not be immediately obvious to the student, and at times students refuse to participate in procedures that are not being performed precisely according to guidelines. They should be exploring how to adapt theories to practice instead.

However, Lakasing and Francis (2005) argue that because a number of health-care profession lecturers are often not active clinicians, this tends to create a theory–practice gap that practice-based supervisors of learning have to redress during student practice placements, unlike medical academics who are also practising doctors. They indicate that practice-based supervisors of learning should therefore be provided with protected time and extra remuneration to enable them to fulfil this demanding role more effectively. Where extra funding is made available for this, the money can be utilised to employ additional pro rata staff to create protected (or supported) time for more effective practice-based facilitation of learning.

CHAPTER SUMMARY

As with other components in this book, creating and maintaining an effective clinical learning environment is also identified as a key dimension of facilitating students learning during practice placement. This chapter has focused on the different ways in which practice settings can be effective as learning environments, and has therefore explored:

- Students' perspectives on practice placements such as their hopes and expectations; a ward orientation or induction programme; advanced preparation of learners; and ensuring that course practice competencies are achieved.
- Research on clinical learning environments, which underpins the development of the tool for annual educational audits of practice placement areas; learning resources (human and material), including inter-professional learning and learning pathways; role models for learners in the practice setting.
- The part played by national guidelines, standards and current policy documents on practice placements.
- What work-based learning is and how it applies to learning nursing and midwifery practice; and how healthcare providers can become learning organisations.
- Some of the main issues related to practice placements for students.

FURTHER OPTIONAL READING

1. For the QAA's stance on effective learning during practice placements, see:

   - Quality Assurance Agency for Higher Education (2008) *Outcomes from Institutional Audit Second Series: Work-Based and Placement Learning, and Employability.* Available at: www.qaa.ac.uk/publications/information-and-guidance/publication?PubID=150#.WZXIsWZK3IU (accessed 15 September 2017).

2. For a number of ways in which learning organisation as an idea applies to health services, see:

   - Akhnif, E., Macq, J. and Meessen, B. (2017) 'Scoping literature review on the Learning Organisation concept as applied to the health system', *Health Research Policy and Systems,* 15(16): 1–12.

3. Expectation 10: 'Commissioners actively seek assurance that the right people, with the right skills, are in the right place at the right time within the providers with whom they contract' (NHS England National Quality Board [NQB], 2014: 54) – for detailed discussion on plans for provision of adequate staffing levels to provide safe care, see:

   - NHS England National Quality Board (2014) *How to Ensure the Right People, with the Right Skills, are in the Right Place at the Right Time: A Guide to Establishing Nursing, Midwifery and Care Staffing Capacity and Capability.* Available at: www.england.nhs.uk/wp-content/uploads/2013/11/nqb-how-to-guid.pdf (accessed 26 January 2018).

To access further resources related to this chapter, visit **https://study.sagepub.com/gopee4e** where a range of learning and teaching materials are provided.

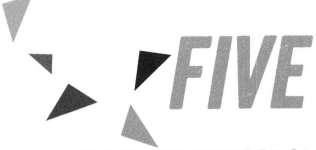

FIVE

PRACTICE SUPERVISORS' LEADERSHIP THROUGH EVIDENCE-BASED PRACTICE AND PRACTICE DEVELOPMENT

INTRODUCTION

One of the preconditions of healthcare registrants undertaking the practice supervisor role is that they have to be proficient in care interventions to the contemporary highest standard. Consequently, practice supervisors have to embody leadership in the quality and effectiveness of their practice, continually ascertaining the evidence base of all care interventions, and of the various factors that influence effective care delivery to health and social care service users.

Being conscious of standards of practice involves being open-minded with regard to novel methods of clinical interventions, of research findings and of developments in one's own specialist field of practice. Codes of professional practice in healthcare often include the requirement that registrants care interventions have to be based on best available evidence (e.g. NMC, 2015a). Furthermore, innovations and practice development are often praised through healthcare professional journals and at conferences. Healthcare policy documents are awash with rhetoric, commendations and recommendations on healthcare leadership. EBP, practice development and leadership apply to all registrants, and therefore also to practice supervisor roles; and leadership applies to the practice assessor role as well.

CHAPTER OBJECTIVES

1. Appraise ways in which forward planning and prioritising work comprise important components of practice supervisors' and practice assessors' leadership.

(Continued)

(Continued)

2. Explain why evidence-based practice (EBP) and clinical practice development are essential components of the registrant's role, in tandem with facilitation of students' practice-based learning.
3. Identify the meanings of the concepts 'effective care', 'EBP' and 'practice development', and demonstrate understanding of the inherent components that they encompass.
4. Ascertain and analyse the extent to which practice supervisors engage in EBP, and disseminate research and project findings.
5. Critically evaluate ways in which practice supervisors are leaders in ensuring practice is evidence based, in practice development and in managing change.

THE PRACTICE LEARNING SUPERVISOR'S LEADERSHIP

Ways in which practice supervisors plan and supervise a range of learning experiences for students on placement, and oversee them accessing pertinent learning opportunities are reflections of leadership characteristics that were alluded to in Chapters 1 and 4 to some extent. 'Prioritising work' is another key feature of the practice supervisor's leadership, which includes designating time for establishing effective working relationships with students and other professionals whom students will encounter during the placement. Leadership therefore also applies to enabling students to focus their learning activities so that they can achieve their placement competencies in good time, and also to acting proactively to pre-empt and avert the likely contemporary problems of assessments, as well as dealing with those that do occur.

Registrants' leadership related to pre-registration and post-qualifying education in healthcare professions has been identified by research for some time (for example, Fretwell, 1980; O'Driscoll et al., 2010). According to O'Driscoll and colleagues, personnel who are in a position to take the lead include clinical nurse specialists, modern matrons, nurse consultants, nurse practitioners, nurse managers and others of similar seniority, but their role in student teaching during practice placements is less well defined. They also found, however, that the ward manager's leadership is crucial in creating an environment for learning in the practice setting, and also that it is the mentor (now practice supervisor) who exercises leadership in facilitation of learning more regularly and fully.

Several definitions of leadership prevail in healthcare literature, most of which emphasise the leader's ability to *influence* the activities, behaviour or actions of their 'followers' towards goal achievement. In the context of healthcare, Gopee and Galloway (2017: 66) suggest that 'leadership comprises the ability to influence the behaviour of the workforce, to motivate, inspire and energise individuals, and to achieve the health and social care goals of the care setting'. These abilities also apply to effective practice supervision. For a thorough analysis of leadership as a concept that applies to most areas of society, the reader is referred to Kouzes and Posner's (2012) *The Leadership Challenge*.

PRACTICE ASSESSORS' LEADERSHIP IN MANAGING ASSESSMENTS

Leadership is also essential in ensuring timely student assessment on their practice competencies. Practice settings are generally informed of the students allocated to them well before the practice placement starts, to which practice supervisors respond by structuring tentative plans of learning experiences for the students for the duration of the placement. However, as discussed in Chapter 7 of this book, research findings (for example, Phillips et al., 2000; Duffy, 2016; Hunt et al., 2016) highlight various alarming issues that could be encountered in the assessment of students' competencies during practice placements. That assessments are conducted 'on the hoof' by registrants that the student 'bumps into' and as part of 'multiple roles', were issues highlighted by Phillips et al. (2000). 'Failure to fail' was the main problem highlighted by Duffy (2016) when sometimes students are awarded a pass without sufficient evidence of their competence in specific clinical skills; and the different, at times unfriendly, ways in which students react to being given a fail is documented by Hunt et al.'s (2016) research findings.

Similarly, O'Driscoll et al. (2010) identify such issues as registrants' workload interfering with facilitation of students' learning during practice placements, and registrants feeling pressurised to take on the practice learning supervisor type role for their career development. The various problems that are likely to be associated with assessments make early and careful planning of assessment imperative. Consequently, the purpose of proactive planning is to prevent issues such as those mentioned above from arising.

Such problems can also be averted by practice supervisors' and practice assessors' leadership through accepting the role as a serious responsibility, and early, careful forward planning of their own workload and the student's practice learning. In their study of mentors' leadership, Adelman-Mullally et al. (2013) identify various ways in which learning supervisors and assessors exemplify leadership, including role modelling, providing vision and challenging the system or status quo. Practice assessors' leadership in relation to assessment of students' practice competencies is also noted in Chapter 7 of this book in appropriate sections.

Nonetheless, ultimately practice supervisors and practice assessors have to be embodiments of professional practice that is evidence-based, and therefore usually agreeable to change practice that improves service user care. They therefore have to be role models of best practice and practice development and service improvement.

PRACTICE SUPERVISORS AS PROFICIENT EVIDENCE-BASED PRACTITIONERS

Evidence-based practice (EBP) is one of the essential components of effective practice and quality assurance in healthcare. It is a concept and practice that has been gradually adopted in all areas of healthcare. 'Safe and effective care' is a phrase that is often mentioned by the NMC in its standards publications (for example, 2010a). Safety of healthcare service users in practice settings is a strand of nursing and midwifery's code of practice (NMC, 2015a) and therefore obligatory. So what does the term 'effective practice' mean?

EFFECTIVE PRACTICE

'Effective clinical practice' is a concept that is closely related to quality of care and treatment, and is also related to such concepts as clinical governance and audits. The word *effective* is an adjective, which, according to the dictionary (e.g. Brookes and O'Neill, 2017: 286), means 'producing an intended or desired result'. It can be used interchangeably with 'efficacious' and 'productive'. Effective practice therefore means that the clinical interventions that healthcare professionals perform do achieve the goals of the care and treatment that are part of the patient's care pathway (or care plan). For example, if certain actions are taken to reduce a patient's body temperature, and after a specified number of minutes the temperature does go down, then the actions were 'effective'.

Ways of achieving effective practice include ensuring that practice is evidence-based and is developed based on new evidence, i.e. practice development, which will be examined in detail shortly. Effective care is therefore a concept that is an integral component of EBP and practice development.

Achieving the goals of care and treatment also belongs to the arena of *patient outcomes*. This term has been explored for several years and is defined according to the research that it is connected with, as documented by the RCN (2004). However, despite the logic in ascertaining patient outcomes, there is a lack of consensus with regard to how patient outcomes are gauged, and it therefore remains in the background as an essential notion warranting further research and refinement.

Related to the practice supervisor role, the word 'effective' therefore signifies that as a qualified healthcare professional the practice supervisor accomplishes the goals in their patients' plans of care and treatment, as intended in their individual care pathways. Effective care and practice development are also part of the work of the NHS England's (2018) *Sustainable Improvement Team* (previously NHS Improving Quality), whose remit is to be one of the driving forces for improvement across the NHS, and to improve quality of care by achieving large-scale transformational improvement and change. Current improvement programmes include those in areas of learning disabilities, primary care, seven-day services, etc.

EVIDENCE-BASED PRACTICE AND RELATED CONCEPTS

As indicated at the beginning of the chapter, EBP is one of the essential competencies of practice supervisors, and it is also usually a component of healthcare professionals' codes of practice, such as the NMC (2015a: 7) and General Medical Council (2013: 8). So, what is EBP?

Evidence-based practice (also referred to as 'evidence informed practice') is closely associated with evidence-based medicine (EBM), for which Archie Cochrane is renowned for being one of its principal initiators (Smith and Rennie, 2014). Sackett et al. (2000) are also well known for being advocates of EBP and, according to them, EBP is the conscientious, explicit and judicious use of current best evidence in making decisions about the care of individual patients. EBP is defined by Polit and Beck (2018: 403) as 'A practice that involves making clinical decisions based on an integration of best available evidence, most often from disciplined research, with clinical expertise and patient preferences'. The key reason for the adoption of EBP in healthcare is the endeavour to ensure that each action taken by the healthcare professional is a 'well-informed' action, that is, it is based on evidence of its effectiveness. It thereby constitutes a shift from traditional or routine procedures to more objective scientific working.

Another term related to EBP is 'evidence-based healthcare' (EBHC), and also evidence-based nursing, evidence-based management and evidence-based education. EBHC is defined by Gray (2001: 9) as 'a discipline centred upon evidence-based decision-making about groups of patients, or populations, which can manifest itself as evidence-based policy-making or management'. Although they overlap substantially, EBHC can be distinguished from EBP in that the former tends to refer to groups of patients, while the latter can refer to single clinical interventions. According to Gray, there are five key elements of EBP, namely:

1. Decisions are based on best evidence.
2. The nature and source of evidence are determined by the problem.
3. Best evidence integrates research and personal experience.
4. Evidence is translated into action that affects the healthcare service user's health.
5. These actions are continually appraised.

REFLECTION POINT 5.1:   BEST EVIDENCE

EBP therefore refers to the use of 'best evidence' and is based on national and international standards. How do we know that every clinical intervention that we perform in our workplace is based on the 'best evidence' currently available?

Research evidence is available from national computer databases. However, Gray (2001) indicates that although the best evidence of the effectiveness of particular clinical interventions comes from well-designed research, other evidence of best practice – referred to as 'best evidence available' – needs to be seriously considered. There are several likely sources of best evidence of good practice, including:

- clinical guidelines (e.g. from NICE) and policy directives (from the Department of Health and Social Care)
- specialist and research conferences
- professional journal articles
- overview of evidence on specific topics on computer databases
- textbooks
- suppliers' information
- unpublished research
- suggestions from patients with a long-term health problem/their family
- colleagues and peer contact – uni- or interdisciplinary professionals
- personal intuition
- trial and error
- personal experience.

HOW DO PRACTICE SUPERVISORS ENSURE PRACTICE IS EVIDENCE-BASED?

There are various ways in which EBP can be achieved. Healthcare professionals can search for evidence of the effect of particular clinical interventions and best evidence on electronic databases such as MEDLINE or Cumulative Index to Nursing and Allied Health Literature (CINAHL), on the internet, or they can do a manual search of targeted literature.

There are also various organisations that store and provide systematically reviewed, meta-analysed or critically appraised research on different healthcare topics. The Cochrane Collaboration (2017: 1) which stores research evidence that has been appraised or systematically reviewed, is one of these organisations. The Cochrane Collaboration (2017: 1) indicates that a systematic review 'summarises the results of available carefully designed healthcare studies (controlled trials) and provides a high level of evidence on the effectiveness of healthcare interventions [which may] inform recommendations for healthcare'.

The strengths of the assembled research literature can be classified as a hierarchy of levels or grades of evidence, in order of validity and significance. Polit and Beck (2018), for instance, classify 'hierarchies of evidence' at eight levels of evidence, from the highest level of evidence being that from systematic reviews to the lowest level being expert opinion, as is shown in Figure 5.1 below.

You would have already encountered some of above-mentioned terminologies. If not, their meanings are easily found on the internet.

Hierarchy of evidence

- *Highest level of evidence*

- Systematic review
- Single Randomised Controlled Trial
- Single Non-Randomised Trial (Quasi-experimental)
- Single Prospective/Cohort Study
- Single Case-Control Study
- Single Cross-Sectional Study (e.g. a Survey) – descriptive, quantitative
- Single In-depth Qualitative Study – for meaning, process, etc.

- *Lowest level of evidence*

- Expert Opinion, Case Reports, etc.

Figure 5.1   Hierarchy of evidence

Other organisations categorise evidence differently, but they are essentially similar. Evans (2003) explored various such classifications and concluded that the appraisal of evidence should also include assessing the evidence's effectiveness, appropriateness and feasibility. Godlee (2014) reminds us that where the evidence comes from just one research study, maybe along with small sample size, and funded by industry, then extra care is required before accepting its findings as evidence. Furthermore, Sackett et al. (1996) and others indicate strongly that RCTs must not be treated as 'gold standards', and should combine research evidence with patient values and preferences. Use of healthcare professionals' personal experience and intuition have also been advised.

Several benefits or advantages of EBP in healthcare have been documented over the years, such as:

- higher quality of care and improved patient outcomes
- increased safety of healthcare service users
- instigate more appropriate and up-to-date interventions
- improved quality of life for individuals
- inform or advise healthcare service users more accurately
- increases healthcare professionals' confidence in the care they provide, makes them adaptable, improves their critical thinking and leads to more informed decision-making
- increases job satisfaction and team cohesion, and consequently promotes job retention
- reduces cost of healthcare compared to care based on traditional or outdated practices
- enables more efficient and effective use of available resources

However, there can be barriers to the implementation of EBP. These barriers are similar to those that present as obstacles to implementation of research findings and are examined shortly. Kopp (2001) suggests that such barriers include a lack of awareness of evidence, and of self-confidence, peer-support or resources. Another perspective is put forward by Sackett et al. (1996), who suggest that in case anyone feels EBP is overplayed, then they should be reminded that although 'practice risks becoming tyrannised by evidence, … without available evidence, practice risks becoming rapidly out of date to the detriment of patients' (ibid.: 71).

The difference between research-based practice and EBP is that research-based practice of clinical interventions usually only allows consideration of findings of quantitative research, while EBP also considers descriptive or qualitative studies, professional experiences, intuition and tacit knowledge (when we know more than we can evidence or tell) (Benner, 2001).

The Health Technology Assessment programme which is funded by the National Institute for Health Research (NIHR) (2017) supports search for evidence that is immediately useful to patients, clinical practice, and policy or decision-makers, and undertakes research on health technology to establish its effectiveness and compares the technology to the current standard NHS intervention to see which works best. It also examines the costs and effectiveness of health technology, and results are made available to NHS workers. Additionally, the York University NHS Centre for Reviews and Dissemination is another resource centre for EBP. There is also the quarterly journal *Evidence-Based Nursing*.

Typical headings for appraisal of a research study are:

- How clear and specific is the research question?
- Was the research funded by a particular organisation and, if so, does the researcher hold any allegiance to them?
- Is the research design the most appropriate to answer the research question?
- Are the sampling strategies the most appropriate?
- Precisely what was measured?
- Precise details and relevance of how the data was collected.
- How researcher effects and other intervening variables were controlled.
- Was the framework or method used for analysing the data the most appropriate?
- Are the statistical tests used appropriate and accurately documented?
- Are the conclusions drawn logically argued and is the generalisability statement justifiable?
- To what extent is the study relevant to clinical practice in the particular practice setting?
- Does the dissemination of the study indicate frameworks for implementation which include resources required, such as costs?

Much more detailed appraisal considerations are quite well publicised, and guidelines for systematic reviews are provided by Gopee (2010), for example. It is in the interest of the implementer of a particular component of EBP to examine closely and carefully the appraisal or systematic review already conducted by established organisations, who in fact are also likely to have accessed and appraised the original study report.

PRACTICE SUPERVISORS' ROLE IN IDENTIFYING, APPLYING AND DISSEMINATING RESEARCH FINDINGS

Identifying existing research on particular healthcare topic areas or components of clinical practice has become increasingly easier with the wide availability of electronic databases such as the Cochrane Library and NHS Evidence. However, the actual dissemination of research findings is often not as effectively achieved. Whether it is the findings of the healthcare professional's own research or those of studies encountered at conferences or on courses, the ultimate stages of research studies entail critiquing the study or studies, implementation, and then systematically disseminating the findings.

Healthcare professionals, including practice supervisors, also need to be aware that dissemination of research findings by a single avenue, such as presenting at a conference, has limited impact. Scullion (2002) suggests that dissemination is a vital yet complex process that aims to ensure that key messages are conveyed to specific groups, which can be done by utilising a wide range of methods so that it results in impact, reaction and preferably implementation. The range of methods of effective dissemination of research findings include:

- journal articles/editorials/short reports
- feedback to research subjects
- in-person support mechanisms
- journal clubs
- seminars, study days
- conference presentations
- poster presentations
- publishing as books/chapters
- inclusion in curriculum
- newsletters
- designing educational materials.

Scullion also suggests that the main barriers to the dissemination process are: poor journal reading habits of nurses resulting in them being unaware of research findings, lack of time, lack of knowledge, negative attitudes towards research and information overload. However, to disseminate new research on innovative practice, the researcher or healthcare professional needs to be focused, for example in planning for the chosen specific audience, identifying objectives for the dissemination session and the use of appropriate artefacts.

Furthermore, even with effective dissemination, there can be obstacles to the implementation of research findings. Two decades ago, Hunt (1997) repeated one of her earlier studies that explored the barriers to research implementation in healthcare and found at the time that these included:

- lack of critical appraisal and research skills
- lack of time to undertake research
- not having access to the right resources
- an organisational and managerial ethos and culture expecting instant answers
- lack of power and financial control to make things happen
- lack of valid research on any one topic, or of user-friendly reviews and guidelines.

REFLECTION POINT 5.2: BARRIERS TO IMPLEMENTING RESEARCH FINDINGS

Consider Hunt's (1997) findings for yourself as a practice supervisor, or discuss with an appropriate colleague, if, and how far, the findings are still prevalent in the context of present-day healthcare settings, both in general and in your own practice setting. Which barriers mentioned by Hunt have been largely resolved?

Williams et al. (2015a) conducted an extensive review of literature to ascertain the barriers to implementation of EBP, and identified the five most commonly occurring barriers as:

- workload
- other staff/management not supportive of research
- lack of resources
- lack of authority to change practice
- workplace/professional culture resistant to change.

So almost two decades after Hunt's study, issues related to implementation of EBP persists, e.g. lack of power to change practice. Education curricula for healthcare professionals have over the years rectified these problems to a good extent by inclusion of research modules in their health profession courses. Of course, undergraduate healthcare education curricula have been required (e.g. by the NMC, 2009; 2010a) to incorporate research appraisal and application of research knowledge and skills to care delivery regularly for more than a decade, and therefore some of the issues discussed by Williams et al. (2015a) may also have gradually been resolved.

Implementing changes to clinical practice is examined later in this chapter. With regard to EBP, Palfreyman et al. (2003) explored nurses' and physiotherapists' perceptions of barriers to EBP, and found that both professions have problems

ACTIVITY 5.1   BARRIERS TO IMPLEMENTATION
OF RESEARCH FINDINGS

Take another look at the barriers to implementation of research findings identified by Hunt (1997) and Williams et al. (2015a) in the preceding bulleted lists, and consider what you see as barriers in your workplace, at ward or trust level, and make some notes on how some of them are, or can be, resolved.

---

overcoming the barrier of time, with nurses also rating themselves as poor in EBP skills. However, some of the ways in which barriers to research implementation can be resolved include:

- making research available and accessible in practice settings
- providing research advice and support to the care team
- enabling healthcare professionals to develop negotiation and management of change skills
- changing registrants' and line managers' attitudes towards research
- establishing self-belief in one's research-critiquing skills.

Furthermore, in their comprehensive analysis of ways of placing research utilisation in healthcare, Pallen and Timmins (2002) concluded their study with a framework for systematic research implementation in practice settings by first considering the four main barriers, namely (1) the healthcare professionals' attitude and knowledge of research, (2) organisational factors such as funding, staffing and education, (3) accessibility to research and databases, and (4) communicating research. In their framework, each item under these four barriers is individually assessed in relation to the extent to which each prevails, plans to overcome them and sets goals, implementing the plans and evaluating them.

Thus, managerial and organisational input and support tend to be as important as individual skills in implementation of research findings, except such implementation needs to be 'managed', as discussed shortly in this chapter.

Research-based practice is an inherent component of practice supervisors' roles. EBP should be a permanent feature, and 'where's the evidence?' sounds like a confrontational question. The healthcare trust's clinical procedure and guidelines, however, almost always include the evidence base for practice. However, consider the following scenario that involves supervising practice-based learning for a student midwife and her perception of EBP.

You do not have to be a midwife to ask relevant questions related to EBP, and in the following case study a number of issues surface when this scenario is put to group discussions. In the context of the discussions in this chapter, all parties will question the strengths of the evidence that Helen seemed to have used during the procedure. They can be explored in the context of levels or grades of evidence available in relation to 'examination of the newborn'.

CASE STUDY 5.1:   EVIDENCE VERSUS BEST PRACTICE

Sarah is the practice assessor for first-year student midwife Helen. A 'triad'* assessment is being conducted with Helen by Sarah and Geraldine, the link lecturer. The topic chosen is the examination of the newborn.

Helen states that she is very nervous. She provides a full clinical picture of the woman and the baby in whose care she has been involved. Having confirmed the woman's consent, she then concentrates on the examination, which she performs in a professional manner. There is, however, little communication with the mother. Helen has to be reminded of the need to complete the relevant documentation. Her hand is shaking as she writes.

Helen then produces and discusses an article regarding examinations of the healthy neonate. She needs some prompting when asked about the NMC's Midwives Rules and Standards and what she would do if she identified a deviation from the norm. When asked about her assessment of her performance, Helen is very self-critical and feels that she did not do very well.

What are the key issues in this assessment situation? What are the ways in which Helen's evidence base influenced her performance, and what are the questions that Sarah and Geraldine might want to ask?

*'triad' refers to a tripartite assessment of competencies in the practice setting that includes the assessee, their practice assessor and a midwife lecturer.

PRACTICE SUPERVISORS' ROLE IN PRACTICE DEVELOPMENT

The two concepts 'effective practice' and 'EBP' both potentially imply making changes to the ways in which care and treatment are delivered if the change benefits the care service user. Such changes are referred to as 'practice development', and this section explores what practice development is, the different reasons for practice development and how these developments are managed, with some basic exploration of the management of change.

WHAT IS PRACTICE DEVELOPMENT?

Practice development (or clinical practice development) implies changing the way in which particular care and treatment interventions are performed for the benefit of healthcare service users. It has to do with improving and enhancing clinical practice where there is scope to do so. It refers to hands-on patient care interventions, that is, patient contact. Which developments in clinical practice are currently happening in your particular area of practice? What changes can be made or have been made recently to specific care and treatments carried out in your practice setting?

ACTIVITY 5.2   PRACTICE DEVELOPMENT

Reflect on how care is currently delivered in your workplace and explore whether any aspect of the way in which care is delivered has changed recently – in the last few months or in the last year or two.

Next, identify an aspect of service user care in your work setting that requires or could benefit from change, either in clinical care, patient teaching or organisation of care. State two examples of such potential changes.

Practice supervisors can be involved in changes in different components or aspects of healthcare delivery, and practice supervisors can influence the nature and direction of these changes. Examples of changes in hands-on clinical practice include:

- adaptation of national early warning systems (NEWS)
- no-lift policy
- a red jug of water next to a patient who is at risk of dehydration
- use of patient-controlled analgesia
- nurse-led specialist clinics
- cognitive behavioural therapy
- nurse prescribing
- using tympanic thermometers rather than glass thermometers
- 'golden hour' in care of patient with sepsis
- cardiac output studies in intensive care units
- bedside handover.

Examples of changes in organisation or management of care include:

- introducing a new shift system
- team midwifery
- outreach work and tele-health
- family-witnessed resuscitation
- open-door availability of influenza vaccines to over-65s at the start of winter
- modern matron role in aspects of care (e.g. who does what to ensure hospital cleanliness)
- allowing parents to be present in the anaesthetic room
- clinical supervision for peer support and CPD (continuing professional development)
- a mechanism for reporting to colleagues from conferences and workshops
- implementing advance care planning in end-of-life care.

Examples of changes in patient teaching include:

- health 'MOTs' conducted by practice nurses or SCPHNs (specialist community public health nurse)

- school nurses' advice to teenagers on sexual activity
- encouraging a person with arthritis to take regular exercise in a gymnasium
- teaching self-relaxation to a patient with heart problems
- teaching dietary control to a newly diagnosed diabetic
- advising older people on how to avoid hypothermia
- smoking cessation support groups meeting.

As practice supervisors, you could think of various instances of changes in teaching students and other learners, such as medical students, healthcare assistants, preceptees and inductees. Practice development is 'a systematic approach that aims to help practitioners and healthcare teams to look critically at their practice and identify how it can be improved ... [and] ... have embedded within them person centred processes, and systems' (Department of Health and Children, 2010: 16). Another helpful definition is provided by McCormack et al. (2013: 4), who states that:

> Practice development is a continuous process of improvement towards increased effectiveness in patient centred care, which is brought about by enabling healthcare teams to develop their knowledge and skills, and to transform the culture and context of care.

According to Bryar and Griffiths (2003), practice development is taken to mean a broad range of innovations that are initiated to improve practice and healthcare services. The term *innovation* differs from practice development in certain respects, especially in that the former refers to implementing something new and unprecedented. The dictionary (e.g. Brookes and O'Neill, 2017: 464) indicates that to 'innovate' means 'to introduce new ideas or methods', implying that a new product, practice or method is being introduced for the first time. Innovations refer to something developed necessarily in response to patient care needs. Innovation implies implementing a relatively radical new practice. 'Development', however, refers to a gradual progressive change and advancement. Change as a concept, however, can mean substituting something with something new, a development, or reverting to an older (but effective) practice.

WHY PRACTICE DEVELOPMENT?

One of the primary reasons for practice development is that, as evidence-based practitioners (NMC, 2015a), all registrants (obviously including practice supervisors) have to be role models of good practice for their learners (e.g. NMC, 2018a), which implies that they should always be reflecting on whether their clinical interventions are of the highest standard known and based on the best available evidence, with a view to making changes that result in their practice becoming even more effective.

The NMC (2015a) clearly indicates that registrants must continually question the evidence base and effectiveness of the care they deliver. However, clinical practice is only one of the components of the practice supervisor's role that can be developed, others being their education and management roles. Another categorisation of healthcare professionals' roles, each of which can be further developed, is by the Department of Health (2004) in the *NHS KSF*, which identifies all patient care activities under six 'core dimensions', namely: (1) communication; (2) personal and people development; (3) health, safety and security; (4) service improvement; (5) quality; and (6) equality and diversity. All categories imply quality assurance, but service improvement in particular relates to making 'changes in own practice and offer suggestions for improving services' (DH, 2004: 70).

Practice development is evolving continually, and the concept is taken further as some healthcare professionals develop their careers to become 'nurse entrepreneurs' (for example, Faugier, 2005b). The term *entrepreneur* of course refers to people who engage in novel, unprecedented ventures on a substantial scale, and implies being innovators. Mooney (2009: 1), amongst others, reports on such developments but indicates that better support from colleagues and peers is required to allow healthcare professionals to innovate and become more entrepreneurial, in addition to the national level support that is already available.

The RN's teaching role starts soon after registering their qualification with the NMC, which is another reason why we need to monitor how up-to-date the evidence base and effective our practice is, but the extent to which we can engage in practice development is variable depending on expertise, experience and clinical circumstances. Becoming a nurse entrepreneur is an even longer-term prospect.

Government directives that promote practice development include *Liberating the Talents* (DH, 2002), a document that encourages primary care nurses and midwives to develop their practice. This was reinforced in various Department of Health documents, including *Towards a Framework for Post-Registration Nursing Careers* (DH, 2008), and currently through new models of care generated under the aegis of NHS England's (2017b) *Five Year Forward View*. These models of care are referred to as 'vanguards', an example of which is reported by Moore (2017) whereby when care home patients are admitted to hospital, they are given a pack which contain details of their health background, which in turn reduces hospital stay by four days on average.

Practice development is also propelled by RNs' expanded or specialist roles as well as via senior nurse positions such as nurse practitioners and nurse consultants. Previously known as 'extended roles', 'expanded roles' refers to those clinical interventions that healthcare professionals engage in following relevant post-registration training and assessment.

With the implementation of the *European Working Time Directive* in 2004 (British Medical Association, 2012) leading to a reduction in doctors' working hours, etc., an increasing range of clinical interventions that were previously doctors' roles are now also performed by other healthcare professionals.

These roles afford healthcare professionals greater autonomy and further scope for decision-making in holistic care, and therefore for creativity and consequent practice development.

However, clinical practice development is often triggered by a need for new actions to resolve a health problem. For example, falls amongst older people have presented as an issue for some time, and one of the actions taken by the predecessors of the Sustainable Improvement Team (NHS England, 2018) was by publishing case studies of good practice on preventing and managing falls, regarding which Ward et al. (2010) also report on novel interventions that are being implemented, namely:

- use of sensor alarms that alert nurses when an 'at risk' patient gets out of bed unaided
- identification of a falls team that is led by a matron, whose role includes staff training on the issue/topic area
- distraction therapy in dementia
- a new observation tool to identify the risk of falls.

Another example is compassionate care (discussed shortly), lack of which was presented in the Francis (2013) Report, and more currently 'person-centred care'.

CONCEPT ANALYSIS OF PRACTICE DEVELOPMENT

Moving on from actual examples of practice development and the two definitions of the term cited earlier in this section, in most instances practice is not developed or improved by individuals (e.g. practice supervisors) acting on their own, as it usually takes team effort to change to new practice. The team can be a small group of colleagues based at a specialist area (for example, day surgery unit, nursing home, intensive care unit), or a hospital level team (when a change is introduced at organisational level), or at national or supra-organisational level (as currently in the development of compassionate care).

Before implementing new ways of working, which is discussed in a later section under 'Managing changes', another two perspectives of practice development need to be considered. One perspective consists of exploring more thoroughly all that practice development entails, and one way of executing this is by a concept analysis.

Garbett and McCormack (2002) undertook a concept analysis of practice development based on an analysis of literature, and on focus group interviews with practice developers and telephone interviews with practitioners. A conceptual framework derived from the study comprises the purposes, attributes and outcomes of practice development (see box).

More contemporarily, McCormack et al. (2013: 5–7) provide a further dimension of practice development in indicating that it should be based on nine basic principles, which include:

PURPOSES, ATTRIBUTES AND OUTCOMES OF PRACTICE DEVELOPMENT

The purposes of practice development are to:

- Increase the effectiveness of patient care
- Transform care and the cultures and context within which it takes place

The attributes of practice development are that it:

- Requires a systematic and rigorous approach
- Is a continuous process
- Is founded on various types of facilitation

The consequences of practice development include:

- For users – improved experiences of care in terms of their sensitivity to the needs of individuals and populations
- For practitioners – increased capacity for thinking creatively and more broadly
- Greater awareness of the impact of organisations on practice

- practice development for achieving person-centred care and EBP
- practice development is gauged by the patient's experience of ways in which healthcare is provided
- it integrates work-based learning
- it integrates free thinking with creativity
- it integrates evaluation that is always inclusive and collaborative.

The above analysis of practice development addresses its various facets, but practice supervisors mustn't be overwhelmed by this range of perspectives. Practice development thus continually aims to enhance the quality of patient-centred care, and to mobilise this Heyns et al. (2017) advocate appointment of practice development facilitators, whereby facilitation involves enabling practitioners to adjust their culture of practice so that changes in practice are sustainable and positive. These facilitators therefore also have to be role models as well as change agents.

COMPASSIONATE CARE AS A RECENT PRACTICE DEVELOPMENT

In addition to various examples of practice development stated in the above discussion, one mode of practice that has recently been vociferously advocated is compassionate care, which is a practice that was identified as lacking in healthcare provision in the Francis (2013) Report. The report is the result of a thorough investigation into suspected malpractice in terms of patients being 'neglected', and concluded with approximately 300 recommendations, one of which refers to strengthening compassionate care in healthcare organisations.

As noted in Chapter 2, compassionate care is one of the essential skills clusters together with a number of competencies that student nurses have to gain a pass in during their pre-registration programme. It is also identified as a requirement in the Department of Health's (2015) *NHS Constitution for England*, and by the NMC (2018b). Compassionate care is further strengthened in a publication by the CNO for England entitled *Leading Change, Adding Value – A Framework for Nursing, Midwifery and Care Staff* (NHS England, 2016).

ACTIVITY 5.3   WHAT DOES COMPASSIONATE CARE MEAN?

Discuss with a colleague/peer whom you trust whether you practise compassionate care in your day-to-day care delivery; and then explain in your own words what it is that you do that comprises compassionate care.

Compassionate care involves caring through a relationship that is 'based on empathy, respect, and dignity – it … is central to how people perceive their care' (DH, 2012b: 13). As a practice supervisor, your ways of providing compassionate care are the ways that your student is very likely to adopt for their future practice as an RN or RM, as your practice supervisor role incorporates being a role model. So, you are likely to incorporate acting with warmth and empathy, actively listening, being sensitive and accessible, respecting dignity and privacy, etc., when interacting with service users, which are characteristics also found by Bray et al. (2014) in their study of healthcare professionals' understanding of compassionate care.

Adam and Taylor (2014) suggest that compassion is developed through understanding patients' experiences, and approaching patients in gentle and respectful ways, and that the prerequisites of compassionate care include the ability to build effective working relationships with patients, and being able to feel secure and trusting of colleagues in the team.

Additionally, Adam and Taylor suggest ways of teaching students the ability to practise compassionate care that includes experiential learning and reflection. However, on exploring the RN's process of professional socialisation, Curtis et al. (2012) found that healthcare profession students' socialisation tends to drift towards the uncertainty of having time to practise compassionate care on qualification as a registrant. Nevertheless, compassionate care does not always depend on time, because it is an inherent component of most clinical interventions and can happen in the briefest of interactions with patients, and this is another instance where role modelling of practice supervisors is so crucial for the student's learning.

MANAGEMENT OF PRACTICE DEVELOPMENTS

Titchen (2003) identifies three themes that form the basis for effective practice development, which she refers to as the practice development diamond. The themes are: (1) changing the practice philosophy; (2) the process of change in practice; and (3) investing in professional development.

The second perspective is that implementing a new way of practice (changing how a clinical intervention is performed), might require new resources in terms of new equipment, medical devices or disposable materials, and a step-by-step procedure for performing the new practice. We also have to be completely clear about the 'purposes' and 'consequences' (Garbett and McCormack, 2002) of the novel practice. This perspective is captured by the Donabedian (1988) 'structure–process–outcome' model of implementing change, as also noted by Gopee and Galloway (2017).

Thinking, for example, in relation to introducing patient-controlled analgesia (PCA), the 'structure–process–outcome' model consists of the following:

- *Structure* refers to the material items required for implementing the new practice, such as new equipment, devices (such as PCA devices) and premises.
- *Process* refers to the step-by-step procedure for the new practice, such as the procedure for utilising the PCA device, and for teaching the patient how to use it, etc.
- *Outcome* refers to identifying clearly the results of the new practice, which in relation to PCA comprise, for example, pain relief in x seconds, saving staff time, quicker patient recovery.

The Donabedian model is a very practical framework for implementing and monitoring or formatively evaluating (see Chapter 9) the progress and effect of a new form of practice. The framework can be introduced or utilised by individual practitioners, at team level, at organisational level (for example, hospital), at supra-organisational level (for example, within a clinical commissioning group's [CCG] healthcare providers) or nationally.

ACTIVITY 5.4   DEVELOPING PRACTICE

Based on the list of developments generated as a result of Activity 5.2, think of two aspects of practice at your work base that could be developed. Consider and make notes on how the framework presented by Donabedian (1988) can be utilised to change these two aspects of practice.

The practice development framework suggested by Donabedian should enable you to take these developments further systematically if you so wish, maybe within the context of management of change (discussed next in this chapter).

Nursing posts for practice development include Neonatal Practice Development Nurse, Lead Nurse for Practice Development, Practice Development Facilitator, etc. The resources that can help healthcare professionals include the journal *Practice Development in Healthcare*, and national conferences specifically on practice development. Several NHS trusts employ Practice Development Nurses or Facilitators. Some have Practice Development Units that conduct experiments on new modes of practice.

EBP, PRACTICE DEVELOPMENT AND MANAGING CHANGES

All healthcare professionals will have encountered changes in the way care and treatment are organised and delivered in various practice settings. EBP implies potential changes in clinical practice, and practice development actually constitutes making changes. It is therefore almost inevitable that practice supervisors will be involved as participants in change, and are also expected to initiate change as and when appropriate. Therefore, the practice supervisor needs to have knowledge and competence in managing change. It is important to distinguish between the concepts of 'managing' change and 'introducing' or 'imposing' change; the latter can be effected at short notice, but managing the change implies longer-term, planned and systematic activities.

Other than EBP and practice development, there are various other reasons for changes in clinical practice, which are identified in the box below.

REASONS FOR CHANGES IN HEALTHCARE

1. Change in medical technology	• New medical devices and equipment; use of computer networks and easier access to information
2. New knowledge	• Research and audit findings; expert guidelines
3. Safer and more effective products	• Consumable materials and hardware being superseded by more efficient ones
4. The nature of the workforce	• Workers of different age groups and with domestic responsibilities; changes in qualified:unqualified staff ratio, e.g. healthcare assistants with different skills
5. Revised policies and strategies	• Use of devices and strategies to prevent injury to staff, or to avoid 'hospital acquired infections'
6. Quality-conscious consumers	• Consumer satisfaction surveys indicating the changes that should be made
7. Funding and budgets	• Availability and distribution of scarce resources

At times change occurs in reaction to dictats from government departments, or as a result of CQC audits, or publication of new clinical guidelines, *National Service Framework* or care pathways; or to improve patient outcomes, or as service efficiency measures.

MODELS OF CHANGE MANAGEMENT

A range of proformas or frameworks for managing change has been published for systematic management of change, such as the NHS England's (2017c) *Change Model*, which is a framework comprising eight elements that should be considered when leading change. These eight elements need to be applied to each individual change being implemented, and they are:

Our shared purpose

Leadership by all

Spread and adoption

Improvement tools

Project and performance management

Measurement

System drivers

Motivate and mobilise

Yet another management of change model consists of a cycle consisting of: Plan–Do–Study–Act (PDSA) (Institute of Healthcare Improvement, 2017). The model is usually presented as a cycle made up of four arcs, each beginning with one of the four steps, and thereby meant to represent a 'complete' circular model. Moreover, a relatively more straightforward but comprehensive framework for change is composed of seven essential and interrelated factors for successful management of change created by Gopee and Galloway (2017), the seven factors being: Recognition, Analysis, Preparation, Strategies, Implementation, Evaluation, Sustaining (RAPSIES) for systematic management of change. The RAPSIES framework entails (in sequence):

1. **Recognition** of the need for change to solve a problem, for instance, or to improve an element of practice.
2. **Analysis** of the available options related to the contemplated change, the environment or setting where change will be implemented, and the users of the change.
3. **Preparation** for the change, such as identifying a change agent to lead the implementation of the change, education, defining intended outcomes and involving relevant colleagues.
4. **Strategies** for implementing the change.

5. **Implementation** of the change, including piloting the change, timing of implementation.
6. **Evaluation** of the impact of the change against the intended outcomes.
7. **Sustaining** the change, i.e. how to ensure the change endures and is mainstreamed.

The change could succeed or fail, depending on the effectiveness of each of the seven steps in the framework. For example, when managing change to flexible-hour rostering, then each of the seven steps needs to be managed effectively. To provide more details of step 4 for instance – the strategies for implementing the change – there are several strategies that can be considered before deciding on relevant ones. One strategy for example is *Lewin's three-stage change process*, which entails unfreezing the situation, implementing the change, and then refreezing it. This is obviously an extremely simplistic explanation of activities that warrant careful planning and conduct. Unfreezing can be achieved by the SWOT or forcefield analyses. The implementation of the change is referred to as 'movement', and 'refreezing' refers to sustaining the change.

Following a SWOT or forcefield analysis, the actions that can be taken entail reducing the weaknesses and strengthening the driving forces. A format like the ones presented in Template 5.1 for introducing flexible hours, and in Template 5.2 for peri-operative visiting can be utilised for this.

The management of change requires a systematic approach and takes time, and a more detailed explanation of management of change is provided at https://study.sagepub.com/gopee4e. Furthermore, full details of the management of change is available in relevant textbooks, e.g. Gopee and Galloway (2017) *Leadership and Management in Healthcare*, Chapter 6.

Template 5.1 Forcefield analysis – introducing flexible hours – and subsequent actions

Probable actions	Driving forces	Restraining forces	Probable actions
	What people want	Long-term staff against	
	Retention issues	Fear of coming off worse	
	Encourage recruitment	'Unfair'	
	Staff morale	Difficulty fitting in with practical routine	
	Maximum use of staff time	Not feeling part of the team	
	Government favours this	Staff morale	
		Lack of communication	

Template 5.2   SWOT analysis – peri-operative visiting – and subsequent actions

SWOT analysis	Probable actions
Strengths • Reduces anxiety • Patient compliance up • Less post-operative compliance required • Patient articulates preferences to nursing staff • More interdisciplinary collaboration • Patient divulges more information • Continuity of care *Weaknesses* • Resources • Time • Possible lack of knowledge • Too many people disseminating information *Opportunities* • Role expansion • Specialist role • Education • Increased cost-effectiveness through patient compliance • Enhanced patient care *Threats* • Lack of continuity of care • Cost – funding • Patient information overload • Elitism – conflict	

PRACTICE SUPERVISORS AS ROLE MODELS OF EBP AND PRACTICE DEVELOPMENT

On summarising the discussion on the registrants' and practice supervisors' role as evidence-based practitioners and practice developers, it is clear that one of the added values or knock-on effects of practice supervisors' activities is that they also embody the qualities of a model healthcare professional. Appreciating that being a model healthcare practitioner also leads to being a role model for colleagues, juniors and learners, this necessarily incorporates being proficient or expert in one's practice as well as having the associated knowledge and appropriate behaviour.

Being amenable to adopting changing modes of clinical intervention, new medical devices, diagnostic techniques, and medicines that benefit or enhance the patient's health is a characteristic of a role model that those open to learning can emulate and adopt.

Price and Price (2009) support the argument that role modelling is an appropriate method or process for enabling students to learn safe and effective practice.

The notion is based on Bandura's (1997) social learning theory that, as noted in Chapter 1, suggests that individuals learn behaviour through observation, mental retention of the procedure utilised, reproducing the behaviour and reinforcement. An analysis of role modelling was also presented in Chapter 1.

CHAPTER SUMMARY

This chapter has focused on registrants' and practice supervisors' leadership, their roles in evidence-based effective practice and practice development, as well as management of change to some extent, and has therefore examined:

- Practice supervisors' leadership in careful forward planning of students' learning during practice placement, and prioritising daily work to accommodate support for them.
- Effective practice and its relevance for the practice supervisor role.
- Evidence-based practice, addressing what it is and how it is achieved; research-based practice, and the practice supervisor's role in identifying, evaluating, applying and disseminating research findings, and how to overcome barriers to implementation.
- Practice development, what the term means, including definitions and a concept analysis of practice development, the reasons for developing practice and how they can be managed effectively.
- Models and frameworks for managing change briefly, practice supervisors as role models of EBP and practice development.

FURTHER OPTIONAL READING

1. For a more detailed account and analysis of leadership in healthcare, see Chapter 3 of:

- Gopee, N. and Galloway, J. (2017) *Leadership and Management in Healthcare*, 3rd edn. London: SAGE Publications.

2. Various detailed examples of innovations (case studies) and practice development in healthcare are available on NICE's website, e.g.:

- National Institute for Health and Care Excellence (2017) *Transforming the Care of Children and Young People in London with Asthma*. Available at: www.nice.org.uk/ sharedlearning/transforming-the-care-of-children-and-young-people-in-london-with-asthma (accessed 17 September 2017).

3. For a basic reminder of what EBP is in healthcare, and how it impacts on practice, see:

- Aveyard, H. and Sharp, P. (2013) *A Beginner's Guide to Evidence-Based Practice in Health and Social Care*, 2nd edn. Maidenhead: Open University Press.

4. An excellent resource for the best ways of critically appraising research papers is:

- Greenhalgh, T. (2014) *How to Read a Paper: The Basics of Evidence-Based Medicine*, 5th edn. Oxford: Wiley-Blackwell.

To access further resources related to this chapter, visit **https://study.sagepub.com/gopee4e** where a range of learning and teaching materials are provided.

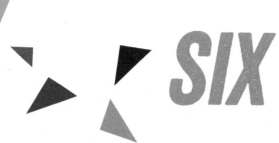

SIX

ASSESSING THE LEARNER'S PRACTICE COMPETENCE AND KNOWLEDGE BASE

INTRODUCTION

One of the fundamental functions of the practice assessor is to assess students' and other learners' clinical skills and associated knowledge. This chapter explores student assessment from the perspectives of what assessments are, the reasons for performing them, at which points in the programme students are assessed, who other than the practice assessor assesses them (e.g. peer-assessment), and the range of methods of assessment that are available. The specified procedures that have to be followed, and the validity and reliability of assessments are other components that are addressed. These points essentially constitute the principles and processes of assessments. The concepts that are inherent within the principles of assessment are therefore essential, and the practical considerations as well as the theoretical base are addressed in both this chapter and Chapter 7. Problems with assessments, as well as past and present criticisms and how they can be averted or resolved, are also components addressed in Chapter 7.

CHAPTER OBJECTIVES

1. Identify what assessments are, and the elements of healthcare courses on which students are assessed.
2. Enunciate a number of reasons for assessment of clinical skills and knowledge of students on healthcare profession courses.
3. Cite instances of various staff members who are involved in assessment, including the roles of self- and peer-assessment.

4. Explain a range of methods of assessment that practice assessors can utilise in the conduct of student assessments, and the various fundamental principles of assessments that they need to abide by to fulfil this function.
5. Explain the role of 'ongoing record of achievement' and the requirements that practice assessors have to fulfil to competently ascertain students' achievement of proficiency.
6. Explain ways in which assessments can meet essential criteria such as validity and reliability.

ASSESSING PRACTICE

Assessment is an integral part of all credit-awarding healthcare courses, and one of the principal purposes of practice assessor courses is to equip course participants with the capability to assess students on their placement competencies and SOP. At the end of each assessment by direct observation, the practice assessor has to make a decision regarding whether the student is competent to perform the assessed skill independently, unsupervised and safely, and signs the appropriate section of the student's competency document as pass or fail. The NMC (2018a) indicates that assessment of nursing and midwifery students is conducted by practice assessors and academic assessors, with input from practice supervisors.

There are a number of factors that practice assessors need to consider to fulfil their assessment duties effectively. Specifically, for nursing and midwifery students, in the *Standards Framework for Nursing and Midwifery Education* (NMC, 2018c: 12) document, under 'Curricula and assessment', the NMC (2018c) stipulates a range of considerations related to student assessment, including that assessment must occur throughout the programme and across practice settings to determine student progression, and that practice assessments are 'evidenced by (direct) observations and other appropriate methods'.

Additionally, in *Standards for Student Supervision and Assessment*, the NMC (2018a: 9) identifies a number of facets of the 'practice assessor' role, such as 'practice assessors conduct assessment to confirm student achievement of proficiencies and programme outcomes for practice learning. These statements identify requirements such as the need for educational preparation (attending a course) for the practice assessor role, and ways in which assessment of students needs to be conducted to ensure the evidence base and effectiveness of the assessment process.

However, the NMC (2018a: 7) also details the new practice supervisor's role in student assessment and progression through four clauses reproduced in the box below.

So, clearly practice supervisors have a fundamental and crucial role in monitoring the development and achievement of the student's care skills, knowledge and attitude. Technically, practice supervisors thus conduct formative assessments (discussed later in this chapter), and their role include recording the student's achievements, and take action if they have concerns that the student is under-performing and underachieving. Practice supervisors providing relevant information about students' progress during practice placement to practice assessors as appropriate.

PRACTICE SUPERVISORS' CONTRIBUTION TO ASSESSMENT AND PROGRESSION

Practice supervisors:

4.1 contribute to the student's record of achievement by periodically recording relevant observations on the conduct, proficiency and achievement of the students they are supervising

4.2 contribute to student assessments to inform decisions for progression

4.3 have sufficient opportunities to engage with practice assessors and academic assessors to share relevant observations on the conduct, proficiency and achievement of the students they are supervising, and

4.4 are expected to appropriately raise and respond to student conduct and competence concerns and are supported in doing so.

The practice assessor role in nursing and midwifery is complemented by the 'academic' assessor's role, the latter normally being a university-based lecturer, who, in collaboration with the practice assessor, determines whether the student has met all NMC's pre-registration education requirements to be able to become a registrant with the NMC.

WHAT ARE ASSESSMENTS?

To begin to examine the principles and processes of assessments, it is useful to establish first what you as the healthcare professional already know about assessments of competencies.

ACTIVITY 6.1   WHAT YOU ALREADY KNOW ABOUT ASSESSMENTS

1. Think of the courses that you have already attended, and any one(s) you might currently be on. Think also of your contact with other learners and students on various programmes of study. What are the various methods of assessment that are used to assess learners' knowledge and skills? Jot down as many methods as you can think of.

2. Consider what else you already know about assessments, which aspects of assessments you are unclear about, and what else you feel that you need to know about assessments. Make written notes of your responses.

So, what do you already know about assessments? In response to Activity 6.1, you may have thought that assessment of clinical skills is best carried out by direct observation of the learner's performance, and some by asking the learner specific questions, or by their reflective write-ups. Essays and written examinations are used for the assessment of theory (also referred to as knowledge base). Most of these will be examined in this chapter under 'how to assess'. In addition to assessment by direct observation of practice-based competencies, other examples of assessments of theory and practice in healthcare education programmes include:

- practical assessments in skills laboratories
- profiles and portfolio, with reflective accounts
- care studies/case studies
- written examination
- OSCE (i.e., Objective Structured/Simulated Clinical Examination)
- objective or multiple-choice tests
- short-answer questions
- structured essays
- seminars and presentations
- individually negotiated projects
- longitudinal studies
- viva voce (previously referred to as oral examinations).

Other assessment methods that usually contribute to summative assessment of students include testimony of service users and carers, peer assessment and student self-assessment. The HEE (2017a: 25) adds storyboards and 'professional conversations' to the methods of assessing nursing associates. Tweed et al. (2010) add that for clinical psychology students, video recordings on digital video discs can be utilised instead of direct observation, with the permission of any service user involved of course, for assessment of students' competencies. Your response to what else you feel you need to know about assessments obviously depends very much on your experience, existing knowledge and understanding of the concept, and it varies between individuals. You might have felt, for instance, that you could do with knowing more about formative, summative, continuous, peer/self-assessment or about practice competencies.

With regard to the final bullet point in the above list, a viva voce is a face-to-face questions and answers examination between the student and the examiner. This is standard practice for PhD student assessments, and several years ago in pre-registration student nurse overall assessment. For nursing associates, the current equivalent assessment is referred to as the end-point assessment.

Furthermore, you might need to know about student assessment in programmes for newer nursing titles such as apprentices, nursing associates, etc. For nursing associates, training competencies are based on the current Skills for Health (2017) *Care Certificate Standards* which are designed mainly for non-regulated vocations, while other customised ones are being piloted before implementation (HEE, 2017a). For nurse apprenticeships, which is an undergraduate programme, the end-point assessments are identified as a reflective essay and a 'professional discussion' that lasts 60 minutes and is scenario-based (*FE News*, 2016).

——————   **ACTIVITY 6.2   ASSESSMENTS THAT I'VE PASSED**   ——————

To explore this area further, first look back to a course that you attended, preferably recently, and make notes on the following:

- A list of assessments that you had to pass in order to complete the course successfully.
- When exactly during the course were you assessed, and on which components of the course?
- Specifically, what was assessed?

WHAT DO WE MEAN BY ASSESSMENTS?

A number of assessment methods such as written examinations, practical assessments and projects have just been identified.

If you were assessed by continuous assessment, then you would have been exposed to a range of assessment components on different occasions, during both practice placements and in university skill laboratories and classrooms.

DEFINITIONS OF ASSESSMENT

The dictionary (Brookes and O'Neill, 2017: 48) states that the word 'assess' originates from the Latin word *assidere*, which means sit by or beside, which implies a close relationship and sharing an experience. The word also means 'estimate the value or worth of someone or something', and 'to judge the worth or importance of'. Based on general current understanding of the term, assessment therefore tends to imply staying by the learner's side and observing them perform a clinical intervention with a view to stating at the end of the performance whether the intervention was carried out competently. It also seems to imply being supportive and identifying subsequent learning needs.

Taking a step back, however, it is important to note that an assessment is not an activity we perform only occasionally to fulfil our work role. We assess life situations all the time before we take any action, whether it is to do with assessing whether to wear a coat when going out based on the perceived weather and temperature outside, whether it is safe to overtake when driving, or whether we can treat ourselves to a delicious cake while bearing in mind the day's calorie intake. Such assessments do not result in someone awarding us a pass or fail but they still involve assessing stimuli or data, and then making a decision.

Assessment is also reflected in health assessment of the health service user, which entails collecting information and identifying actual and potential patient problems from the data, from which decisions are made regarding the actions to be taken. Student assessment, however, is related to collecting information as evidence of the student's ability to perform particular clinical skills or competencies and their critical thinking skills. Some of the core skills necessary for assessing patients' needs and problems are also relevant for assessing learners. These are observing, measuring, interviewing and making decisions. So, these skills also apply to assessment of students' knowledge and skills.

For assessing health profession learners' clinical competencies and related knowledge, assessment can be defined as the purposeful observation and questioning undertaken to ascertain the learner's ability to perform particular care interventions in precise accordance with approved guidelines, and their knowledge of rationales for each action. Curzon and Tummons (2013) suggest that assessments involve collecting, measuring and interpreting information related to students' responses to the process of instruction.

Assessment is also a measurement of the quantity of learning, as well as the quality. While quantity of learning implies the number of skills or part-skills that the learner has already learnt, quality of learning refers to how thoroughly the skills (or knowledge) have been learnt. The two elements also provide a measure of progress, and thereby also form the basis for identifying areas of further learning.

WHAT DO WE ASSESS?

As noted in Chapter 2, acquiring professional competencies involves learning in all three domains – cognitive, psychomotor and affective. That means learning the professional knowledge base required to perform our healthcare duties, the skills required for performing care interventions, and also having the appropriate attitude. Attitude in this context is also referred to as values and behaviours.

The NMC's (2018b) *Standards of Proficiency for Registered Nurses* and NMC's (2010a) *Standards for Pre-registration Nursing Education*, identify the exact learning outcomes that pre-registration students need to achieve to gain registered nurse status on the NMC's professional register. The NMC (2018b) standards, as noted at the beginning of Chapter 2, are detailed under seven 'platforms', and also under 'Communication and relationship management skills' (Annexe A of NMC, 2018b) and 'Nursing procedures' (Annexe B). These standards apply to all four fields of nursing and students have to be competent in them at the point of registration.

In addition to the NMC's (2010a) generic and field competencies, essential skills clusters (ESC) (NMC, 2007a) are incorporated into all pre-registration nursing education programmes. The specific ones that form part of particular practice placement objectives to be achieved by students are discussed with them and their practice supervisors and practice assessors before students embark on the particular placement. For the NMC (2018b) based pre-registration programme, practice assessors assess students on all competencies stated in the competencies documents (often known as PAD – Practice Assessment Document) that have been designed from the outcomes under the seven 'platforms'.

As for the NMC (2010a) standards for pre-registration nurse education, it contains 'generic' and 'field' (previously known as 'branch') (mental health, adult, child and learning disabilities) competencies under four 'domains': (1) professional values; (2) communication and interpersonal skills; (3) nursing practice and decision-making; and (4) leadership, management and team-working that each student needs to achieve for entry to the professional register (NMC, 2010a), as also noted in Chapter 2.

The NMC's (2010a) standards apply to the 'Degree Apprenticeships – Registered Nurse' programme (Institute for Apprenticeships, 2016a), but the methods of student assessment are largely prescribed by the Institute for Apprenticeships (2016b).

Similarly, the HCPC publishes separate standards for pre-qualifying different AHP courses. These standards and competencies are reflected in the course's and modules' aims and learning outcomes, in theory and in practice components. There are also 'specialist practitioner outcomes' for SCPHNs (NMC, 2004a).

As we shall see later, it is absolutely vital for the practice assessor to establish very early on during the practice placement exactly which specific competencies that students on the particular practice placement are expected to be assessed on. Otherwise, the assessment may not meet the curriculum's requirements. In the notes that you made in response to Activity 6.2, you may have mentioned that the NMC or the associated university has already laid down the components that we need to assess in the form of competencies, but more detailed information can usually be found in a range of documents such as the practice assessment document, the assessor's handbook and the course curriculum.

All assessments of the pre-registration curriculum are mandatory, and those in the first year of the programme are set at academic level 4 (higher education certificate level); those for the second year are set at level 5 (higher education diplomas and foundation degrees); those for the third year are set at level 6 (Bachelor's degrees with or without Honours); and those set at level 7 are for Master's degrees, Postgraduate diplomas and Postgraduate certificates (QAA, 2014a: 17). Various other ways of differentiating between academic levels have also already been developed (for example, Steinaker and Bell, 1979; Krathwohl, 2002).

The competencies PAD that students bring with them to the practice placement contains other useful information such as the process of assessment, the roles and responsibilities of the practice supervisor and the practice assessor, those of the student, and the university support available to them. Furthermore, at a number of university–trust partnerships, an electronic version of the PAD and assessment record is now being utilised, referred to as the Online Practice Assessment Record and Evaluation (PARE) (Council of Deans of Health, 2017b). PARE can be accessed by practice supervisors, practice assessors, students, lecturers and other appropriate personnel such as PEFs.

In addition to constituting a record of practice assessment for each student in their electronic PAD, advantages of PARE include the ease of access to these records from anywhere via computers, which saves time, markedly reduces paperwork, is potentially more accurate and reduces the risk of cross-infection through paper-based PAD being handled several times and across practice placement areas. It also facilitates student evaluation of placements and the resulting appropriate actions taken.

The competencies are usually available in a 'learning resources' folder for students in your practice setting but it might prove useful to obtain a photocopy of this for yourself for revisiting if required.

ACTIVITY 6.3 PRE-REGISTRATION
STUDENT ASSESSMENT

Find out from your partner university all the assessments that the pre-registration student needs to pass for the field-specific part of the programme while on placement in your practice setting. You could access this information via the link lecturer, for instance, for your practice setting, or the PEF.

In addition to the placement competencies or practice objectives set by the university, students are encouraged to achieve as many other competencies as the placement can offer and thereby maximise learning. A number of clinical areas have their own clearly identified competencies or learning objectives that can be achieved during placement. A number of them are optional for pre-registration students but compulsory for newly appointed qualified healthcare professionals on induction or preceptee programmes.

ACTIVITY 6.4 PRACTICE PLACEMENT
COMPETENCIES

Obtain a copy of the staff induction pack for your practice area, one that contains all the clinical skills or practice competencies that RNs or RMs in your practice setting need to be able to perform to fulfil their duties effectively after the induction or precepteeship period, and consider:

- Are these practice competencies separate from ward or team aims and objectives? If so, why?
- How far do the ward or team aims and objectives give a clear indication of all competencies that students can learn during the placement?

In addition to the regulatory bodies' standards of proficiency, professional bodies (or colleges/societies) such as the Chartered Society of Physiotherapy (CSP) publish further specific standards, such as those in the publications *Physiotherapy Framework: Putting Physiotherapy Behaviours, Values, Knowledge & Skills into Practice* (CSP, 2011 – updated Sept 2013), and *Learning and Development Principles* (CSP, 2017). The *Physiotherapy Framework* comprises four elements with substantial details that constitute professional practice, which are:

Professional values

Physiotherapy knowledge

Physiotherapy practice skills

Generic behaviours, knowledge and skills.

The *Learning and Development Principles* publication (CSP, 2017) indicates a further 17 elements that contemporary pre-registration physiotherapy programmes should incorporate, such as: physiotherapy's role in public health; quality and quality measurement/evidence of benefit; self-management of long term conditions; etc.

Furthermore, the practice assessor may also be required to assess non-regulated care workers, such as healthcare support workers (HSW). In terms of what to assess, the information will be provided by educators responsible for the HSW's learning programme, which leads to a 'Care Certificate' being awarded. National standards for Care Certificate programmes are identified by the Skills for Health (2017). As for the nursing associate role, the required standards are still underdeveloped and currently being piloted under the guidance of Health Education England's (2017a) curriculum framework.

WHY DO WE NEED TO ASSESS OUR STUDENTS?

We have already referred to some of the aims of assessments. Most individuals have mixed feelings about being assessed as, on the one hand, it creates anxiety but, on the other hand, on passing the assessment, the learner can be given permission to practise the particular clinical skill with less supervision. To begin our discussion on why we need to assess, consider what the range of purposes of assessments is, in addition to the NMC's (2018a) requirement for practice assessors to assess learners.

ACTIVITY 6.5   PURPOSES OF ASSESSMENTS

Think of all the methods of assessment that you noted during Activity 6.1, and of the reasons for assessing students and other learners. Make notes of these reasons for assessment. What did each assessment test?

According to the NMC (2018a: 9) the nominated practice assessor in partnership with the nominated academic assessor must indicate whether the student has achieved the NMC (2018b) standards for pre-registration nurse education and therefore whether they are safe and effective in practice, and thus the practice competencies are designed to test the student's ability to perform service user care interventions safely. Structured essays test the student's knowledge and understanding of concepts in nursing, but practice assessors are not involved in marking essays as this is the remit of the HEI (including the academic assessor). In addition to these, assessments also ascertain learning in the affective domain (Bloom, 1956; discussed in Chapter 3), that is, values and attitudes. Several purposes of assessments are identified by different researchers. In summary, we assess learners in order:

- To establish and then authorise learners as developing health professionals to practise specific clinical intervention with some autonomy.

- To inform the learner of their level of achievement at that point in time.
- To determine the student's progress with the learning programme.
- To ascertain the learner's overall competence and fitness for practice.
- To motivate the learner towards new components of learning.
- To judge the level of professional learning in the psychomotor (dexterity with clinical skills), affective (attitude) and cognitive (knowledge and thinking) components.
- For the student to identify further learning needs based on self-assessment and practice supervisor and practice assessor feedback.

As assessments also constitute an opportunity for identifying learning needs, this suggests that learning is an integral component of the assessment process, and not simply a means of measuring attainment. Students are encouraged to undertake self-assessment and to reflect on their learning. It could be argued that all assessments are learning situations, in that if the learner makes any error, then they are likely to be aware of it, or the assessor will point it out to them and identify learning needs. This notion also suggests that even if the student performs the skill competently, there is still scope for progressing from 'competent' to 'proficient' levels, for instance on Benner's (2001) skill acquisition continuum.

From the teacher's perspective, assessment also provides a measure of teaching effectiveness. It provides some feedback on the practice supervisor's and their colleagues' effectiveness at teaching particular competencies during practice placements. Naturally, the student will normally have had some teaching related to those competencies at the university beforehand. Assessments of theory also provide nurse lecturers with a fair measure of their university-based teaching.

In addition to the aims of assessments already mentioned, another function of assessments is to fulfil one of society's needs directly, in that they identify which healthcare professionals have acquired the necessary repertoire of knowledge and competencies for safe and competent practice, as a primary practitioner initially, and probably as a specialist later.

WHO ASSESSES LEARNERS?

As to who assesses learners, obviously it is qualified healthcare professionals who have completed a practice assessor or equivalent course who are given 'a licence' to

REFLECTION POINT 6.1:   WHO ASSESSES?

Think about assessments that you and your colleagues have been involved in recently. Spend a few minutes thinking about who conducted the assessments, on what, on whom and how. Is it only the practice assessor who assesses the learner's competencies, or are other individuals also afforded this responsibility?

assess learners' competencies. However, it is pertinent to consider the broader question of who else are the relevant personnel who assess competencies.

Perhaps an immediate response to this Reflection Point is that it is the practice assessor who assesses students in the practice setting. In fact, you might have concluded that all qualified healthcare professionals, including doctors, are involved in assessments, albeit often informally or indirectly. So, the answer to the question 'Who assesses?' could be everyone in the practice setting, and includes students' self-assessment, peer assessment and assessment by care service users. However, as in the role of practice supervisors, the majority of these personnel 'contribute' to the assessment process, with final decisions being the remit of practice assessors and academic assessors. These are now discussed.

STUDENT SELF-ASSESSMENT AND PEER ASSESSMENT

Self-assessment is one of the most valuable forms of assessment for students. It is almost always formative and therefore a learning exercise. As implied, the student uses a set of criteria or a checklist, written or mental, to self-assess their knowledge of a sub-topic area or of a specific competency. It also enables them to own the learning and to control the way they meet their needs. Self-assessment may be performed informally or more formally by the use of profiling documents or reflective diaries.

Much informal or subconscious self-assessment carried out by learners is based on their own individual aspirations, values and beliefs. These could be influenced by their views on patient care based on their own personal and professional experiences.

ACTIVITY 6.6   SELF-ASSESSMENT

Take a critical look at the idea of self-assessment by students, and of the strengths and weaknesses of self-assessments, and identify as many of these as you can think of.

WHAT IS SELF-ASSESSMENT?

According to Boud (2016), self-assessment is characterised by involvement of students in identifying standards and/or criteria to apply to their work and making judgements about the extent to which they have met them. On examining the concept with groups of post-registration students, a number of areas of strengths as well as weaknesses were identified (Gopee, 2000). Strengths of self-assessment are seen as including:

- inspires a conscious effort to be honest with self
- opportunity to identify limitations of own knowledge, and of learning needs

- identifies where more practice/knowledge gain is required
- is less traumatic than traditional methods of assessment such as examinations.

Furthermore, Siles-González and Solano-Ruiz (2016) argue that self-assessment can promote reflection-on-action and critical thinking. As for the weaknesses of self-assessment, it was felt that some students can be too self-critical while others can be too lenient in their judgement of their own performance. Some, however, may not be capable of gauging the effectiveness of their own performance sufficiently accurately, and thus self-assessment could worsen a student's poor self-image. Based on the diversity of individual student's values, motivations, interests and aspirations it seems advisable to implement self-assessment gradually and cautiously in education programmes.

PEER ASSESSMENT

The value and impact of peers' and colleagues' impressions of our competence in various aspects of our roles cannot be underestimated. This is often informal, with colleagues, friends and even family members having different perceptions of our capability, based perhaps on their different professional experiences. Peers can assess how well a student conducts a seminar, a short teaching session, or certain non-invasive clinical intervention in simulated situations.

Because of its value to the student, increasingly peer assessment is being built into formal assessment processes. In distance and e-learning modes of education delivery, facilitators often encourage students to form their own 'learning sets' for the purposes of learning together, for discussions and questioning each other. In this case, peer assessment is not formal in that other students or colleagues do not usually award a summative 'pass' or 'fail' to the peer assessed. They do, however, provide valuable opinions, thoughts and feedback on the individual's knowledge, which can be formally incorporated into a profile or a record of reflective learning. In this way, peer assessment usually presents an opportunity to verbalise uncertainties and reservations about one's learning without having to deal with the anxiety of examinations and pass or fail situations.

Assessment by peers, formal or informal, is increasingly becoming accepted as an educationally sound activity (e.g. Ohaja et al., 2013; Ashenafi, 2017). Many of us may find assessing our peers uncomfortable. We either do not wish to appear to be over-critical, and therefore tend not to assess or voice our views fully, or we feel that as we have such good rapport with our peers, we could damage their self-confidence with our 'criticisms'. It is also important to recognise that being assessed by our peer group can be more daunting than being assessed by a qualified assessor. If it is done badly, peer assessment can quickly destroy students' confidence or make them feel unable to face their peers again, and therefore it is an activity that needs to be supervised or facilitated.

Peer assessment, therefore, just like any other form of assessment, can benefit from the expertise of a facilitator if it is to be effective and help the student.

Thus, peers who are doing the assessing, as well as the person being assessed, are helped by the facilitator to recognise the parameters of their roles. When one group of post-registration students were asked to list the advantages and disadvantages of peer assessment, they felt the advantages included (Gopee, 2001):

- it can confirm previously held belief in skills or lack of them
- it is a chance to share colleagues' perception of the performance
- it is an opportunity to identify one's weaknesses, which can later be worked on, to improve
- feedback from colleagues/students of equal status has impact
- it is usually formative, so will not result in a pass or a fail for the course.

However, as with self-assessment, there can well be problematic areas related to peer assessment in that some students can find it hard to take any criticism from equals; someone could be over-critical and destructive; the individual might not accept peers' views; it could destroy self-confidence and lead to deserting the course altogether; and there could be complete disagreement between peers.

Another related term is *peer review*, which involves seeking the views and impressions of peers in a structured or semi-structured way. When clinicians design a new protocol or audit tool or patient assessment tool, for instance, they might ask an uninvolved colleague who works some distance away but in the same clinical specialism to comment on it prior to finalisation for use. Lecturers usually engage in peer review by asking a colleague to observe their teaching on specified occasions and provide feedback against standardised criteria, which makes the exercise a review rather than an assessment. Similarly, in relation to students' peer reviewing each other's work, Duers (2017) discusses a set of student-designed peer review criteria which Duers claims to be more credible and effective.

SERVICE USER INVOLVEMENT IN ASSESSMENT OF STUDENTS' COMPETENCIES

One of the judges of how competently a healthcare profession learner performs a clinical skill could be the healthcare service user. User involvement in learner assessment and provision of feedback on how competently the learner functioned in particular care interventions is increasingly advocated (e.g. NMC, 2018c: 12; Mott Macdonald and NMC, 2017: 33, 36). In recommending user involvement in assessments, HEIs are advised to explore ways in which lay people (including service users and carers) can be involved in the assessment of practice and supply evidence of this involvement, and that of clinical practitioners in Programme Boards/Boards of Study that establish the requirements for practice learning and assessment (Mott MacDonald and NMC, 2017).

So, what are the specific ways in which practice supervisors and practice assessors can do this? Usually, the practice supervisor or practice assessor gauges how content the care service user is with the care that they receive, by observation and even by casually asking them. The service user can provide feedback to the practice supervisor or practice assessor about the learner's communication skills, or injection-giving skills, for example, which are competencies under the NMC (2010a) domains *Communication and interpersonal skills* and *Nursing practice decision-making* respectively; and also the *Communication and relationship management skills* and relevant 'platforms' identified by the NMC (2018b).

User involvement in assessment of competencies related to professional values and attitude can be achieved by the practice supervisor or practice assessor asking the patient or service user if they felt that their consent had been obtained by the student prior to the clinical intervention, if they felt that they were treated with dignity and whether confidentiality was maintained in the presence of others. These actions are also consistent with the current definitions of person-centred care.

Service user feedback or testimony is recorded in the student's PAD by the practice supervisor, and to make the feedback even more useful, the student is advised to write a short reflection on this, which include stating why they think what they did were the correct actions with reference to any relevant publication, and the learning actions that they are going to engage in subsequently.

Evidence of effective service user involvement in students' learning and assessment is readily available (for example, Stickley et al., 2010; Haycock-Stuart et al., 2016), although it is acknowledged that it is a time-intensive activity that also requires additional infrastructure.

HOW ARE ASSESSMENTS CONDUCTED?

Broadly, pre-registration healthcare students' knowledge base (cognitive learning) is assessed at the university, and professional skills and attitude are assessed in the practice setting during practice placements. Learners deemed competent in performing a particular clinical skill can move on to learn other skills identified in their practice competencies booklet for the placement. In this major section on how to assess, further principles of assessment are addressed, and comprise:

- ensuring the learner has learned the clinical skill
- the assessor's essential interpersonal skills
- dimensions of assessment
- assessing different levels of competence
- fairness of assessment
- assessment criteria and pass or fail decisions
- accurate ongoing recording of process and outcomes of assessment.

Additionally, the process of assessment of competencies has to be managed, decisions made and feedback given to the learner. These latter points, along with how the practice assessor averts and resolves problems of assessment, are examined in Chapter 7.

ENSURING THAT THE LEARNER HAS LEARNED THE CLINICAL SKILL

An important prerequisite of assessment of a learner is to ensure that they have been taught the clinical skill systematically and given the necessary practice opportunities over time and under supervision prior to the point of assessment. Which care intervention skills, competence and competencies students are required to learn was discussed in Chapter 2, and how learners acquire the required competencies, including stages and levels of skill acquisition (for example, Fitts and Posner, 1973; Steinaker and Bell, 1979; Benner, 2001), in Chapter 3. But crucially and logically, before the student is asked to demonstrate that they are competent in any care intervention, they naturally need to learn to perform the skill according to approved procedures, and under the guidance of a registrant. The learning also has to be in the context of eventualities in the practice setting (i.e. situated learning).

THE ASSESSOR'S ESSENTIAL INTERPERSONAL SKILLS

Assessment is a role that has to be executed responsibly by the practice assessor, and, to do so effectively, certain specific personal and interpersonal skills are essential to enable the student to feel at ease when they are being assessed performing clinical interventions. These skills are subsets of the concept 'Establishing effective working relationships' that was discussed in Chapter 1 of this book.

ACTIVITY 6.7   INTERPERSONAL SKILLS
IN ASSESSING A STUDENT

Make a list of what you consider to be the general communication skills required in all assessment situations, and then a list of the more specific communication skills required by the practice assessor for conducting assessments effectively.

Several communication skill items emerge when exploring in detail what and how practice assessors communicate with the learner. The box lists many of the essential interpersonal skills required during assessments that were identified by just one group of registrants on a previous mentor course.

COMMUNICATION AND INTERPERSONAL FACTORS RELATED TO ASSESSMENTS

Generic communication skills	Specific interpersonal skills
• Non-verbal communication – e.g. eye contact, facial expression • Body language – posture, body orientation, proximity, attitude, behaviour, space • Being non-judgemental – warmth, empathy, respect • Always remaining calm • Openness • Questioning – open or closed questions • Reflecting • Active listening • Verbal communication – pace, volume, tone, clarity • Diplomacy • Considering environmental factors • Being enthusiastic, interested • Making time, using silence • Constructive criticism/advice • Approachable and friendly, non-intimidatory	• Putting the learner at ease • Enabling learner to relax if anxious so that they can perform the skill to their potential • Building confidence by positive feedback if necessary • Giving clear directions • Continuous feedback • Being non-judgemental by not criticising verbally or non-verbally • Giving prompts/clues if student's mind goes blank • Allowing enough time for the learner to perform the care intervention fully, including appropriate documentation • Making time to listen, and to maintain rapport • Preventing observer bias and observer effect • Ascertaining level of understanding of terminologies/jargon • Confidence – in the student/in self • Reinforcing what has been discussed

DIMENSIONS OF ASSESSMENT

There are a number of other essential facets of assessments that we need to consider to gain a more comprehensive picture of how to assess. Hughes and Quinn (2013: 245) and others identify what are generally known as 'dimensions of assessments'. Particularly relevant is whether assessments are:

1. continuous or episodic
2. formative or summative
3. criterion-referenced or norm-referenced.

CONTINUOUS OR EPISODIC ASSESSMENTS

Until the latter half of the 1980s, the assessment of pre-registration students used to take place at predetermined points during their course. The student on the general nursing course was assessed on their ability to administer medications in Year 1 of the course, and to use aseptic techniques and organise the total care of an individual or a group of healthcare service users on specific subsequent occasions. They also had to pass written examinations at the end of the course. These were episodic assessments, with those identified at the end of progression points referred to as summative assessments. For current healthcare apprentices and trainee nursing associates assessment of competencies are undertaken by continuous assessment and 'end point' assessments (Institute for Apprenticeships, 2017: 1; HEE, 2017a: 25) (sometimes referred to as 'terminal assessments').

Obviously, students had to learn numerous other care intervention skills necessary to function as a healthcare professional, which were identified in a competencies booklet and signed as appropriate. However, these snapshot assessments were not seen as representing the wide range of skills acquired during placements, nor were they seen as a genuine representation of how students usually delivered care, and they therefore fell into disfavour. They were replaced by continuous assessment and subsequently by modularisation of preparatory programmes, involving assessment of practice and theory on numerous occasions throughout the course.

Episodic (or intermittent) assessments therefore involve testing the student at specific times or occasions during an educational programme, such as at the end of a module, a placement or year. Continuous assessment aims to increase the quality and quantity of evidence gathered in relation to achievement of competencies by each individual student. It involves a continuing awareness by the practice supervisor of the student's level of knowledge and competence, and is thus a cumulative judgement about progress and achievement.

ACTIVITY 6.8   ADVANTAGES AND DISADVANTAGES OF CONTINUOUS AND EPISODIC ASSESSMENTS

Consider what you think might be the advantages and disadvantages of episodic and continuous assessments, and make some notes.

The principal reason for episodic assessments being discredited in nursing and midwifery in the past is that decisions about the student's competence were being made on the basis of one-off performances. These performances, be they excellent or otherwise, might be atypical. Another disadvantage is that some key skills can remain untested if they do not present themselves during the identified assessment episode.

Subsequently, following extensive previous consultation, the NMC (2010a; 2009) has identified 'progression points' in the pre-registration nursing and midwifery education curriculum when students are assessed and have to achieve a 'Pass' on several key competencies before progressing to the subsequent stage of their education programme. These assessments can also be examples of episodic assessment, and students are required to demonstrate that they are competent in those competencies to be able to register subsequently with the NMC as an RN or RM, or with the HCPC.

FORMATIVE OR SUMMATIVE ASSESSMENTS

Another dimension of assessment is whether the assessment is formative or summative. In common with the context of evaluation (which we discuss in Chapter 9), 'formative' relates to the developmental and improvement stages of something (for example, a clinical skill). The primary aim of the formative assessment of a professional practice skill is to promote learning so that the learner can perform the skill safely and effectively, and knows the rationales for each step of the intervention. The student's capability is thus developed under conditions in which they can reflect-in-action and think creatively without being too concerned about final pass or fail grades. The student also has the opportunity to take time to learn the skill thoroughly with the support of practice supervisors.

Formative assessment applies to assessment of theory as well as to practical skills. For the theory component of education programmes, the student thereby obtains feedback on the evidence they are presenting to the marker or lecturer on how far they are demonstrating knowledge of the subject area, critical analysis, general presentation of the paper, etc. Formative assessments are therefore instituted to provide feedback to the student on their progress, and their aims are to:

- maximise learning
- identify strengths/weaknesses
- inform the student of how they are progressing
- allow for individual development.

As a concept and an activity, formative assessment has been advocated for decades, but implementation proves erratic even today, which could be due to it being yet another extra requirement to create time for in busy day-to-day professional activities in both the practice setting and HEIs. Thus, it has resource and efficiency implications. It is, however, an educationally sound concept and students tend to be grateful for the feedback that they receive from it.

Pla-Campas et al. (2016) report various benefits of formative assessment in social work education. Bijol et al. (2015) provided students with free access to formative web-based quizzes as a form of self-assessment and found that those who did participate in the quizzes performed much better (statistically significantly better) at final examinations than those who didn't engage with the quizzes. The researchers argue that the quizzes promoted learning and improved the student experience.

'Summative' relates to a point in time during a unit of learning, for example a practice placement, when the practice assessor makes a decision about whether to declare the learner competent or otherwise on a specific component of learning.

Summative assessments are conducted to determine whether the learner is now competent to work without direct supervision and, if so, then this is recorded in their competencies' document.

Summative assessments also constitute a periodic record of the student's achievement of the aims and outcomes of a course or module. The grade awarded for these assessments, along with those for coursework and examinations, contributes to the final classification of the student's university award.

It might prove useful to ask your student, or to look back on any long course you have done in recent years, to identify the range of formative and summative assignments incorporated in the programme. As to assessment in the practice setting, the student learning part-skills (for example, some of the skills required for administering an intramuscular injection) itself constitutes a formative assessment. The 'professional discussion' at the end of apprenticeship programmes, and dissertations for university degrees are summative assessments.

In healthcare courses, summative assessments are concerned with healthcare service user safety and standards of practice. They are also concerned with justice for the student and credibility of the university's awards. They must therefore meet the highest standards of reliability and validity, which are discussed in some detail later in this chapter.

CRITERION-REFERENCED OR NORM-REFERENCED ASSESSMENTS

The third dimension of assessment we consider is norm referencing and criterion referencing. In norm-referenced assessment, the student's score, marks or grades are determined to an extent by those of other students in a given group or cohort. Programme Assessment Boards (also known as Award Boards) have the discretion to adjust the marks required by a particular cohort to achieve a particular grade if unusual circumstances have prevailed. Criterion-referenced assessments are more straightforward in that the score or mark given to a particular student for a particular piece of coursework is decided entirely on the basis of a predetermined set of marking criteria. Students will have been informed of these criteria long before the assessment date.

> ### REFLECTION POINT 6.2:   NORM- OR CRITERION-REFERENCED ASSESSMENTS
>
> Think about some of the assessments that you have mentioned for Activity 6.1 and decide whether they are norm-referenced assessments or criterion-referenced.

Occasionally, a criterion-referenced assessment can be marked on a norm-referenced basis at the discretion of the appropriate Programme Assessment Board.

The approved detailed procedure or clinical guidelines used in healthcare trusts to perform clinical care safely and effectively also constitute the pass/fail criteria for student assessment for the specific intervention.

ASSESSING DIFFERENT LEVELS OF COMPETENCE

Student nurses tend to be taught and assessed at different academic levels during Year 1, Year 2 and Year 3. The NMC's (2018b) SOP for example are configured at different academic levels in the competencies booklets that students take to practice placements. Healthcare assistants studying for national vocational qualifications are also assessed differently at different levels.

To teach and assess competencies at different levels of learning, a number of current nurse education curricula tend to use Steinaker and Bell's (1979) model (or taxonomy) of experiential learning. This taxonomy consists of exposure level, participation, identification, internalisation and dissemination. A broad guide to how the experiential taxonomy levels can equate with the QAA's (2014a) academic levels is:

- Certificate level/academic level 4 – exposure, participation
- Diploma level/academic level 5 – participation, identification and internalisation
- Degree level/academic level 6 – identification, internalisation and dissemination.

This is a very simple classification and just a general guide that underpins specific wording of competencies to reflect the different levels. Alternatively, some programmes use Benner's (2001) stages of skill acquisition model, which was discussed in Chapter 2. Others use Bondy's (1983) five levels of competency, namely dependent, marginal, assisted, supervised and independent, usually in post-registration courses.

The assessment of theory at different levels in healthcare professions, however, is usually based on Bloom's (1956) taxonomy of cognitive learning, which was discussed in Chapter 3. You may wish to look back to the appropriate section to remind yourself of the details of this model, which comprises knowledge, comprehension, application, analysis, synthesis and evaluation. In both models of assessment, the first points, that is, exposure and knowledge, represent lower-level learning and the last points represent the higher levels.

FAIRNESS OF ASSESSMENTS

In practice assessments, we are measuring the performance of the individual student on particular competencies. Wouldn't you agree, however, that assessments have to be as objective as possible and must be fair and unbiased for every student? The NMC (2018c: 12) states that assessments must be 'fair, reliable and valid'. So, what does fairness of assessments mean?

_____   **ACTIVITY 6.9   BARRIERS TO 'FAIRNESS'**   _____

Think about your own experiences of assessment (either assessing or being assessed) and consider instances when students' practice assessments might, or could, have been 'unfair', and how we can ensure that they are 'fair'. Identify all factors that you feel interfere with the fairness of the assessment, using the three headings: (a) student factors; (b) assessor factors (practice supervisor or practice assessor); and (c) environmental (the practice setting) factors. If you can't remember being assessed, then make some notes of your own ideas of aspects that we should be aware of during an assessment to ensure that it is being conducted fairly.

It is conceivable that, on occasion, the demand being made on a student during assessment or the questions being asked may seem beyond the boundaries of what would generally be expected. Fairness of assessment refers to being aware of external circumstances that could influence the student's performance of the clinical skill. There are several factors that could hamper fairness of assessments. An unfair assessment could also mean that it might not be a valid assessment. Student factors that can make an assessment unfair include:

- expected level of knowledge is too high
- theory–practice disjunction/gap
- not enough opportunities to practise the competencies
- last-minute delays or changes
- undeclared physical illness or fatigue.

You should be able to think of other student factors, including personal circumstances. Assessor factors include practice supervisors not working with the student on a sufficient number of shifts, bias towards or against the student, not having had valid educational preparation to become a practice assessor, overpowering attitude and lack of knowledge of the student's course. Some of the factors in the clinical environment that might unfairly affect assessments are interruptions, lack of resources in the practice setting (for example, equipment), suitability of placement and low staffing levels.

ASSESSMENT CRITERIA AND PASS OR FAIL DECISIONS

Following a fairly conducted assessment, the practice assessor has to decide whether it's a pass or a fail for the particular competency. This decision may well depend entirely on whether the student closely followed the trust's approved procedure to perform the clinical skill, or the written (or unwritten) protocol. The items in the procedure are the actual 'assessment criteria'.

The term *assessment criteria* refers to the predetermined set of components that are used for deciding whether the learner performed the clinical skill competently.

They can therefore constitute a checklist of the step-by-step actions taken by the learner when performing the care intervention. These step-by-step actions are normally the trust's approved procedure or clinical guidelines for that intervention and are set down in two columns as 'actions' and 'rationales', and are usually supported by references to make them evidence-based. They are normally kept in the practice setting's 'Policies and Procedures' section for use and for reference purposes. There is likely to be a separate folder for clinical guidelines or protocols that refer to expanded role competencies.

The significance of having specified assessment criteria is also recognised by Helminen et al. (2017), who indicate that it ensures a good quality process in practice assessments. However, for those nursing activities for which there is no identified step-by-step approved procedure, the performance criteria can be established by asking the skilled practitioner to describe to someone in detail everything that they would do to perform the intervention competently. For instance, there might not be a procedure for assessing communication skills, for bed-making, for taking body temperature using tympanic thermometers or, say, for doing patient handovers. A set of performance criteria for patient handovers (or 'reporting on patients' progress') is presented in the box.

ASSESSMENT CRITERIA FOR ASSESSING COMPETENCY – PATIENT HANDOVERS

- Have the right documentation, e.g. care plan/pathway, to refer to
- Have a good understanding of the patient's/service user's health conditions
- State the interventions that have been performed, e.g. removal of drains, sutures
- Keep the information concise and focused
- Use appropriate English and technical words

(Continued)

(Continued)

- Pitch the amount of information imparted to the level of knowledge the handover recipients already have, e.g. more detailed information may need to be imparted if new staff or if students are present
- Ensure that information that must be given, is given
- Inform about individual service user's overall progress
- Note any relevant communication from the service user's family or from members of the multidisciplinary team
- State any investigation results received, and any subsequent action required
- State any changes in medication, and service user's reaction to them
- State the plan of care for the rest of the day
- Include service user's awareness of own condition, e.g. in mental health
- Observe confidentiality issues, especially for bedside handovers

The criteria for handover listed in the box are generic and are likely to vary to some extent depending on when and where the handover is being given. It is however not merely a daily ritual, because it is a necessary medium for communicating the effects of care and treatment to staff on the next shift, but also very much a teaching and learning opportunity, encompasses patient safety, and has several other benefits. A more detailed analysis of handover itself can be found in Ballantyne (2017) for example, and various other publications. Another way of conducting structured and effective handovers is by the use of the four components of the SBAR (situation, background, action / assessment, recommendation) tool. As a means of effective communication, SBAR has been advocated for some years now, and Kirkham (2018) and Stewart and Hand (2017) suggest that the SBAR can make inter-professional communication more concise, complete and consequently enhance patient safety.

For competencies for which there are no written assessment criteria in the practice setting in the procedures or clinical guidelines folder, they might be found in, for instance, *The Royal Marsden Hospital Manual of Clinical Nursing Procedures* (Dougherty et al., 2015). The criteria or procedures might also be available from NICE, the World Health Organisation, Scottish Intercollegiate Guidelines Network and other reputable authoritative organisations via their websites, especially clinical guidelines, or from manufacturers' instructions. However, from the time that a book or clinical guideline is written to the time it is available for use, adjustments may have been made to the procedure, based on more up-to-date evidence or research. Trust-based procedures tend to have an addendum to reflect this.

As to keeping the information concise, handover reports are naturally time limited as they could be seen as keeping healthcare staff away from caring for patients or service users. On noticing ineffective patient handover practices, Davies and Priestley (2006) suggest that conversation on irrelevant topics should be excluded from this activity.

Depending on the clinical specialism, further specific information may need to be imparted during handovers, for example resuscitation status or mobility levels in rehabilitation services. Very importantly, often teaching and learning points arise from patient handovers, for both students and clinically based unqualified staff and registrants. Thus, the assessment criteria for passing or failing a student on their ability to do patient handovers can be quite involved.

STUDENTS' RECORD OF ACHIEVEMENT

From one of its periodic reviews of pre-registration education curricula, the NMC (2007b) concluded that supervisors of practice-based learning and assessors of practice competencies would benefit from having access to their students' progress documentation of preceding practice placements as evidence of skills that they are already deemed competent in, prior to establishing the student's learning requirements and needs in their current placement. The NMC subsequently issued guidelines for universities to implement a systematic way of establishing a mechanism to achieve this.

This mechanism was initially termed a 'passport' but due to different interpretations of this term, it was changed to 'ongoing achievement record' (OAR) (it retained at least one element of passports which is to have the student's photograph included in the document). With the information in OAR and the placement's competencies document that the student brings with them, a 'diagnostic assessment' of competencies is made at the initial meeting with the student at the beginning of the placement so as to establish the student's specific learning needs and objectives. The OAR has been a requirement for all students who commenced on pre-registration nurse education programmes since September 2008, but see reference to the Online Practice Assessment Record and Evaluation (PARE) earlier in this chapter.

The NMC (2007b: 2) notes that the OAR is necessary for documenting continuity of assessment, to ensure safe and effective practice and 'enable judgement to be made on the student's progress'. Finally, the pre-registration student is assessed by the practice assessor and academic assessor whose roles essentially are to ascertain and vouch that the student has achieved all practice competencies and the NMC's (2018b) SOP, which they do by a combination of means, and sign and date the appropriate pages of relevant documents, or not.

The combination of means includes a review of requirements in the OAR document; the student's practice competencies documents from all preceding placements; any other relevant skill achievement document; certificate of attendance from additional study days/workshops, etc. The practice competencies document tends to have a section where the supported learning time is recorded – see Template 6.1 for an example of this.

Accurate recording of supported learning time with the student has several advantages. When evidence of this NMC requirement is asked for, then the record will be proof of this provision. Recording supported learning time is also likely to act as a trigger to ensure that this contact time happens which can also mean increased support for the student to achieve the necessary competencies. The contact must however be recorded straightaway, and not retrospectively.

Template 6.1 Recording supported learning time for supervision and practice placement

Week 1	Notes on learning during this week:	
	Signature of student:	Date:
	Signature of practice supervisor:	Date:
Week 2	Notes on learning during this week:	
	Signature of student:	Date:
	Signature of practice supervisor:	Date:
Week 3	etc. …	

The reasons for assessment of competence and ensuring proficiency during the final practice placement include ensuring safe and effective practice, and must achieve validity and reliability of assessments and fairness of assessments. Final documentation needs to be carried out by a practice assessor and the academic assessor who are on the same part or sub-part of the NMC's professional register as that which the student is aiming to enter. When all evidence has become available to indicate that the student has successfully completed all theory and practice requirements, then the HEI informs the NMC accordingly, leading to the student applying to have their name entered on the NMC register as an RN.

Protected learning time for supervisor and student to work together, however, has often proved difficult to achieve in a number of very busy practice settings, or during particularly busy periods, as was also found in research conducted by Rooke (2014) and by Hutchison and Cochrane (2014). Furthermore, in midwifery practice, on reviewing prevailing modes of practice assessment, Passmore and Chenery-Morris (2014: 92) conclude that there is no need for tripartite assessments (lecturer, mentor and student midwife) of students anymore, because sign-off mentors (now practice assessors) are now 'much better prepared to undertake this role'.

Moreover, if a student is awarded a fail on this final placement, then this can raise questions about the quality of practice supervision and assessment of competence that the student has experienced over the preceding two-and-a-half years of their education programme. To resolve the 'challenges' of time, workload, responsibility related to the role and practicalities of the assessment of competence, Rooke's study participants suggested various possible solutions, including more concerted proactive forward planning of the work roster to ensure that students and their supervisors and assessors work together in collaboration.

ASSESSING SUPPORT WORKERS AND OTHER LEARNERS

Registrants periodically gets allocated students for practice placement who are on other health or social care profession programmes than the one they are themselves qualified in. This is of course fully acceptable especially in the current ethos of inter-professional learning, and endeavour towards a health and social care seamless service. This is also so that the underlying principles of supervising learning comprise core healthcare knowledge and skills that apply to all registerable professions. However, logically registrants might be required to undertake further information sessions or to attend relevant workshops, in particular to comprehend the technicalities of their role towards learners from other specific healthcare professions.

To supervise and assess support workers on NVQ courses, for example, they would need to have successfully completed and achieved the A1 Assessor Award (previously D32 and D33). If the nurse is facilitating practice learning for a medical student, then they have to acquaint themselves with the competencies that the medical student has to achieve by the end of the placement.

VALIDITY AND RELIABILITY OF ASSESSMENTS

The principles of assessment constitute further key considerations that are usually referred to as attributes or essential factors. There are four attributes that are absolutely crucial in all assessments of competencies. These are validity, reliability, discrimination and practicability (or usability) of assessments.

VALIDITY

'Validity' is the most crucial aspect of an assessment in that it refers to the extent to which the assessment measures what it is expected to measure. A valid assessment is one that assesses the competency or learning outcome(s) it sets out to assess and does not target other competencies that might not have been learnt adequately by the learner at that point in time. The five main types of validity are: content validity, predictive validity, concurrent validity, construct validity and face validity. However, some of these apply more to the overall curriculum and not necessarily to assessment of competencies in practice settings.

CONTENT VALIDITY

'Content validity' refers to the extent to which the assessment adequately covers the content of the whole curriculum. Do the assessment questions and assignment guidelines assess all the learning outcomes of the curriculum? Note that, for various reasons, not everything that the student learns during the course can be assessed. Content validity is primarily addressed by the structure of the assessment in the endeavour to assess all module or course outcomes and is monitored by the programme manager for the course.

PREDICTIVE VALIDITY

The extent to which the result of assessments can predict the future performance of the student is referred to as 'predictive validity'. It is important for the assessor to determine if the student's performance during, say, a particular practical assessment, can predict how far he or she will perform to the same standard in future situations, and also whether the student can adjust the performance to different practice settings, for example from a ward setting to community care and to service users of different age groups, etc.

CONCURRENT VALIDITY

The extent to which the assessment results correlate with those of other assessments administered at the same time is referred to as 'concurrent validity'. In other words, if two different assessments are designed to measure the same learning outcomes, then the student should do equally well in both, for example asking a student to talk through how they would perform a skill, and actually to demonstrate it.

CONSTRUCT VALIDITY

Validity that refers to the extent to which the results of the assessment are related to impressions or evidence gained from observations of the individual's behaviour with regard to their attitudes, values and intelligence (which are also known as 'psychological constructs') is referred to as 'construct validity'.

FACE VALIDITY

'Face validity' involves stopping to consider the overall impression of how competently the clinical skill was performed, and whether the student actually demonstrated the complex array of observational, analytical, interpersonal and technical skills required for the competency.

> ## REFLECTION POINT 6.4:   TYPES OF VALIDITY
>
> A first-year student is being assessed on a surgical ward changing a patient's dressing using aseptic technique. The purpose of this particular episode of assessment is specifically to do with changing a dressing using aseptic technique skills. However, during the procedure, the patient makes some statements that clearly reflect marked disorientation, and the student is unable to respond therapeutically to disorientation. The aseptic technique is performed correctly. Should the assessor pass or fail the student? Which decision is the valid decision?

RELIABILITY

In addition to validity, another key consideration of any assessment is its 'reliability', which is a term that is used to indicate the consistency with which an assessment measures what it is designed to measure. This means that if the assessment is conducted again, the same level of performance should produce the same result, provided other variables remain similar.

To take this a step further, reliability has to do with consistency in the grade or result awarded for a particular piece of work:

1. between different assessors
2. between different occasions on which the work is done, and
3. between different methods of assessment.

In all cases, the result or grades awarded should be almost, or preferably exactly, the same for the test to be deemed 'reliable'. Consistency in assessment of student competencies in this way is referred to inter-assessor reliability and is discussed in detail in Chapter 7.

> ## REFLECTION POINT 6.5:   RELIABILITY OF ASSESSMENTS
>
> Think about assessments you or your colleagues have been involved in recently. Then spend a few minutes thinking about how reliably the assessment was conducted. Decide why you think that the assessment was or was not reliable.

Generally, there are certain factors that might negatively affect reliability being achieved. These are practical issues, such as:

- individual biases
- halo effect

- insufficient time allocated for the assessment
- ambiguity of questions being asked
- competence as an assessor
- whether more than one assessor was involved, as two assessors could mean less subjectivity
- whether the assessment criteria had been agreed.

DISCRIMINATION

Discrimination in assessment refers to the ability of assessment to differentiate between different levels of competence demonstrated by students, such as Year 1, Year 2 or Year 3 students. Steinaker and Bell's (1979) taxonomy of learning is generally used to differentiate between these levels of competencies. However, by and large, learners should be given the opportunity to demonstrate their true level of ability, regardless of the level that they are expected to reach at the particular stage of the course.

Discrimination also refers to the distinction between all learners. A healthcare assistant would be assessed against different criteria for a particular care intervention from a medical student or from a student nurse, for instance, mainly because the level of theoretical knowledge expected of each is different.

PRACTICABILITY (OR USABILITY)

The concept 'practicability' refers to whether the assessment can be conducted within the time, and with the resources, available.

Practice assessors could encounter problems of practicability of assessment when practice placements are too short, or when for some reason the assessments have been left until the last few days of the placement. In the study of assessment of competence by Phillips et al. (2000) several problems of practicability of assessment were identified, the more crucial ones of which will be explored in Chapter 7. However, despite effective assessments being complex and challenging, the validity and reliability of assessments remain the benchmark of rigour in the assessment of health and social care competencies (for example, Lafave and Katz, 2014; Moniz et al., 2015).

A study conducted by Norman et al. (2002: 143) that examined the validity and reliability of different methods of assessment of competence of pre-registration nursing and midwifery students concluded that 'no single method is appropriate for assessing all clinical competence of nursing and midwifery students', and that a 'multi-method approach' should be taken. See https://study.sagepub.com/gopee4e for a scenario/case study in which Adam, who is a student on a practice assessor course, performs a supervised student assessment.

POLICIES AND STRATEGIES FOR ASSESSMENTS

Overall, each university identifies clearly in their course documents exactly which assessments students have to pass to complete the course successfully. The assessments to be conducted in practice settings are documented in the placement competencies document/PAD, and also in the approved curriculum document. The documentation is supported by further assessment guidelines and specifications in the module and course documents.

Specific requirements for assessing practice competencies are also detailed in students' PAD. These and other requirements for the course will have been planned before students start on the course, under the scrutiny of the university's quality assurance guidelines and protocols for designing courses and modules. They will have gone through a rigorous course approval process before being offered to students. They would then have been approved by an assembled panel of experts, which usually includes representations from the NMC, probably the HCPC, and subject specialists from other universities.

During the planning stages, the modules will have been fully discussed by the Course or Module Curriculum Planning Teams. There are specific assessment strategies within each course and module. The pass marks for assessments may vary by a few points between different universities, as may the weightings between practical and theoretical assessments, or different assessment components. The number of assessments may vary, as may the number of formative assessments related to the summative ones. Each course and module is assessed on its learning outcomes and/or competencies.

Overall monitoring of module or course assessments are conducted by designated university committees and Boards, which do so by following the university's protocols, such as the university's Assessment Parity Rules. Finally, each student's assessment results are scrutinised and ratified by the Subject Assessment/Examinations Board.

So, for assessment of practice, students' PAD clearly identifies the procedure for assessment of competencies. This entails an initial supervisor–student interview when the competencies to be achieved are ascertained, and often a learning contract constituted. Approximately halfway through the placement, a mid-placement interview takes place so as to ascertain the student's progress with the contracted competencies. During the last week of the placement, a final interview is conducted, and the nominated practice assessor makes a final decision on which clinical competencies have been achieved, and those that have are signed and dated accordingly.

A case study of a student for whom an action plan had to be constituted after the mid-placement interview follows on the next page.

If Kayleigh had not managed to achieve any of the objectives in the action plan, then she would have failed the practice module. However, students are usually allowed a second attempt at any fail component, which in this case could constitute

CASE STUDY 6.1:   A SUCCESSFUL ACTION PLAN

Kayleigh is a 33-year-old third-year mental health student nurse who is a new mother, and whose return from maternity leave was delayed due to medical reasons. On her return, she had two theory modules and the final practice module to pass in order to complete her pre-registration programme. For the practice module, Kayleigh was placed for 12 weeks at a 9–5 day services centre for working-age adults with mental health problems and who have been referred to secondary mental health services for further therapy and rehabilitation.

Although an initial interview with the practice supervisor and practice assessor took place in the first week, and the required supported learning time was utilised to monitor progress with practice competencies, Kayleigh struggled to re-engage after the break from the course, and in subsequent weeks found it difficult to achieve the agreed competencies and was unable to express why this was so to her practice supervisor. Both practice supervisor and the day services manager were very accommodating and supportive. The student failed various objectives at the mid-placement interview and an action plan was compiled in the presence of the student, practice assessor, link lecturer and day services nurse manager. The competencies that were identified in the action plan, which were related mainly to 'interpersonal skills', included:

- Be consistently on time for shifts and planned activities, and thereby demonstrate reliability, punctuality and good time management.
- Take responsibility for meeting professional codes of practice and organisational policies whilst prioritising care of service users, and work with team members to promote health with high standards of practice, whilst acting with integrity.
- Take responsibilities that are appropriate for Year 3 students by demonstrating the ability to take the lead in reviews, admissions and group work.

The student felt disappointed but had anticipated being given fails during the mid-placement interview and needing an action plan. The support that would enable Kayleigh to achieve the action plan objectives were identified as the practice supervisor and the manager, and resources included the NMC's guidelines and codes of practice, as well as the trust's policies and procedures. The PEF would regularly contact the practice supervisor to check on progress and offer any further help and advice required and made himself available during the subsequent weeks for further support.

The student composed herself and, with the above-mentioned support during subsequent weeks, put the required time and effort in, and went on to achieve the competencies in the action plan and the remainder of her practice competencies, and subsequently passed the practice placement.

extending the placement by four to six weeks or changing to another placement for a similar period of time.

To assess students' competence during practice placements, various assessment strategies are advocated, such as direct observation of skill performance, writing a reflective account and questions and answers. It is usually up to the practice assessor to decide which NMC competency area can be assessed by each strategy. For example, direct observation can be utilised for assessing care intervention, attitude, communication skill; and questions and answers for the rationale for each action taken, knowledge of the effects of medication, etc.

A variety or 'diversity' of assessment strategies is also recommended by the QAA (2013: 17) to enable students to demonstrate their capabilities and achievements of module or programme outcomes, as does the Skills for Health (2017: 5). For assessment of theory components, critical analyses of key concepts and seminar presentations, written examinations are utilised. It is, however, well known that some assessment methods, for example written examinations, enable some students to demonstrate their capabilities more effectively, whilst other methods suit other students better. Garside et al. (2009) explored the feasibility and outcome of allowing students a choice of assessment methods, and found that this is achievable, as some students chose to be assessed by seminar discussions, others by poster presentations, others by essays, etc., to good effect.

Consequently, curriculum planners should be able to justify which mode of assessment tests which module or programme outcome more effectively, and complementarily the NMC (2018c) under 'student empowerment' indicates that students are assessed utilising a range of different assessment methods. Research on the effective use of assessment by a combination of assessment methods is limited. However, in a study that explored the extent to which nurse assessors use different assessment strategies in Ireland, McCarthy and Murphy (2008) found that a limited range of these was in use, and recommend further education of assessors on their use.

All aforementioned proceedings are documented as evidence of progress with continuous assessment, for the final summative assessment of the practice module and for legal reasons. The practice competencies documents also identify the exact roles and responsibilities of the practice assessor and those of the student before, during and after the placement. They also contain a set of components related to the student's professionalism, attitude and their team-working, and which the student must demonstrate at a satisfactory level (related to construct validity). Usually there is also a section on actions to take regarding underachieving students, which is explored in Chapter 7.

CHAPTER SUMMARY

This chapter has focused on the assessment of learners' clinical knowledge and competencies, taking the approach of what assessments are, why we conduct them, who assesses, when and how, which encompassed:

- What the term 'assessment' means in the context of assessing professional knowledge and competence. This involved considering various definitions of assessments, and the exact competencies to be assessed.

- Why we need to assess our students and learners, that is, the exact purposes and aims of assessments, and at which particular points in students' programmes of study to assess.
- Who assesses learners, including student self-assessment and peer assessment, and service user involvement in the assessment of competencies.
- How assessments are conducted, which includes ensuring that the learner has learned the clinical skill, the use of essential interpersonal skills, the dimensions of assessments, namely continuous or episodic assessments, formative or summative and criterion-referenced or norm-referenced assessments.
- Assessing different levels of competence, fairness of assessments and the use of performance criteria.
- Validity, reliability, discrimination and practicability as essential aspects of assessments; and the role of approved assessment policies, procedures and strategies.

FURTHER OPTIONAL READING

1. For an analysis of the problematic aspects of assessment, the recurring danger of which usually looms, see:

   - Rowntree, D. (1987) *Assessing Students: How Shall We Know Them?* London: Kogan Page.

2. Access online and maybe print the *Standards of Proficiency* document published by your regulatory body (e.g. HCPC, NMC) that is constituted for your healthcare profession, either to gain an overview or for more detailed scrutiny of the standards and outcomes that pre-registration students have to achieve in order to be able to register in the relevant part of the Professional Register, e.g.:

   - Nursing and Midwifery Council (2018b) *Standards of Proficiency for Registered Nurses*. Available at: https://www.nmc.org.uk/standards/standards-for-nurses/standards-of-proficiency-for-registered-nurses/ (accessed 19 May 2018); or

   - Nursing and Midwifery Council (2010a) *Standards for Pre-Registration Nursing Education*. Available at: www.nmc.org.uk/globalassets/sitedocuments/standards/nmc-standards-for-pre-registration-nursing-education.pdf (accessed 30 January 2018).

To access further resources related to this chapter, visit **https://study.sagepub.com/gopee4e** where a range of learning and teaching materials are provided.

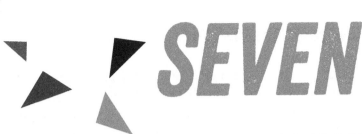

SEVEN

MANAGING STUDENT ASSESSMENT, ASSOCIATED CHALLENGES AND ACCOUNTABILITY

INTRODUCTION

Having discussed the nature and different facets of student assessment in Chapter 6, including validity and reliability of assessments, this chapter focuses on the significance of careful planning and management of student assessment, on ways of managing various problematic areas related to assessment of health and social care students, and the assessor's accountability.

CHAPTER OBJECTIVES

1. Explain specific ways in which forward planning and prioritising work are important components of management of student assessments.
2. Identify likely challenges or problems of assessment of student competencies, and ways in which the practice assessor averts or resolves them.
3. Present an analysis of the responsibilities and accountability of practice assessors in the assessment of practice competencies, along with related ethical and legal aspects of student assessment.
4. Cite various ways in which practice assessors achieve and monitor intra- and inter-assessor reliability in the decisions that they make in relation to the assessments they conduct.
5. Establish the practice supervisor's role in supporting the struggling or underachieving student, and the use of various lines of support that can be available to them, including resources and guidelines.

MANAGING STUDENT ASSESSMENT

Practice assessors have a professional duty to comply with the underlying principles of assessment identified in Chapter 6 of this book. Forward planning of assessments also reflects the practice assessor's leadership in terms of prioritising, supporting and giving feedback.

At the end of the placement, the practice assessor has to inform the student of their levels of achievement, and of a decision to award the student a pass or fail for those assessment components. It is in relation to assessment of competence that many of the challenges of practice placements arise.

Assessment of competencies at times involves one-off short episodes of direct observation of the learner performing clinical skills, but mostly it is a continual process occurring throughout the practice placement. One danger associated with this is that if interruptions do occur during episodes of assessment, then the practice assessor could miss vital steps in the performance of the care intervention, incorrect or unsafe practice can also be missed, and a pass decision (or fail) could be made, wrongly, with incomplete information.

MANAGING THE PROCESS OF ASSESSMENT IN THE PRACTICE SETTING

ACTIVITY 7.1   PLANNING AND MANAGING THE PROCESS OF ASSESSMENT OF PRACTICE

This activity asks you to explore in detail how to manage an episode of assessment of students' practice competencies or clinical skills by direct observation. To do this, focus on the specified outcomes or competencies of a specific practice module of the pre-registration course for your healthcare profession, or the NMC's (2018b or 2010a) competencies for, say, second-year students in your field of nursing, or the outcomes of a post-registration healthcare course. Practice competencies are normally found in the student's practice competencies or practice assessment document (PAD).

You might choose to work on this activity with a colleague or course peer who is in a similar specialism as you. Identify in detail everything that needs to be done from arranging to completing the assessment of these competencies by direct observation, from the time that the student starts on the practice placement to when the student is signed as competent for the particular competencies. Include everything, such as how you would ensure that the skills have been learnt, as well as the organisational aspects that have to be considered to ensure the assessment proceeds as planned.

From your response to Activity 7.1, you would have verbalised various preparations needed to ensure that assessment of competencies is completed effectively and efficiently. Maybe the practice supervisor can compile a teaching and assessment schedule that identifies which competencies will have been learnt by the student by the end of week two, three, etc., and at which points the practice assessor will have assessed the student on each of them. The learning and assessment schedule of course needs to be flexible enough to allow for opportunistic or incidental learning, otherwise it needs to be adhered to as planned, and can form part of a 'learning agreement' (as noted in Chapter 2), and an assessment plan.

For all assessments, there are usually certain curriculum regulations that need to be adhered to, such as submission dates for PADs/practice competencies documents, and the procedure to follow if the student fails a competency. A number of key points specifically related to managing practical assessments using the 'direct observation' method are identified in the box below. They relate to any of the specific nursing standards identified in the NMC's (2010a) document and inherent outcomes, as well as to the standards of proficiency under seven 'platforms' in the NMC's (2018b: 14–15) document, two examples of which under platform 3 are:

3.5: demonstrate the ability to accurately process all information gathered during the assessment process to identify needs for individualised nursing care and develop person-centred evidence-based plans for nursing interventions with agreed goals.

3.12: interpret results from routine investigations, taking prompt action when required by implementing appropriate interventions, requesting additional investigations or escalating to others.

PLANNING AND MANAGING THE ASSESSMENT PROCESS

Prior to the assessment (mostly practice supervisor input)	• Agree, during Week 1 of placement, the objectives/competencies that need to be achieved and assessed. • Ensure that the learner has learnt the skill, allocate registrants to teach the skill in accordance with agreed procedure or clinical guidelines. The skill is taught at the appropriate academic level. The learner is given sufficient practice opportunities and has been formatively assessed during the placement. • Practice assessor feels: (a) up to date with interventions being assessed; (b) competent to assess/has attended practice assessor updates; (c) takes a supportive and positive approach.
	• Day of assessment – ensure that the student feels ready for the assessment, set time of day, consider 'practicability' and fairness of assessment issues. • Obtain consent of patient/service user, if any involved. • Colleagues aware if and when they can interrupt (if necessary), give bleep/pager to another person. • Agree assessment criteria.

(Continued)

(Continued)	
During the assessment	• Use appropriate communication skills (see box in Chapter 6 titled 'Communication and interpersonal factors related to assessments'). • Create a climate that enables the student to relax so that they can perform the skill to the best of their ability. • Indicate to the student to start the clinical intervention(s) when ready. • Safety issues – if the learner makes a mistake, consider the seriousness of the mistake, and intervene, ask questions about next step, or provide prompt/clues, as appropriate. • Responsive assessment – taking into account the patient's changing healthcare needs. • Situated assessments, i.e. in the context of available resources and clinical activities, for instance. • Consider predictive validity of assessments, i.e. whether the learner can perform as well in future and in other patient care situations.
After the assessment	• Need to exercise professional judgement throughout. • Decide on whether to award a pass or fail for each skill or competency assessed. • Give feedback according to established good practice (discussed shortly). • Ensure documentation is completed – for care intervention performed, student competency and of feedback given. • If fail is given, then the practice assessor needs to follow the university's procedure for subsequent actions to take, which normally includes informing the link lecturer or the PEF.

For examples of specific student competencies related to allied health professions, and to midwifery, see Chapter 8 of this book.

ASSESSING STUDENTS' ATTITUDE, VALUES AND INTERPERSONAL BEHAVIOUR AND SKILLS (THE AFFECTIVE DOMAIN OF LEARNING)

As noted in Chapter 2, each healthcare profession competency consists of three domains of learning, namely (1) a comprehensive knowledge of the competency (cognitive domain), (2) the capability to perform the care intervention safely and effectively (psychomotor domain), and (3) reflecting the appropriate attitude towards the performance and the recipient of the intervention.

The earliest advocates of these domains were Bloom (1956) and Krathwohl et al. (1964), and were more recently examined by Anderson, et al. (2014b). These domains of learning are very widely applied in several professional learning programmes, be they training programme or educational. The knowledge base and the psychomotor skill have been discussed already in Chapters 2, 3 and 6 of this book. As for the affective domain, this can be less easy to assess.

The affective component of a clinical intervention refers to the performer's (learner's) attitude and behaviour towards the service user, the service user's health problem, and the intervention itself. It refers to the learner's, or professional's, values and the demonstration and utilisation of compassion, for example. Healthcare professionals' values tend to refer to the individual's acceptance of the service user, truthfulness, equality, dignity, care, compassion, self-discipline, etc., and are closely linked to the profession's code of practice and ethics.

A case study relating an instance of underachievement in the affective domain by a second-year ODP student illustrates this, and is also a situation that creates extra demands on practice supervisors' and practice assessors' time.

CASE STUDY 7.1:   AN UNDERACHIEVING SECOND-YEAR ODP STUDENT

Jade is a second-year student on an Operating Department Practitioner (ODP) programme on a 12-week placement block in the Day Surgery Unit of a large teaching hospital. She had an uneventful first year of training. However, during the Day Surgery placement, she was involved in an incident alleging the use of unprofessional communication with a senior surgical colleague, and a complaint was made that was immediately dealt with by that trust's Theatre Manager, and Jade's personal tutor was informed.

Four weeks into Jade's placement in the Day Surgery Unit, a placement visit was undertaken by Jade's personal tutor. The tutor was asked to speak to one of Jade's practice learning supervisors, Lisa, who discussed the student's progress in detail, and expressed concerns for her student, noting that Jade's understanding of the role of the ODP was poor and she had a limited base of knowledge from which to develop despite being a second-year student. Jade was not able to meet the criteria for clinical competencies due to this lack of knowledge and the supervisor had grave concerns about her progress, despite them consistently working together.

Allied to this were further concerns about Jade's professionalism. The concern raised was that she was overly familiar with senior colleagues, using first names instead of professional titles, made ill-timed jokes during clinical interventions, and discussed personal matters with patients. Senior clinical staff stated that Jade was unaware of the potential problems this would cause and was unfocused.

Given the nature of both her unprofessional interactions and lack of knowledge related to the role, the personal tutor and supervisor felt it necessary to address the issues and had a formal meeting with Jade.

After discussion, it was found that Jade's situation was neither acceptable nor beneficial to her progression and an action plan was drawn up. The action plan incorporated agreed practice outcomes and included behaviour observations to aid Jade's development. The practice outcomes therefore cover all three domains of healthcare activity, and the action plan for Jade included the following:

(Continued)

(Continued)

ACTION PLAN		Student's name: Jade		Practice supervisor's name: Lisa	
Student's learning needs	Specific objectives to be achieved	Who will help student achieve the objectives and how?	Other resources required	Achieve-by dates	Evidence of achievement of objectives
1. Understanding professionalism	Ability to display professionalism in clinical practice	Practice supervisor, clinical team and theatre manager		13 February 2018	Displays professionalism in individual attitude, communication and interactions
2. Assisting the Anaesthetist	Be able to assist an Anaesthetist in achieving safe endotracheal intubation	Practice supervisor, clinical team, Anaesthetists	Local policies, procedures and clinical guidelines related to patients undergoing general anaesthesia	7 February 2018	Displays the ability to assist an Anaesthetist in the delivery of endotracheal intubation, understanding the underpinning knowledge related to the procedure.
3.					

AGREEMENT OF ACTION PLAN

Practice supervisor's signature: .... Date: 9 January 2018

Student's signature: .... Date: ....

ACHIEVEMENT OF OBJECTIVES

Practice assessor's signature: .... Date: ....

Jade's action plan presented above constitutes a template for action plans that is widely utilised, and another one is presented at https://study.sagepub.com/gopee4e in the section referring to this chapter – it is often laid out in landscape format.

Examples of practice competencies that ODP students can be required to achieve based on HCPC (2014a) standards for ODPs, include:

- Demonstrates the ability to correctly identify the patient on admission to operating departments, checking documentation in accordance with hospital policy.
- Demonstrates ability to assist the anaesthetist during the induction, maintenance and emergence from general anaesthesia.

The competencies constitute learning healthcare activities in all three domains of learning. Examples of SOP (HCPC, 2014b) for ODPs from which practice competencies are translated and which ODP students need to achieve by the end of their pre-registration programme are noted in the box below.

EXAMPLES OF STANDARDS OF PROFICIENCY FOR ODP STUDENTS

14.2 be able to conduct appropriate diagnostic or monitoring procedures, treatment, therapy, or other actions safely and effectively

14.5 be able to undertake appropriate anaesthetic, surgical and post-anaesthesia care interventions, including managing the service user's airway, respiration and circulation

14.9 be able to assess and monitor the service user's pain status and as appropriate administer prescribed pain relief in accordance with national and local guidelines.

In view of the above case study of an underachieving ODP student, it is of course necessary for practice supervisors (or practice educators) to be up-to-date with actions that they are required to take and those that are recommended for such situations. Accordingly, the HCPC (2017a: 44) states, 'We expect that all new practice educators are trained and that this is followed up with regular refresher training and support.'

Returning to a person's values, these also include sincerity, respect, individuals' freedom to make own decisions, morality, etc. Attitudes on the other hand are influenced by the person's positive and negative feelings about certain things, or certain behaviours. For example, if a service user is admitted to hospital with Type 2 diabetes, and is also grossly obese, the healthcare professional's values and attitude might be that people in general must maintain a healthy body weight. Towards those who don't, the healthcare professional might harbour negative feelings that may surface spontaneously in their attitude towards the service user, or in their behaviour.

As a professional, such negative behaviour is not acceptable, and breaches the healthcare profession's code of practice (e.g. NMC, 2015a), and therefore the healthcare professional must develop self-awareness of their personal feelings and values, and not allow them to interfere with safe, effective and high-quality care delivery.

Whenever assessing a student's ability to perform a clinical intervention, the practice assessor will also gauge the student's practical knowledge to a good extent, and their attitude. In many PADs, the attitude and behaviour (affective) component is assessed by a list of 'interpersonal skills and attitude' (or 'interpersonal interaction profile') which are therefore not assessed separately, but as integral components of performing service users' care interventions.

The affective domain is enshrined implicitly within SOP under all seven NMC's (2018b) 'platforms', as well as under 'Professional values' in NMC (2010a). An example of competence addressing the affective domain of care delivery is: 'Provide and promote non-discriminatory, person centred and sensitive care at all times, reflecting on people's values and beliefs, diverse backgrounds, cultural characteristics, language requirements, needs and preferences, taking account of any need for adjustments' (NMC, 2018b: Clause 1.14). Practice assessors have to be confident that pre-registration students are competent in these SOPs before signing the corresponding practice outcome in their PAD as a pass.

The above-mentioned competence can be translated into practice competencies to be achieved during practice placement, such as 'Ensures the service user's care is their primary priority, and therefore treats them as individuals and respects their dignity'. The student's activities that will demonstrate this include:

- communicates with people (service users, their carers/family and colleagues) appropriately, including listening
- maintains people's privacy and dignity
- is respectful and courteous and non-judgemental
- uses their skills of empathy and is sensitive to the needs of others.

However, as noted above, assessing students in the affective domain is probably less straightforward than assessing psychomotor skill or the knowledge base. This is because interpreting interpersonal and attitudinal aspects is likely to be clouded by subjectivity, different interpretations and assumptions. Realising this difficulty in relation to paramedic students and learners, Tanner (2014) examined this component and suggests a 12-item framework for this activity which includes assessing the student's listening skills, body language, appearance, etc., in addition to demonstrating compassion, verbal communication, etc.

Furthermore, the affective aspect of care delivery seems to have been deficient in pre-registration healthcare courses, or not valued by registrants, as it came to the fore through the Francis (2013) report which highlighted service users' concerns that healthcare staff lack care and compassion towards them, and that their behaviours and values are inappropriate. The actions taken to prevent such complaints include the new NMC (2018b) standards of proficiency, NHS England's (2016)

Leading Change, Adding Value – A Framework for Nursing, Midwifery and Care Staff, and Health Education England's (2014) *Values Based Recruitment Framework* publications.

For examples of specific student competencies related to allied health professions, and to midwifery, see Chapter 8 of this book.

MAKING DECISIONS AFTER ASSESSING THE STUDENT AND GIVING FEEDBACK ON THEIR PERFORMANCE

Following assessment of competency, the practice assessor has to indicate to the learner whether they have passed or failed after giving them feedback on their performance. Feedback is also a means of justifying the pass or fail result. Feedback can be: (a) *intrinsic feedback*, which occurs within the performer through self-assessment and reflection (the student often knows how well or not so well they did); or (b) *extrinsic feedback* (or augmented feedback), which is given by the assessor or peers and done concurrently during the skill performance and/or on completion of the performance. Some practice assessors might find it difficult to give honest feedback on a weak or faulty student performance. This could be tricky for the learner as well, but feedback has to be given honestly, and is generally accepted more readily if given constructively.

It is useful to ask the learner how they felt they performed straight (or soon) after completion of the clinical skill, instead of telling them first how well or badly they performed. The benefits of asking the student first are that this is likely to make them put aside any anxiety that they might still have about their performance, think more objectively and be more receptive to feedback. So, the practice assessor could ask, 'How do you think you did?' This constitutes self-assessment by the learner (which was discussed in Chapter 6), albeit usually only briefly, which should also give the practice assessor an indication of the learner's insights into their level of competence.

It is noteworthy that written feedback is also provided by practice supervisors and others on students' learning, behaviour and values in students' PADs. However, at times, teachers' time pressures and administrative issues could negatively affect the nature of the feedback provided. Furthermore, as Houghton (2016) notes, at times students are given feedback on their clinical performance at end-points such as at the end of a placement, or at mid-placement interviews. Such occasional feedback is of limited benefit to the student who should instead be provided with feedback regularly as and when new skills are learnt and formatively assessed. Comprehensive and timely feedback can also lead to enhanced student engagement with their learning.

Good practice guidelines for giving feedback that is comprehensive and timely to students are listed in the box below.

GUIDELINES FOR GIVING FEEDBACK TO THE STUDENT AFTER CLINICAL SKILL PERFORMANCE

- Ensure privacy and that adequate time is allocated.
- Use the sandwich method, which entails starting with comments on the positive points or strengths, discussing areas for improvement, and ending on positive notes.
- Give feedback constructively, as the aim of feedback is to enable the learner to learn and improve.
- Try to be honest and fair but never be destructive.
- Be clear and concise.
- Allow the recipient of the feedback time to discuss and ask for clarification.
- Do not allow anxiety levels to increase unduly.
- Gauge the impact of your feedback on the student's feelings and self-esteem throughout the exercise.
- Respect and treat the recipient as an individual and focus on behaviour and skill performance rather than personality traits (i.e. it mustn't be perceived as a personal remark).
- Acknowledge good practice.
- Suggest measures to correct inappropriate practice.
- Remain calm and objective; do not respond in kind to anger, aggression and defensiveness.
- Motivate the recipient to consolidate strengths and address limitations through strategies such as action plans.
- Be empowering through encouragement of the recipient to comment and explain issues discussed.
- Advise student to develop a positive and open-minded attitude towards feedback despite the mark or grade awarded, so that they can build on their achievement.

Good general communication skills are essential when giving feedback, including non-verbal communication such as maintaining eye contact. Following feedback, action plans or learning points can be constituted and mutually agreed, as also suggested by the RCN (2017b). However, in an ethos of self-directed learning, ultimately it is up to the receiver of the feedback to decide how much of it to heed and act upon, and when, and to be accountable for their decisions.

Various viewpoints discussed so far suggest that appropriate documentation is vital to practice assessor activities. Furthermore, the documentation should be in line with the section on record-keeping in the NMC's (2015a) code of practice. In fact, documentation of assessments is crucial, considering the NMC's (2010c) position that recording constitutes documentary evidence of actions taken.

ACTIVITY 7.2   THE STUDENT'S
PRACTICE COMPETENCIES

Look through your copy (practice assessor's copy) or the student's copy of the practice competencies booklet and read the sections where it identifies the roles of the practice supervisor, the practice assessor, the link lecturer and personal tutor, and of the student during the placement.

A clause in the booklet usually states the actions that the practice supervisor needs to take if the student is perceived as underachieving or 'failing'. They tend to entail drawing on the expertise of colleagues if deemed appropriate, of the link lecturer, the PEF or the student's personal tutor. There may also be a section on the appeals procedure. However, for each new course or module being offered, there would have been briefing sessions for prospective practice supervisors and practice assessors to familiarise themselves with the course requirements and the specific competencies to be achieved by students, and to discuss potential issues.

If you are on a practice assessor course yourself, it is very important that, on completion of the course, before you conduct any student assessment, you acquaint yourself with the student's placement competencies and preferably with the overall assessment strategy for the course. Furthermore, you should fully understand the particular summative assessments that you are going to conduct. The action to take in case of 'failure to achieve required standard' by the learner is discussed later in this chapter.

However, despite careful planning, unfolding day-to-day events could still disrupt the smooth running of assessments. The patient could refuse consent to students performing clinical interventions on them, staff sickness, unexpected emergency admissions or referrals might present as obstacles. Nevertheless, these do not always present as problems, as Neary (2000) for example recommends 'responsive assessment', which entails taking into account situational contexts such as the patient's current physiological or psychological state, and prevailing resource issues.

ACTION PLANNING

An example of an action plan was presented earlier in this chapter in relation to behaviour issues manifested by ODP student Jade. Often action plans are constituted at the mid-placement interview during the practice placement, which is in fact itself an important component of assessment of students' progress with their placement competencies. The competencies to be achieved will have been agreed at the beginning of the placement and might be in the form of a learning contract. The mid-placement interview can technically be a formal formative assessment point, which involves dedicated time for a discussion on, and documentation of, the student's progress with placement competencies.

If the student has been progressing mostly as expected, then this is documented, and the student continues as agreed in the learning contract. If the student has not been achieving as expected in the knowledge, skills and attitudes components, then a negotiated action plan needs to be constructed, which the practice supervisor, the practice assessor and learner mutually agree on and sign. A PEF or an academic such as the link lecturer might also be present and sign the action plan accordingly.

In addition to Tanner's (2014) observation regarding assessing interpersonal and attitudinal aspects as being more problematic than assessing psychomotor skill or knowledge base, Jervis and Tilki's (2011) qualitative research also revealed difficulty with assessing students' attitude and behaviour towards service users and team members accurately, with the undesirable consequence that some practice supervisors or assessors could pass students who are in fact not competent in the attitudinal component of student competence.

Action planning involves specifying all components identified at the top of the template related to ODP student Jade. If such an action plan was not constituted, then the student could have grounds for complaint and appeal if they were subsequently deemed a 'fail' for the placement. This point also indicates the importance of documentation of progress with achievement of placement competencies.

While there are some similarities between learning contracts and action plans, there are distinct differences between them in that the former are more learning centred and the latter are more assessment centred. The learning contract is a systematic but speculative plan of learning based on practice competencies to be achieved and projected learning opportunities, and may be adjusted during mid-placement progress discussions. The action plan is a 'must-achieve' device that identifies competencies that need to be achieved by an identified date during the practice placement, non-achievement of which would lead to a 'fail' mark being awarded.

RE-ASSESSING THE LEARNER

Once the action plan has been agreed, it must be adhered to, in that the practice supervisor (or the PEF) and the student jointly ensure that the competencies are being acquired, continuous assessment is occurring and, when ready, the student is re-assessed summatively and the documentation signed as and when competencies are achieved. The action plan is regularly reviewed and on the agreed date a review is conducted, which incidentally can lead to subsequent actions if the student does not achieve the competencies in the action plan.

The components discussed in the preceding sections addressed mostly the duties of practice supervisors and practice assessors with regards to assessing students' achievement of their practice competencies. Assessments have to meet the essential criteria of validity and reliability, as discussed in Chapter 6 of this textbook. The next section explores another dimension of the concept reliability namely intra- and inter-assessor reliability.

INTRA- AND INTER-ASSESSOR RELIABILITY

On the practice assessor course, at practice assessors' update sessions and at course reviews, on and off, the question is asked as to how we know that practice assessors are consistent in their assessment of students' competencies. That is, how do we know and monitor how consistent each practice assessor is in assessing how students perform specific clinical interventions, and that they are consistent in their expectations and decisions when assessing how different students at the same stage of their professional education perform that particular clinical intervention; and also how consistent different practice assessors are when assessing how students perform the clinical intervention? This is the arena of intra- and inter-assessor reliability, the latter being referred to by Mott Macdonald and the NMC (2017: 37–38) as inter-rater reliability of assessment of competence.

Increasingly, the quality of student performance in practice competencies is graded (for example, Andre, 2000), and although grading practice normally requires further appropriate educational preparation for practice assessors, this activity should also enable the achievement of intra- and inter-assessor reliability with more ease.

Furthermore, it is only fair to students that practice assessors are consistent in their expectations of the standard to which students perform care interventions, the highest standard being the healthcare organisation's approved procedure, protocol or clinical guidelines for performing the particular intervention.

Thus, the term intra-assessor reliability refers to how consistently the practice assessor assesses particular categories of students on a particular clinical intervention, that is, that they consistently use the same identified criteria for deciding on whether to give a pass or a fail for that particular intervention, within a responsive assessment approach. Inter-assessor reliability refers to the consistency with which all practice assessors assess a particular category of student on each clinical intervention.

Practice assessor preparation courses and update sessions usually also incorporate an exploration of ways in which intra- and inter-assessor reliability is achieved and can be monitored after qualifying as a practice assessor.

REFLECTION POINT 7.1:   INTRA- AND INTER-ASSESSOR RELIABILITY

Think of ways in which practice assessors can achieve and monitor intra- and inter-assessor reliability. What are the informal and more structured situations or opportunities that they can utilise to explore these?

As you would have sensed, achieving and maintaining intra- and inter-assessor reliability is a feature of the professionalism of practice assessors. There are various ways of monitoring intra- and inter-assessor reliability. The practice assessor update study days and trust-based update workshops provide suitable opportunities to explore how far consistency within and across practice assessors is achieved. Assessment case studies can be examined in small groups, or these groups can be invited to discuss consistency in the context of situations that they have personally encountered as practice assessors. In these groups, conclusions can be drawn on consistency in assessments conducted, and, with the help of the facilitator, bench-marks of good practice can be established.

However, monitoring intra- and inter-assessor reliability must not wait for update study days. Informal monitoring is undertaken continuously through discussions with peers or team members in the practice setting or unit, with one's line manager, the academic assessor or the assessor's clinical supervisor. So, further ways of achieving intra-assessor reliability are by:

- consistently using approved protocols/clinical guidelines
- ascertaining that approved procedures and clinical guidelines are up-to-date
- ensuring that their own competence and skills are up-to-date
- informal monitoring of their own pass/fail rates of learners
- ensuring an appropriate environment for assessing (so that the learner is relaxed when performing the clinical procedure)
- ensuring that the learner is being taught to the same standard and protocol/procedure by different registrants/associate practice supervisors
- student feedback such as evaluating how the student feels about the assessment process and decisions
- external feedback, from colleagues through reflections on assessments conducted
- ensuring that learners are aware of the level of performance expected of them
- reflection-on-action on assessment just conducted
- ensuring being aware of halo effect, being non-judgemental, for instance about the learner as a person; objectivity
- being consistent in own standard of clinical practice.

In addition to the above-mentioned ways of achieving reliability of assessments, inter-assessor reliability is achieved by:

- assessor meetings within ward/unit team – formal and informal
- involving PEF when uncertain
- consulting colleagues on same ward/unit as appropriate
- auditing practice assessor's performance of assessments (e.g., by negotiating peer assessment)
- student feedback on practice assessments
- feedback from university following student evaluations
- monitoring attendance at practice assessor updates, trust-based or university-based
- knowing and consulting/informing link lecturer

- exploring assessment issues at clinical supervision meetings
- monitoring and recording whether practice supervisors and practice assessors are up-to-date with clinical guidelines/protocols.

AVERTING AND RESOLVING PROBLEMS OF ASSESSMENTS

Having discussed intra- and inter-assessor reliability of student assessments, this section now examines potential problems of assessment of practice competencies. Problems of assessment can be averted by careful planning, and this is the component wherein practice supervisors' and practice assessors' leadership is absolutely essential. However, problems with assessments do occur and, when they do, they need to be resolved relatively quickly and efforts made to learn how to avoid them in future.

POTENTIAL PROBLEMS OF ASSESSMENT OF COMPETENCE

The aims or purposes of assessments are quite clearly identified by several writers on nurse education, as noted under 'Why do we need to assess our students?' in Chapter 6. However, how far and how smoothly these aims are achieved in reality varies. We also need to consider exactly what types of problems practice assessors actually encounter in the assessment of students, and what the criticisms directed at assessments are, including those of written examinations.

ACTIVITY 7.3   CURRENT PROBLEMS OF ASSESSMENTS

1. Think of the weaknesses of assessments and the reasons why assessments, even written examinations, are unpopular with students (assuming that they are). Make brief notes.
2. Identify the actual problems that tend to occur with student assessment of theory and practice in your healthcare profession, ones that you have experienced or observed, or that you feel could occur.

Practice supervisors and practice assessors and learners could encounter various difficulties with assessment of practice competencies. For assessment of theoretical knowledge (for example, of human physiology) and numerical skills as in drug administration and nurse prescribing courses, written examinations remain a favoured method, particularly in higher education. The likely solutions to the problems that you have identified will be explored shortly. A range of problems with assessment was identified by just one group of students on a previous mentoring course. Many of these are presented in the box.

PROBLEMS WITH ASSESSMENT

- Leaving things to the last minute (i.e. poor time planning)
- Difficulty with integration of theory and practice, or ineffective application
- Personality problems/clashes
- Problems of organisation in the practice setting
- Lack of time
- Student disagrees with practice assessor
- Attitude problems – student's or practice assessor's
- Structure of learning programme (e.g. placement is too short)
- Practice assessor accountable and responsible for how student performs the clinical intervention
- Inconsistency of student performance
- Student absence
- Practice assessor's low morale
- Practice assessor changes or is absent
- Student appears indifferent
- Student's level of knowledge
- Lack of resources (e.g. equipment)
- Non-cooperation or refusal of consent by the healthcare service user

One of the most cited difficulties encountered in the past has been insufficient time for student supervision activities. Cognisance of this recurrent problem necessitates more robust leadership on the part of practice supervisors and practice assessors in terms of forward planning, prioritising and proactive actions. The substantial empirical study on assessments by Phillips et al. (2000) highlighted various problems encountered by assessors, which include (see also Chapter 1 and case studies at https://study.sagepub.com/gopee4e):

- The quality of assessment varies enormously, depending on staffing levels and workload in the practice setting.
- Difficulty in understanding different levels of practice.
- Few assessors feel well prepared for doing assessments and most express a desire for continuing support after initial preparation, and consideration of adequate infrastructure for valid and reliable assessments.

Other problems with assessments have been identified, for example by Rowntree (1987), Lankshear (1990), Duffy (2003, 2016) and Gainsbury (2010). Rowntree discusses some of the 'side-effects of assessments', referring to concepts such as 'self-fulfilling prophecy', whereby students who are expected to achieve low grades tend to achieve low grades, which might not necessarily be a reflection of their innate ability.

Gainsbury (2010) reports on a problem with assessment referred to as 'failure to fail' that was identified two decades earlier by Lankshear (1990), and also later by Duffy (2016), and therefore still prevails. Gainsbury's report reminded universities and their partner healthcare trusts of their accountability with regard to passing students signifying fitness for practice. Furthermore, Duffin (2005) reported some time ago that the NMC also has remained concerned about the range of clinical expertise in the armoury of the newly qualified nurse, midwife or SCPHN.

However, many of these weaknesses could occur in healthcare courses, although actions have since been taken to rectify some of them. The findings of Duffy's research are discussed shortly with regards to the 'underachieving student'.

DIFFICULTIES WITH ASSESSMENT OF CLINICAL SKILL PERFORMANCE

ACTIVITY 7.4   DIFFICULTIES WITH STUDENT ASSESSMENT

Think about current day-to-day potential problems of assessments and, considering them in the context of your own current place of work, first identify at least one clinical assessor who has already conducted quite a few clinical assessments. They do not need to be based solely in your workplace but should work broadly within your specialism. Your task is then to approach the assessor and ask them to explain precisely what steps they take in preparation for, and in actually conducting, assessment of competence with learners. Find out also from the assessor how they anticipate potential problems and avert them. Ask about some of the actual problems encountered, and the options that they had for resolving them.

At the same time or afterwards, reflect for yourself on such problems and decide how you would go about dealing with them if they occurred in your own practice setting.

Alternatively, think for yourself of all the problems that you might encounter in your assessment function as a practice assessor, and then the options that will be available to you to resolve each of them.

Problems of assessment include differences in the interpretation of the exact meaning of placement competencies. There might be problems in conveying the depth of knowledge expected, or level of skill demonstration. Issues like these can be rectified by open discussion between all personnel directly involved.

RESOLVING PROBLEMS WITH ASSESSMENT

ACTIVITY 7.5   RESOLVING DIFFICULTIES ENCOUNTERED BY PRACTICE ASSESSORS

Refer back to the box titled 'Problems with assessment' and work on the difficulties encountered by practice assessors by identifying a number of problems of assessment you could encounter with a particular group of students, and the probable solutions for each of them. This can be done by completing Template 7.1.

Template 7.1   Criticisms or difficulties with assessments, and actions that can be taken to resolve them

Criticisms/difficulties with assessments	Actions that can be taken to resolve them
Leaving things to the last minute	....
Difficulty with integration, or ineffective application, of theory and practice	....
Personality problems/clashes	......
Problems of organisation	....
Lack of time for conducting assessments	....
Student disagrees with practice assessor	....
Attitude problems – student's or practice assessor's	
The service user or patient not consenting to student assessment	
Lack of resources (e.g., equipment)	
Structure of learning programme: variation of experience, e.g. allocation too short	
...... (etc. – add others you have identified)	

Chances are that you will be aware of or have thought of yet other problematic situations encountered by practice assessors in the assessment of students, for which similar steps can be taken. They might include passing a student because the practice assessor likes the student or failing the student because they dislike them (at times referred to as 'halo' and 'horns' effects respectively), unqualified trainee practice assessors signing up clinical competencies or misinterpretation of wording of practice competencies.

With some of these problem areas there could be instances when a practice assessor passes a student on a specific competency when they should be awarding a fail. This cannot be condoned, but failure to fail students has already been identified over the years. If a student is failing, the practice assessor's decision-making comes into play, and action plans are constructed.

Furthermore, in their research related to students who fail practice competencies, Hunt et al. (2016) found that some students react negatively to feedback that they have not performed to the required standard in their practice assessments, as also noted by Jervis and Tilki (2011). In such situations some students become upset, and others even become angry and threatening. Some say they will take grievances against their assessor. Other students become manipulative by either being charming and obliging or coercive, some blame external factors for failing, while others express open hostility and make personal threats to the assessor.

Hostile student attitude leads to breakdown in supervisor–student relationships and trust. However, all practice supervisors and assessors are accountable practitioners, and therefore simply have to abide by the assessment protocol laid down in the students' course curriculum, as well as by their code of practice. The next section considers the ethical aspects of student assessment particularly in terms of the assessor's accountability.

THE PRACTICE ASSESSOR'S ACCOUNTABILITY RELATED TO ASSESSMENTS

All registrants have to comply with their professional body's code of practice, and this applies to practice assessment, and supervising juniors and colleagues' learning. 'Being an accountable professional' is one of the seven platforms in the NMC's (2018b) *Standards of Proficiency for Registered Nurses*, that directly addresses ethical aspects of the nurse's role and responsibilities. The platform lists the outcomes that students have to demonstrate competence in for gaining entry to the NMC's professional register. Similarly, 'Professional values' is one of the 'domains' that addresses ethical and legal aspects of the NMC's (2010a) standards.

Thus, practice assessors should already be knowledgeable about ethical aspects of professional practice through their pre-registration preparation, while their students will be developing these through theirs. On exploring the ethics of practice learning supervision and assessment, Brown (2005) suggests that practice supervisors need to be well aware of their own values and ethical interpretations of clinical practice to enable students to develop 'ethical competence'.

'Ethics' refers to the social behaviours, morals and values of individuals and groups in relation to doing good for the greatest number, and to the impact, or end results, of clinical interventions (adapted from Brown, 2005). One widely accepted set of principles of ethics that applies to many spheres of life, including medicine, business and education, has been formulated by Thiroux and Krasemann (2014).

These principles are:

- the value of life
- goodness or rightness
- justice or fairness
- honesty and truth-telling
- individual freedom.

These principles apply directly to instances of practice assessment in the following ways:

- *The value of life* – can refer to ensuring that students develop the necessary competencies for effective clinical interventions that would restore health and well-being. It can also refer to ensuring that students acquire the necessary knowledge, skills and attitudes to register as a nurse so that they can earn a living.
- *Goodness or rightness* – refers to the practice supervisors doing good to students and healthcare service users, and doing the right things.
- *Justice or fairness* – refers to ensuring that all students acquire the knowledge, skills and attitudes in appropriate detail and depth.
- *Honesty and truth-telling* – ensuring that incorrect information is not given.
- *Individual freedom* – means that students have some freedom in deciding on the amount and type of learning, and care service users have a say in the clinical interventions available, where possible.

Other principles of ethics include: (1) being trustworthy; (2) autonomy; (3) beneficence (doing good); (4) non-maleficence (doing no harm); and (5) self-respect. Furthermore, the British Association for Counselling and Psychotherapy's (BACP) (2016) 'ethical framework' for counselling encompasses values, principles and personal moral qualities. Values refer to respecting human rights and dignity, alleviating personal distress and suffering, and fairness. Personal moral qualities include empathy, sincerity, humility and competence.

The codes of practice of healthcare professional regulatory bodies usually incorporate ethical principles that registrants have to follow. As for practice assessors' ethical practice related to assessment of competence, they should, for instance, not award a pass to a student for any particular competency if they are not completely sure that the student can perform the clinical intervention competently and safely.

The previous NMC (2008) standards for supporting practice learning emphasised ethical aspects under the domain 'Assessment and accountability' for example, and also specified the imperative for being competent to 'manage failing students so that they may enhance their performance and capabilities for safe and effective practice' (ibid.: 52–53). This competence implicitly suggests compliance with ethical and legal aspects to ensure care service users' safety, in particular in relation to the facilitation of learning for students and assessment of competence.

Furthermore, the NMC's (2018a) *Standards for Student Supervision and Assessment* also identifies effective practice assessment practices in that it indicates for example that practice assessors need to 'receive ongoing support and training to reflect and develop in their role' (2018a: clause 8.2), which implicitly suggests that practice assessors have to be fully aware of the knock-on effects of 'pass' decisions on care service users' health.

Consequently, if an inexperienced practice assessor finds dealing with the under-performing student a challenge, then they need to recognise this, and seek guidance and support from more experienced practice assessors, or the PEF or link lecturer, as per local guidelines (see Figure 7.1 later in this section). Other sources of practice assessor support might be:

- Student's personal tutor
- Practice assessor's clinical supervisor
- Practice assessor's line manager
- The university's disabilities support officer
- Specific guidelines or protocols on ways of managing problematic situations
- Retrospectively at assessor update workshops
- Employers' and university's intranet
- In practice supervision team meetings
- Own emotional resilience.

One of the legal implications of assessments is that, on being awarded a pass, the individual is being given a licence and the legal right to practise the skill unsupervised when they register with their professional body. Awarding a licence to practise to someone who is not competent is in breach of the law, and the NMC's (2015a) code of practice clearly indicates that all registrants must keep to the laws of the country (Clause 20.4).

A feature that frequently surfaces when the legality of the actions of registrants is questioned is the documentation of the actions taken. Molle and Durham (2004: 146) and various others clearly believe and assert that 'if it is not documented, it was not done'. Alternatively, Kendall-Raynor (2007) reports on the case of a registered nurse who had allegedly failed to supervise a student adequately, which resulted in the wrong dose of medication being given to a service user, who subsequently died. The case was dropped by the Crown Prosecution Service (CPS) 'because of insufficient evidence'. Evidently, this was a situation of unethical practice on two counts, firstly because the wrong dose of medication resulted in harming a patient, and secondly incompetent documentation led to injustice and unfairness.

The three professional bodies most directly involved in health and social care, namely the HCPC, NMC and GMC, either explicitly or implicitly incorporate into their codes of practice such ethical components as respect for care service users as individuals, obtaining consent prior to clinical interventions, protecting confidential information, and identifying and minimising risk to patients or service users.

The principles of ethics translate into current healthcare practice by addressing accountability, informed consent, confidentiality (including record keeping), professional misconduct, delegation and supervision.

RESPONSIBILITY AND ACCOUNTABILITY OF PRACTICE SUPERVISORS AND PRACTICE ASSESSORS

All healthcare professionals are accountable for delivering care competently (NMC, 2018b; 2010a), and also for other components of their roles such as enabling healthcare learners and colleagues to develop their clinical skills. We are accountable to our patients, ourselves, our employers, our professional regulatory bodies, and in fact also to the general public.

To be responsible implies being answerable for one's actions, and it is a component of accountability. However, before the health or social care professional can be held accountable for particular clinical interventions or their overall professional competence, they must already have acquired educational preparation in the knowledge, skills and attitudes that underpin their clinical actions. In addition their employment endows them with the authority and responsibility to perform those clinical actions.

One of the main thrusts of practice assessors' accountability is that it is related to the rules, regulations, policies and scope of practice that govern assessments. These are usually detailed in the appropriate practice assessor's handbook issued by the partner HEI, and briefly in the student's practice competencies booklet for the placement. It is also related to specific eventualities in the assessment of professional competence, to implementation of assessment strategies, to personal and professional responsibilities, and to the relevant legislation. You would need to refer to the student's placement competencies booklet and to your professional regulatory body's code of practice for further clarification when needed.

ACTIVITY 7.6   TEACHING AND LEARNING AS COMPONENTS OF PROFESSIONAL CONDUCT

Refer to your professional regulatory body's code of practice and the partner HEI's practice learning and assessing handbooks for your own profession, and ascertain how they express your responsibilities in terms of teaching and assessing learners and colleagues.

You will have noticed that a few clauses in the codes of practice directly identify registrants' teaching and their own CPD responsibilities and roles. This is usually also a component of the healthcare professional's job description (or contract of employment) for the post they occupy.

Registrants may not transfer or delegate their accountability to another person. Practice supervisors and practice assessors also function under legal obligations to know the student's course curriculum and built-in assessment procedures and regulations set out by the relevant HEI, and the appeals system that the student needs to follow if they feel that they are being unjustly treated. Students have a right to appeal against the conduct of the assessment, but not against the practice assessor's decision to pass or fail, or their professional judgement about safe practice.

In accepting the role of practice assessor, the registrant is implicitly accepting responsibility and accountability for maintaining standards of supervision and assessment. Practice supervisors must ensure that students gain the necessary clinical experiences to develop their professional competence and that students do 'no harm' to healthcare service users, by teaching them the correct way of performing clinical interventions.

Moreover, making professional judgements about the performance of students and their ability to provide professionally competent and safe care, also constitutes an endeavour to achieve predictive validity and reliability in assessments of competence.

However, Rowntree (1987) indicates that there are times when assessors might intentionally give permission to the learner to perform clinical interventions while supervising them unobtrusively, which can be expected, but at the same time assessing their performance without having specified this to them beforehand. This is sometimes referred to as 'hidden assessment' and could be another instance of unethical action by the assessor.

The NMC (2015a) affirms that the interests of the care service user are paramount, that is, accountability to the service user is more important than accountability to the student. However, the legal perspective can be, depending on individual situations, that the student is also answerable for incompetent interventions. Lack of experience or knowledge is not an acceptable reason for incompetent care.

On not being awarded a pass for a clinical intervention that was not performed competently, the learner might feel either merely disappointed or emotionally distraught. The practice assessor then needs to contact the PEF or link lecturer if further help and support are needed but might also have to use basic counselling skills to help the learner. As for all professional skills, if practice assessors have not had training in counselling skills, then they should refer the learner to an appropriate professional or department that does have those skills.

SUPPORTING THE UNDERACHIEVING STUDENT

As mentioned earlier in this chapter, practice supervisors' leadership includes careful planning of practice placement to ensure practice competencies are achieved. However, it is well appreciated that, for a number of reasons, some students could be seen as struggling or even failing to show consistent learning and progress during the placement. So what are the different reasons for a student failing to achieve as expected?

REFLECTION POINT 7.2:   THE UNDERACHIEVING STUDENT

From your own experience of students who struggle to achieve their clinical competencies, think of the different reasons for this happening during practice placements.

Some students genuinely experience obstacles that intervene in their achievement of placement competencies. Could this be because they are working extra shifts to supplement their income, and are therefore unable to find sufficient time to work on their practice competencies? There can be work-based reasons, or personal or domestic reasons. The signs that suggest that a student might not progress as expected with the placement competencies can appear very early during the placement. Limited interaction with clinical staff, lateness, sickness, absent-mindedness, inconsistency in standards of care delivery are just a few of them, but when such signs are detected, prompt action should be taken.

ACTIVITY 7.7   FAILING TO FAIL STUDENTS

So, for one reason or another, a student might not be progressing as expected, and the practice supervisor is not convinced that particular competencies will be achieved. However, in the past mentors have on occasion still decided to award a 'pass' to such students on their practice competencies, as found by Duffy (2016) for example.

Consider the whole spectrum of reasons why you think that a practice assessor might award a pass to a student for a particular competency, even if the student has not demonstrated competent performance. List as many reasons as you can think of.

You should have been able to think of various day-to-day circumstances that might lead to the practice assessor awarding a pass to a failing student, none of which is likely to be a justifiable reason. These could include, for instance, pressure from the student, who indicates that it is the last week of placement and that they have passed all previous placement competencies, and that insufficient time was allocated for assessing competencies.

As indicated earlier, 'failure to fail' has been identified as a dilemma over a number of years and can occur in various health and social care professions (for example, Furness and Gilligan, 2004). At times, the practice supervisor may have done all the planning for the student to achieve competencies, and yet on assessment they might find that the student has not reached the level of competence required to award them a pass for particular competencies. This could mean failing the practice placement. Consequently, the student's placement may have to be extended to allow them more time to achieve the competencies, and their course extended.

Individual HEIs usually provide their own specific guidelines on the actions to take to support the struggling student. The necessary steps in such guidelines are sketched out as a simple algorithm in Figure 7.1, and include: meeting with the student as soon as possible to discuss this issue; informing other practice supervisors and the designated PEF; clarifying the area of weakness and advising on how to progress; constituting a realistic action plan; making provision for any extra support; and keeping careful notes of all discussions and incidents.

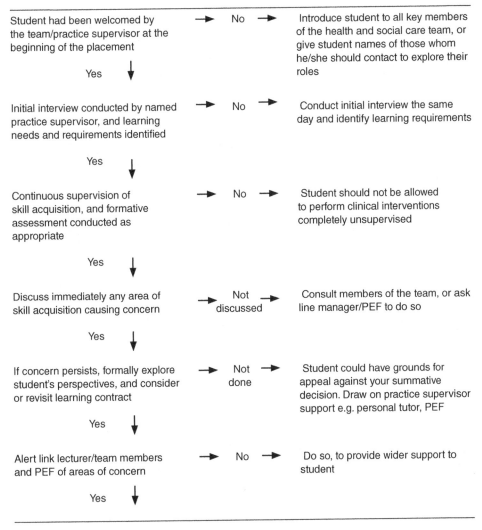

Student had been welcomed by the team/practice supervisor at the beginning of the placement	→ No →	Introduce student to all key members of the health and social care team, or give student names of those whom he/she should contact to explore their roles
Yes ↓		
Initial interview conducted by named practice supervisor, and learning needs and requirements identified	→ No →	Conduct initial interview the same day and identify learning requirements
Yes ↓		
Continuous supervision of skill acquisition, and formative assessment conducted as appropriate	→ No →	Student should not be allowed to perform clinical interventions completely unsupervised
Yes ↓		
Discuss immediately any area of skill acquisition causing concern	→ Not discussed →	Consult members of the team, or ask line manager/PEF to do so
Yes ↓		
If concern persists, formally explore student's perspectives, and consider or revisit learning contract	→ Not done →	Student could have grounds for appeal against your summative decision. Draw on practice supervisor support e.g. personal tutor, PEF
Yes ↓		
Alert link lecturer/team members and PEF of areas of concern	→ No →	Do so, to provide wider support to student
Yes ↓		

(Continued)

Figure 7.1   (Continued)

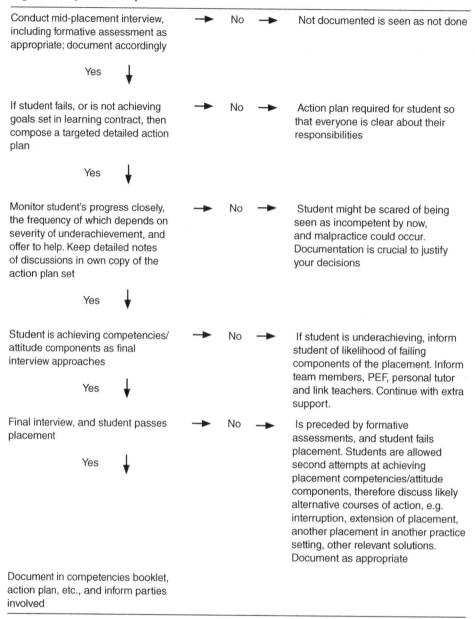

Conduct mid-placement interview, including formative assessment as appropriate; document accordingly	→ No →	Not documented is seen as not done
Yes ↓		
If student fails, or is not achieving goals set in learning contract, then compose a targeted detailed action plan	→ No →	Action plan required for student so that everyone is clear about their responsibilities
Yes ↓		
Monitor student's progress closely, the frequency of which depends on severity of underachievement, and offer to help. Keep detailed notes of discussions in own copy of the action plan set	→ No →	Student might be scared of being seen as incompetent by now, and malpractice could occur. Documentation is crucial to justify your decisions
Yes ↓		
Student is achieving competencies/attitude components as final interview approaches	→ No →	If student is underachieving, inform student of likelihood of failing components of the placement. Inform team members, PEF, personal tutor and link teachers. Continue with extra support.
Yes ↓		
Final interview, and student passes placement	→ No →	Is preceded by formative assessments, and student fails placement. Students are allowed second attempts at achieving placement competencies/attitude components, therefore discuss likely alternative courses of action, e.g. interruption, extension of placement, another placement in another practice setting, other relevant solutions. Document as appropriate
Yes ↓		
Document in competencies booklet, action plan, etc., and inform parties involved		

Figure 7.1   The underachieving student – action that the practice supervisor should take

Although appearing to be a compact whole-story process, Figure 7.1 does constitute the actions that practice supervisors and practice assessors should take to facilitate learning and achievement for the underachieving student, each step or stage constituting a concerted intervention that needs to be handled carefully and professionally. Houghton (2016) and Vinales (2015) also detail the general actions that need to be taken when a healthcare student is underachieving.

However, the question arises as to how confident practice assessors feel in their judgement and skill at giving a fail for a competency if the student is unable to perform the intervention competently. It is noteworthy that a study conducted by Mead (2011) using a convenient sample of conference attenders as the subject of the study, revealed that mentors had no problem with failing students if the latter could not demonstrate competence in particular service user care skills. They felt that they had 'sufficient training to enable them to fail nursing students' (ibid.: 23).

However, Hunt et al.'s (2012) study findings were the opposite to Mead's in that they concluded the preparation and support that mentors receive is not adequate for them to be able to fail incompetent students confidently. Nonetheless, Heaslip and Scammell's (2012) research on this issue revealed that just over half of the 112 mentors who participated in the study indicated that they felt confident to fail students, and also recommended that grading practice may contribute to making it easier because, instead of a pass/fail result, the assessor can give a better indication to the student as to whether their fail was borderline or a more serious fail.

Nonetheless, on conducting a literature review of 'failing to fail', Hughes et al. (2016) found that there were various facets to the concept, and that it was still a real major issue. The review resulted in five themes related to 'Failure to fail', and the authors recommend more focused research on the topic area. The themes are:

- Failing a student is difficult
- Is an emotional experience
- Confidence is required
- Unsafe student characteristics
- University support is required to fail students

Still, some students are likely to become upset or ashamed at failing the placement, or maybe they did all that they could but still did not achieve. The practice supervisor will then need to draw on their helping skills to help the student further. Some registrants on practice supervisor courses may find the idea of having to use helping skill anxiety-provoking, and therefore need to know where they can seek advice and guidance if required (as discussed later in this chapter).

HELPING AND COUNSELLING THE STRUGGLING STUDENT

The general and specific communication skills needed to establish a relationship and support the student develop and achieve competencies were explored to some extent in Chapter 1. In particular, the 'communication continuum' and related purposes and skills, and who uses them detailed by Scammell (1990) (also in Chapter 1) suggest that specific communication skills are needed to help students who are struggling to achieve their clinical competencies, or who may be struggling with the nursing course as a whole and are even in danger of failing in their chosen career.

It is suggested at this point that you refresh your understanding of the communication skills (for example, those discussed in Chapter 1). In addition to the generic communication skills that are necessary for all effective relationships, specialist communication skills are also required by the practice assessor to deal with more problematic situations.

The special skill of 'counselling' is one of the essential roles of supervisors of learning and teachers (Hughes and Quinn, 2013: 374). However, it is well recognised that for counselling to be effective, the process should be entered into voluntarily by the person who is the counsellee (in this instance, the health profession student). Indeed, it is generally agreed that unless counselling is actively sought by the student, the interaction might not be as effective, even if the helper uses most of the skills used in counselling. Second, counselling is a therapeutic technique, requiring specialist training. Persons not skilled in its use will, at best, not help the student, and at worst potentially compound the student's problems. Therefore, unless they are fully qualified as counsellors, supervisors and other teachers in healthcare are more likely to use helping or 'basic' counselling skills. For more intense student problems, referral should be made to specialist services such as the university's counselling service, which is often a section of student services provision.

CASE STUDY 7.2:   THE FAILING STUDENT

Bina is a pre-registration student on an eight-week placement at the end of the first year of her course. Her practice learning supervisor has varied roles as part of their managerial functions and has to cover extra shifts on days and nights due to staff sickness. However, Bina's placement has been marked by her frequent absence from the practice setting due to sickness and occasional tearfulness, claiming to feel depressed. She has been advised to seek help from the trust's Occupational Health Department and has been made aware that she can access the university's counselling facility if preferred.

Shortly after the placement started, the PEF went on maternity leave, and it took a few weeks to install a replacement for her. The acting PEF contacted Bina's personal tutor to explain Bina's circumstances and was advised that, among other things, a mid-placement interview needed to be conducted to ascertain Bina's progress with practice competencies and be documented accordingly. In particular, if these competencies were not achieved, then Bina would fail the first year and not progress to the field-specific part of the programme. The student was described as lacking in motivation and as 'a real struggle' by the acting PEF.

Due to Bina's continuing absence and health problems, the mid-placement interview only took place quite late in the placement, and an action plan was instituted as various practice competencies had still not been achieved.

Consider what would be the specialist helping or counselling skills that could be utilised in regular supervisor–student contact if both Bina and her practice supervisor were more available.

The most important factor within a counselling situation is the relationship between the counsellor and the counsellee (for example, the practice supervisor and the student). This was identified initially by Rogers (1983) and later by Rogers and Freiberg (1994). Both identified three key qualities (also known as 'core conditions' of helping) that are required for effective counselling. These key qualities, as detailed under student-centred teaching in Chapter 3, are: genuineness, trust and acceptance, and empathic understanding.

In addition to the generic communication skills, verbal and non-verbal, key helping skills include: self-awareness, attending, active listening, summarising, reflecting, questioning, and using silence. This set of skills can be used as a framework for checking how thoroughly you feel you dealt with these situations. By analysing your interactions with others, you will develop a greater awareness of how far you, as a professional, are able to help others.

Dedicated time is required for a systematic approach to counselling. This is done by utilising a model of helping, such as Heron's (2009) six-category intervention analysis. This model indicates six possible interactions between the two parties as detailed next.

In the aforementioned case study, for instance, the practice supervisor could help Bina by utilising components of Heron's framework. Instances of responses by the practice supervisor to the student's account of his or her perception of the situation would therefore be as follows:

- *Prescriptive* – advise Bina to reduce less important life activities to concentrate on working to achieve her placement objectives as a priority.
- *Informative* – give information on professional and personal matters as appropriate (e.g. location of Occupational Health Department).
- *Confrontational* – ask Bina directly what she is doing or how she could behave differently for a more satisfactory placement experience.
- *Supportive* – allow Bina time and silence to think over the practice supervisor's questions and suggestions.
- *Cathartic* – allow Bina to verbalise and explain in ample detail why she is struggling in this placement.
- *Catalytic* – the practice supervisor acts as facilitator to enable Bina to meet her learning needs.

ACTIVITY 7.8   AN UNDERACHIEVING STUDENT WHOM YOU HAVE ENCOUNTERED

Think of a student whom you have known to have failed to achieve required practice competencies resulting in the student being disappointed, upset or distressed. In case you haven't encountered such a student, think of a situation that you might encounter. Describe the situation in up to 75 words. Then, utilising Heron's (2009) six-category intervention analysis framework, identify the specific actions that you could take, using each of the categories to help the student.

Alternatively, consider Mel Alexis' situation cited in Chapter 1, and follow the above instructions.

One perspective on how practice supervisors manage underachieving students comes from a study by DeBrew and Lewallen (2014) that explored the thought processes that assessors go through in deciding whether to pass or fail a student on specific competencies. The researchers concluded that when practice assessors encounter these situations, they might still be wondering afterwards if they have made the right decision. To resolve this feeling, DeBrew and Lewallen recommend that they should afterwards engage in 'deliberate, intentional reflective practices' as a means of checking on the correctness of their decisions and, possibly, professional development. This sounds like a useful recommendation, although such reflective discussions may need to be facilitated by someone who is not closely involved with the practice supervisor's work setting, and of course the name of the student being discussed should be withheld.

Hawkins and Shohet (2012) suggest taking an inter-subjective approach that focuses on the relationship between practice supervisor and student. This notion largely implies using empathy. Universities usually provide a counselling service for any student who is distressed about any issue that is affecting their progress with their course. To become a skilled counsellor, especially for dealing with particular psychological problems, requires several years of structured educational preparation. However, Hawkins and Shohet also provide a number of pointers on how supervisors can help, such as by developing 'the qualities of a good supervisor' in themselves, which are noted in the box.

QUALITIES OF A GOOD SUPERVISOR

- Flexibility with use of different concepts and intervention methods
- A multi-perspective view (i.e. being able to see the situation from different angles)
- A solid knowledge of the profession and orientation in which they supervise
- The ability to work transculturally
- The capacity to manage and contain anxiety, their own and that of the supervisee
- Openness to learning from supervision situations
- Sensitivity to the impact of wider contextual issues on the supervision process
- Ability to handle power appropriately
- Humour, humility and patience

Source: Adapted from Hawkins and Shohet (2012: 52)

Proctor's (2011) 'supervision alliance model' is widely accepted as a suitable framework for systematic supervision. As a model of helping that is also acknowledged by Hawkins and Shohet, it comprises three main functions or roles of the helper, namely: normative, formative and restorative (see Chapter 1 of this book for a discussion on Proctor's model of supervision).

Although practice assessors are expected to exercise professional judgement and make pass or fail decisions on particular student performances, there are support networks that they can draw on whenever they are unsure. Informal or formal team supervision and peer consultation frameworks might already be in place but, as indicated in this chapter, the practice assessor's copy of the practice competencies document normally contains full details regarding the procedure to follow in these circumstances, such as contacting the PEF.

This chapter has explored ways in which practice supervisors and practice assessors exercise leadership in managing assessments. However, it is useful to note that the leadership role is not just about taking action to avert problems. It is also about taking action to achieve aims and good practice. Sines et al. (2006) report on joint action taken by an NHS trust and the partner university in order to ensure that student nurses achieved fitness for practice by the end of the three-year undergraduate course. Most of the mechanisms instituted were not unknown, and several of them were planned in substantial detail. These mechanisms include:

- identifying core skill clusters
- adapted OSCEs
- enhanced clinical skills laboratories
- an additional training programme in assessment of skills for existing practice assessors
- regular assessor updates
- appointment of PEF.

GOOD PRACTICE GUIDELINES FOR ASSESSMENTS

This final section on student assessment completes the focus on the principles aspect of assessment that were discussed in Chapter 6 and in this chapter by identifying good practice guidelines. The 'principles of assessment' are generally identified by universities and other education providers. They tend to recognise the Assessment Reform Group (2002) ten principles of assessment, but these principles usually constitute assessment at course level and in academic settings. For health and social care profession students, deriving from the above general principles, together with the profession specific guidelines (e.g. NMC, 2018c; DH, 2001; Rowntree, 1987) a comprehensive set of good practice guidelines related to practice assessment is presented in the box below.

GOOD PRACTICE GUIDELINES FOR PRACTICE ASSESSMENT OF HEALTH AND SOCIAL CARE STUDENTS

- Practice supervisors and practice assessors ensure that they are fully familiar with the student's practice competencies and standards prior to the start of the practice placement.

(Continued)

(Continued)

- Allocate registrants for teaching specific care intervention and associated knowledge to the student.
- Agree times and dates for student assessment, diary them, and treat it as 'supported time' (e.g. NMC, 2018a).
- Inform other staff to ensure that they do not interrupt during student assessment.
- Be aware of any crises in the practice setting, e.g. staff sickness, stress, emergencies.
- Inform service user and obtain permission for student assessment.
- Ensure that all equipment is available.
- Ensure that the learner has had sufficient practice opportunities prior to assessment of the skill.
- Ensure that you are fully available and accessible as the assessor.
- Plan the assessment, ensuring availability of procedures and guidelines.
- Assessments are conducted in collaboration between practice supervisors, practice assessors, and academic assessors, when needed.
- Assessments are also informed by service user feedback and other registrants who have worked with the learner being assessed.
- Most care interventions are assessed by direct observations, other competencies by other methods.
- Utilise opportunities for formative (or mock) assessments.
- Incorporate continuous assessment records from practice supervisors and other registrants.
- Consider levels of assessments based on the stage of the pre-regristration course the student is at.
- Ensure the assessments you conduct are valid, reliable and fair to students.
- Create the opportunity for the learner to talk through the procedure, if necessary.
- Be sensitive to the student's self-confidence or lack of it.
- Always remain calm and use appropriate interpersonal communication skills.
- If the learner displays awe of the assessor, give confidence.
- Be and look enthusiastic and motivated.
- Keep the assessment situated (in the context of the practice setting) and responsive.
- Allow the student to work at their own pace as long as this doesn't cause undue discomfort to the service user.
- Allow for holistic/person-centred care.
- Intervene appropriately if unsafe practice is about to occur.
- Ensure that the learner knows the assessment criteria for the skill.
- Encourage self-assessment, allow room for reflection and give feedback as you feel appropriate.
- Incorporate professional judgement when making pass/fail decisions.
- Heed previous criticisms of assessments, e.g. research findings such as 'failing to fail' (Duffy, 2016) and 'on-the- hoof' assessments (Phillips et al., 2000).
- Do not be biased by occasional polarised instances of exceptionally thorough or poor practice during continous assessment.
- Beware of other factors, e.g. the learner being preoccupied with other course assignments.
- Document results in practice competencies booklet, etc.
- Take prompt supportive and remedial actions if the student is given a fail.

CHAPTER SUMMARY

This chapter has focused on the practice supervisor's and practice assessor's role in the assessment of student competence, the challenges that these roles can present in relation to assessments, and has therefore explored:

- The importance of practice supervisors and practice assessors exercising leadership through careful scheduling and planning of student assessments.
- Current difficulties and potential problems of assessment of learners' clinical skills, resolving these problems, including action planning and re-assessment of the learner, and how these problems are averted.
- The responsibility and accountability of practice assessors in ensuring that pass or fail is awarded appropriately, and relevant subsequent action taken.
- Use of professional judgement, and how intra- and inter- assessor reliability can be monitored and achieved; and the ethical and legal aspects of student assessment.
- How underachieving students can be supported using basic communication and helping skills, and more specialist communication skills, including counselling. They constitute skills that would also apply to student assessment situations, and include time management and proactive actions, and the use of support networks with peers, PEFs and academic staff.
- Good practice guidelines for assessments.

FURTHER OPTIONAL READING

1. For more details on the Duffy (2016) report on 'failure to fail', see:
   - Duffy, K. (2016) *Failure to Fail – A Systematic Review of Where we Are Now*. Available at: www.rcn.org.uk/professional-development/research-and-innovation/research-events/rcn-2016-research-conference (accessed 27 April 2017).

2. For further guidance on the ethics of practice supervision and assessment, see:
   - Gopee, N. (2008) 'Assessing student nurses' clinical skills: The ethical competence of mentors', *International Journal of Therapy and Rehabilitation*, 15(9): 401–407.

To access further resources related to this chapter, visit **https://study.sagepub.com/gopee4e** where a range of learning and teaching materials are provided.

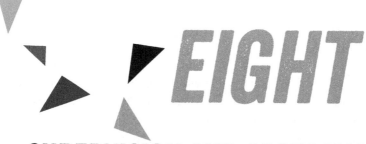

SUPERVISION AND ASSESSMENT OF ALLIED HEALTH PROFESSION AND MIDWIFERY STUDENTS

WITH NATASHA TAYLOR AND COLLETTE CLAY

INTRODUCTION

All allied health profession (AHP) students' pre-registration programmes incorporate a substantial proportion of learning in practice settings, comprising practice education in caring for care service users, as required by the NMC, HCPC and other healthcare profession regulators. For nursing and midwifery students the NMC (e.g. 2018e: 13) states that practice education should consist of at least half of the minimum 4600-hour pre-registration programme, which incidentally can include an agreed percentage of time in simulated learning in skills laboratories, as noted in Chapter 2 of this book. For physiotherapy students, as an example of programme requirements for allied health professionals' practice education, the Chartered Society of Physiotherapy (CSP) (2017) indicates that students should undertake approximately 1000 hours of learning in the practice environment.

As the title of this chapter and the chapter objectives below suggest, this chapter explores key aspects of practice education requirements for AHP students, with specific focus on those for paramedic students; and the second half of the chapter determines specific practice education requirements for student midwives. It therefore examines supervision of learning and assessment of competence of AHP and midwifery students.

CHAPTER OBJECTIVES

1. Identify the HCPC's standards of proficiency and competencies that allied health profession students need to achieve during their pre-registration programme, including during practice placement.

2. Examine the specific requirements for paramedic students during practice placement, and the assessment of paramedic students' practice competence.
3. Specify standards of proficiency and competencies that student midwives have to achieve during practice placement, and the unique ways in which they are assessed in practice, including grading clinical practice.
4. Recognise the challenges involved in supervising practice-based learning for AHP and midwifery students during clinical practice, and some of the ways of resolving them; and the support that practice-based learning supervisors, practice educators and practice assessors can draw on when needed.

SUPERVISING PRACTICE-BASED LEARNING FOR ALLIED HEALTH PROFESSION STUDENTS, AND THEIR STANDARDS OF PROFICIENCY

Enabling students and learners to acquire skills for safe and effective practice is a crucial component of all health and social care profession programmes. In addition to knowledge gained from own research as well as the planned activities drafted by practice learning supervisors to enable learning, professional and regulatory bodies provide informed guidance on how clinical skills can be learnt. For instance, several healthcare profession organisations publish separate profession-specific standards for practice learning supervisors (referred to as 'practice educator' by the HCPC [2017]), such as the College of Operating Department Practitioners' (CODP) (2009) *Standards, Recommendations and Guidance for Mentors and Practice Placements*.

The HCPC's (2017a) *Standards of Education and Training Guidance* provides recommendations for the design of pre-qualifying AHP education curricula, which is supported by specific standards of proficiency (SOP) for each of the 16 allied healthcare professions (HCPC, 2017b) that it currently regulates. The standards of proficiency determine the professional competence that each profession's pre-registration students have to achieve for their name to be entered on the HCPC professional register. Consequently, the HCPC has published SOP for:

1. Arts therapists
2. Biomedical scientists
3. Chiropodists/Podiatrists
4. Clinical scientists
5. Dietitians
6. Hearing aid dispensers
7. Occupational therapists
8. Operating department practitioners
9. Orthoptists

10. Paramedics
11. Physiotherapists
12. Practitioner psychologists
13. Prosthetists/Orthotists
14. Radiographers
15. Social workers in England
16. Speech and language therapists

Other healthcare professions – such as clinical perfusion scientists, dance movement therapists, sports therapists and complementary therapists, who are not yet regulated by the HCPC and generally already have their own separate professional bodies – can join the HCPC at some point through a formal process of application and approval, and thereafter their standards of proficiencies can be identified.

The HCPC indicates that all 16 professions have at least one professional title (e.g. Clinical Psychologist, Therapeutic Radiographer) that is protected by law, and include those shown in the above list. This means, for example, that anyone using the title 'Physiotherapist' or 'Dietitian' must be registered with the HCPC; and that it is a criminal offence for someone to claim that they are registered with the HCPC when they are not, or to use any of the HCPC's protected titles. If anyone does, the HCPC intend to prosecute them for this (HCPC, 2017b: 1). Since 2013, social work in England has also been instituted under the regulation of HCPC.

AHP students have to demonstrate competence in each of these SOP enroute to becoming a registrant in their chosen profession. The SOP define the scope of practice for each profession at the point of registration, and therefore constitute areas of knowledge, skills, behaviour and values to enable the registrant to 'practise lawfully, safely and effectively'.

For physiotherapists for example the SOP are detailed in *Standards of Proficiency – Physiotherapists* (HCPC, 2013). All SOP incorporate 15 generic statements that all HCPC SOP are based on, along with a number of profession-specific standards. Profession-specific standards for physiotherapists, for example, under generic statement 4, 'be able to practise as an autonomous professional, exercising their own professional judgement' (2013: 8), include:

4.1 be able to assess a professional situation, determine the nature and severity of the problem and call upon the required knowledge and experience to deal with the problem

4.2 be able to make reasoned decisions to initiate, continue, modify or cease techniques or procedures, and record the decisions and reasoning appropriately

4.3 be able to initiate resolution of problems and be able to exercise personal initiative

4.5 be able to make and receive appropriate referrals.

As you may have noted, all above selected SOP are skills or competence-based, that is, abilities that pre-registration student physiotherapists will have learnt by the point of registration with the HCPC. As for the paramedic profession, the specific SOP are detailed in *Standards of Proficiency – Paramedics* (HCPC, 2014a), which as mentioned above is also based on 15 generic statements. Examples of profession-specific standards for paramedics under the statement 'be able to draw on appropriate knowledge and skills to inform practice' (statement 14) include:

14.4 know how to position or immobilise patients correctly for safe and effective interventions

14.5 know the indications and contra-indications of using specific paramedic techniques in pre-hospital and out-of-hospital care, including their limitations and modifications

14.12 be able to conduct a thorough and detailed physical examination of the patient using appropriate skills to inform clinical reasoning and guide the formulation of a differential diagnosis across all age ranges.

ACTIVITY 8.1   SOP FOR YOUR ALLIED HEALTH PROFESSION

Unless you have done so already, access the HCPC SOP for your allied health profession, and peruse them in detail to ascertain your understanding of them. Then think from the stance of the pre-registration student and ask yourself whether the student's understanding of these standards will be exactly the same as yours.

PRACTICE EDUCATION FOR AHP STUDENTS

Generally, AHP students acquire professional knowledge in the academic setting, along with a range of practice skills mainly by simulation, as is the case with most healthcare professions. However, most service user intervention skills are learnt while 'in the field' or practice placement under the guidance of practice educators, or practice supervisors (or mentors). The HCPC identifies the 'practice educator' as: 'A person who is responsible for a learner's education during their practice-based learning and has received appropriate training for this role' (HCPC, 2017a: 52).

To fulfil the role of practice educator, the HCPC (2017a: 44) requires that practice educators 'are trained and that this is followed up with regular refresher training and support'. The HCPC adds that if 'practice educators are involved in assessing learners, they should be prepared to do so through training in a way that is consistent across all practice-based learning on the programme'.

The practice educator role is akin to the practice supervisor role in nursing and midwifery, which, as noted in Chapter 1, comes under different titles in different healthcare professions. Fundamentally, it requires the practice educator to perform patient care duties safely and effectively, that is, in accordance with the procedures and clinical guidelines approved by the healthcare employer; to facilitate learning for specific AHP students; and maybe to assess students' competence, unless a designated assessor does this. Each of these three practice educator roles comprises several functions. However, there is some inconsistency in the title of the role in allied health professions, with practice educator and mentor titles used interchangeably at the moment. Certainly, this is the case in national and global emergency care systems, with inconsistency therefore in the use of the role titles.

Additionally, in radiography and other AHP practice educators can opt to undertake a short programme to become 'accredited' practice educators, as noted in Chapter 1 of this book. Furthermore, as is the case with all HCPC registrants, practice educators have to comply with the HCPC's (2016) *Standards of Conduct, Performance and Ethics*.

The next section examines in some detail specific ways in which AHP students learn practice competencies during practice placement and are assessed on these and on SOP, by referring to paramedic students as an example; and the latter half of the chapter examines the nature of supervising midwifery students' learning and assessing them during practice placements.

PRACTICE EDUCATION FOR PARAMEDIC STUDENTS DURING PRACTICE PLACEMENT

Paramedicine as a profession is relatively new. Until the beginning of the twenty-first century, 'ambulance drivers' followed an apprenticeship-type model with learning from teaching occurring whilst carrying out emergency duties with a more experienced member of staff. However, with the increasing evidence supporting more invasive procedures and pharmacological interventions, a greater need for better educated out-of-hospital practitioners was deemed necessary. This led to registration for paramedics with the HCPC, with the associated move to a higher education threshold qualification.

All paramedics in the United Kingdom must adhere to SOP as set out by the HCPC. Student paramedics pass the programme's formative and summative assessments on their journey to (and beyond) registration. These encompass a wide range of cognitive, psychomotor and behavioural learning, both in the university setting, and during practice placement. Of course, most of the practice placement learning that a student paramedic undertakes is in the ambulance environment.

However, there are no specific national standards required for supervising paramedic students and the literature on paramedic student supervision is scant. Although the need for standardised and qualified practice educators is outlined, no standard currently exists, as observed by Armitage (2010) and Lane (2014), and as noted in the HCPC's (2017a) standards of AHP education. Armitage suggests that paramedic 'mentors' used to mean the practice educator-type role, and for such a pivotal role it is worth establishing the standards that are expected of all practice educators.

Depending on the ambulance service, the student's learning may be supervised by:

- A named, qualified practice educator or mentor for the duration of the placement hours.
- A named, qualified practice educator or mentor for some of the placement hours, with some hours working with a qualified member of staff.
- A qualified member of staff, but not a qualified practice educator or supervisor, for the duration of the placement hours.

It is accepted that there are difficulties in out-of-hospital supervision of practice learning. Unlike other health professionals, ambulance staff typically work as a two-person team, in a mobile ambulance, with little or no base station visits. This means that the practice educator or supervisor of learning must go in an ambulance with a student, away from a base. Ambulances are difficult spaces to work in, with little room, so any additional staff will reduce the space available in the back of a vehicle for attending to the service user.

ASSESSING PARAMEDIC STUDENTS' PRACTICE COMPETENCE

Practice educators can assess the competence of students on each of the paramedic standards during practice placement in a number of different ways, using some of the different methods of practice assessment identified in Chapter 6. However, for standard 14.4 ('know how to position or immobilise patients correctly for safe and effective interventions') above, for example, the practice educator requires the student to demonstrate their ability to do so, and the practice educator observes the student performing this intervention directly (i.e. by direct observation).

A number of paramedic standards can be assessed by continuous assessment, but many of them logically lend themselves to assessment by direct observation. The PAD or practice competencies document usually requires the practice educator to assess students on each competency by two or three different assessment methods. The PAD identifies the specific competencies that comprise service user clinical interventions that must be assessed by direct observation, whereby the learner performs the clinical intervention while being closely monitored by the practice educator.

For assessment by direct observation, there can be several practicalities that need to be considered and instituted for episodic and end-point formal assessment to be conducted effectively. The practicalities for assessing student nurses are detailed in the first box in Chapter 7 of this textbook.

ACTIVITY 8.2   THE PRACTICE ASSESSMENT DOCUMENT (PAD)

If you are a student practice educator, try and gain access to an up-to-date PAD as it contains competencies that students in your allied health profession must achieve by the end of a specific practice placement, either for year one, two or three of the course.

To become a practice educator, paramedics initially need to have consolidated their learning from their pre-registration education (e.g. by shadowing or being supervised) and acquired the responsibilities and further competence related to the responsibilities that they have in the practice area where they are employed.

Following preparation for the practice educator role, they will be able to facilitate students' learning and teach them. Learning occurs in a variety of clinical settings, such as in the patient's home, the ambulance hub, at the roadside, in a vehicle and at the ambulance station or whilst on a standby position, and includes planned and opportunistic learning. However, teaching and learning for students need to be planned in advance, and with creativity, and where possible every opportunity used wisely to enable students to learn more widely and effectively, and be assessed for competence to practise. Student practice educators as relatively new registrants gradually assimilate further new roles and responsibilities and also adopt various teaching and learning methods.

What this generally means then is that some assessments are typically carried out during placement hours, 'shadowing' a student during usual working hours, and some assessments occur in the university setting (see box below).

EXAMPLES OF PLACEMENT VERSUS UNIVERSITY ASSESSMENT

Placement assessment:

Communication skills	Communication skills can be assessed during placement hours. This is because an assessor can view the actual interaction with a patient.

University assessment:

Advanced Life Support	More invasive skills are typically assessed in a simulated environment in the university.

**REFLECTION POINT 8.1:   STUDENT ASSESSMENT RELATED
TO INVASIVE INTERVENTIONS**

Why do you think more invasive procedures are more likely to be carried out in a simulated environment rather than on an actual patient? What do you think are the ethical implications? What do you think are the moral implications?

In response to the above action point you may have thought that anyone who hasn't yet demonstrated and proved their competence at an invasive procedure, should not perform the procedure on an actual service user as they can potentially, maybe unknowingly, harm the service user, i.e. it is unethical, and also in breach of the HCPC (2016) code of practice.

So, the student paramedic will be assessed through a mixture of assessment episodes and instances, to ensure not only competency but also consistency, for example on one or multiple occasions, based on their clinical practice competencies document.

As for the pass/fail assessment criteria, there are generic ambulance service 'clinical practice guidelines' in the UK published by the Joint Royal Colleges Ambulance Liaison Committee (JRCALC) (2017). The aim of these guidelines is to 'ensure uniformity in the delivery of high quality patient care' (2017: 1) and therefore also underpins the pre-registration paramedic programme. However, different ambulance services and organisations may still have different guidelines, drug protocols for different treatment and care pathways, and paramedics in the United Kingdom work within a scope of practice specified by their employer.

Conversely, it is noteworthy that for nursing the PAD is being widely standardised, such as the cross-London PAD, which essentially means that the translation of NMC's SOP for nurses is identically implemented by all London healthcare settings where students have practice placements (e.g. Fish et al., 2016). Additionally, for the majority of healthcare professions, there are clinical guidelines published by other UK authoritative organisations such as NICE, Resuscitation Council UK, etc. which are relevant to paramedic practice.

**REFLECTION POINT 8.2:   PROTOCOLS, GUIDELINES FOR
PARAMEDIC INTERVENTIONS**

Why do you think there are differences in scope of practice between different ambulance services? What could be the advantages of all paramedics working to exactly the same protocol, and what could be the disadvantages?

Commenting on the introduction of the *UK Ambulance Services Clinical Practice Guidelines 2016* (Association of Ambulance Chief Executives and Joint Royal Colleges Ambulance Liaison Committee, 2016), Irving et al. (2016) indicate that quite a few new guidelines have been included, and others significantly revised, since the 2013 edition, such as end-of-life care, but much needed guidance for some situations as sepsis have not been included. However, hopefully they will be in later editions of the publication.

As noted earlier in this chapter paramedicine is a relatively new health profession, and good practice for various service user interventions is still emerging. However, you are likely to agree that concerted effort must be made to establish communication between different paramedic services as this can create a medium for identifying more effective practices, and therefore benchmarking good practice.

CASE STUDY 8.1:   PARAMEDIC STUDENT'S PROBLEMATIC ATTITUDE

Andy is a paramedic student. He is very clever and passes all his written exams with very high marks and is consistently good in his practical assessments. Andy is polite and helpful to the teaching staff and is popular among his fellow students.

However, informal feedback is received by the course team that, during practice placement, Andy appears rude with patients he doesn't deem require an ambulance. This is more in terms of body language (putting his hands in his pockets when speaking to patients) and appearing uninterested if the person is not acutely unwell.

What questions might you want to ask yourself to help formulate an action plan for Andy?

So, what does the organisation say about this type of behaviour? Most organisations will have a policy or procedure about such behaviours, which usually includes an example of inappropriate and unprofessional behaviours, and the need to initiate an action plan. The practice educator is aware that the intention of action plans for unprofessional behaviours is to formulate a corrective plan rather than a punitive one.

Is there an informal route or is this serious enough to warrant a formal plan? It depends how the terms formal and informal are defined by the organisation. However, these types of behaviours are enough to cause concern and should always be noted. If these behaviours are noted by a crewmate, they are usually also noted by service users and relatives and need to be addressed as soon as possible.

In conclusion, it's clear that the future of paramedic student supervision during practice placement is somewhat cloudy (e.g. Jones et al., 2012; Lane, 2014). No set standards exist in the United Kingdom, although some paramedic academics are going some way to highlight this issue.

Furthermore, there has been a shift in innovations in facilitation of learning such as a recent evaluative study of peer-learning, with some evidence to suggest that it is well regarded by students (Williams et al., 2015b). The findings of this study can also be incorporated into ambulance-based practice learning in the future because peer-teaching is found to be effective in the education of the paramedic students in developing teaching and supervision skills during their pre-registration programme, which can be further developed in their future career as a registered paramedic.

On the other hand, Lane's (2014: 198) research also identified at the time that there were 960 technicians who could accept the practice educator role, despite some existing practice educators showing a lack of interest and motivation in the practice educator role partly because they felt unsupported. Consequently, such situations and attitudes can negatively affect students' learning experience.

Highlighting the above concerns contributes to arguing for a joined-up approach in healthcare practice learning but consideration must be given to the unique nature of paramedicine. What is clear from the emerging evidence is that this must be a three-way process, involving not just the staff and students but the organisation too, as illustrated in Figure 8.1. Similarly, Jones et al. (2012) note that all paramedics should act as supervisors of learning, but healthcare organisations need nationally approved processes and structure to accommodate this requirement.

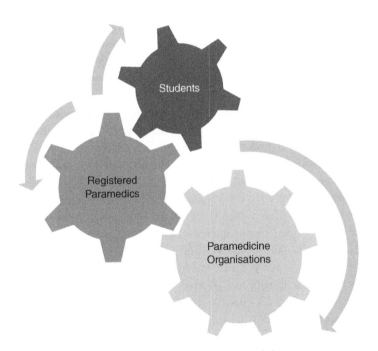

Figure 8.1   A co-ordinated approach to student supervision

Mallik and McGowan (2007) completed a scoping exercise on the nature of practice education in five healthcare professions, namely dietetics, nursing, occupational therapy, physiotherapy and radiography, and concluded that although there are areas of good practice, 'these do so against the provision of well-supported, clearly supervised and adequately quality-assured practice education' (ibid.: 58). They recommend that such issues should be resolved by the various healthcare professions and need to be recognised and rewarded, and that collaborative work across the professions should be enhanced for achievement of more well-rounded practice education.

In contrast, Hinton (2009) reports on her experiences of mentoring Operating Department Practitioner (ODP) students in which she indicates that it is an activity that is beneficial not only for students, but for ODP practice learning supervisors as well.

MIDWIFERY STANDARDS OF PROFICIENCY AND COMPETENCIES

Preparing the next generation of midwives is a critical role undertaken in the practice setting by midwifery practice supervisors. They play a vital role in ensuring that students are prepared appropriately for safe and competent practice, and within healthcare settings this is fundamental for their development and education. Practice supervisors are thus an essential component in preparing students for registration with the NMC, the professional body that governs midwifery. The NMC's (2018a) *Standards for Student Supervision and Assessment* applies to midwifery students as well as nursing, and comes into force when the NMC approves its implementation for each university individually at approval events.

The NMC (2009) sets the standards of education, training and conduct that midwives need to deliver high-quality healthcare consistently throughout their careers. As the health and care landscape has evolved and transformed the way that care is delivered, the NMC is currently undertaking consultations that will renovate the standards for midwifery education and ultimately prepare them to deliver a more contemporary and responsive standard of healthcare to meet the future needs of the public.

Until the new standards have been reviewed during the consultation period to reshape midwifery education in the United Kingdom (UK), midwives and students will continue to be guided by the current standards for pre-registration midwifery education (NMC, 2009) and be conversant with circulars that impact upon preparing a workforce that is fit-for-practice and fit-for-purpose at the point of registration. These standards include European Directives (European Parliament and the Council, 2013) and the essential skills clusters for midwifery education. Student midwives have been required to spend at least 50% of their time in clinical practice (NMC, 2009), working with a sign-off mentor for at least 40% of this time (NMC, 2008).

At varying stages of midwifery education students require different types and levels of support. It is essential that practice learning supervision incorporates giving support, assistance and guidance in learning new skills, and also in adopting new behaviours and acquiring new attitudes. Research on practice learning supervision in midwifery and nursing demonstrates that positive student–supervisor relationships influence students' self-esteem, their sense of belonging, confidence and the quality of the learning achieved in the practice setting (Frazer et al., 2014).

Furthermore, there are many components involved in the process of practice supervision that are dependent upon each other for success. The relationship between practice supervisor and student midwife, the HEI and practice setting within which the practice-based learning occurs, can present potential challenges for all parties involved.

It is essential that midwives from the practice setting and midwifery lecturers from the HEI have a partnership approach to meet the needs of the student and ensure that they have continuity of supervision during practice placement. The current support for student midwives in the practice setting in conjunction with the HEI can be one of the following:

- Personal tutor/Academic advisor
- Midwife practice supervisor
- Link lecturer (also known as Academic in Practice)
- Midwifery placements co-ordinator

Students are allocated a personal tutor who provides personal, professional and educational support during their pre-registration programme. Within clinical placements, each student is allocated a practice supervisor who provides support and is involved in the student's learning and continuous assessment. There are also link lecturers allocated to each NHS Trust who are able to provide support throughout the placement.

Whilst on practice placements, students work with practice supervisors who are suitably experienced and who have been formally prepared to undertake this role (NMC, 2009: Standard 11). Practice supervisors are required to attend regular update sessions, which include any changes to the curriculum, and to highlight issues experienced by students.

The organisation and management of practice placements for all midwifery students is the remit of the Midwifery Placements Co-ordinator. Students and nominated midwives in the practice setting receive programme plans at the commencement of the programme and details of individual placement allocations at the beginning of each academic year. All placements are carefully monitored to ensure they are not overloaded with students from a number of different courses and that there are a sufficient number of practice assessors to support the students across the practice settings.

Examples of competencies that student midwives usually need to achieve during their pre-registration programme include:

- Recognise the signs of labour
- Participate in midwifery assessment to establish maternal and foetal well-being
- Participate in parent education to ensure health, safety, protection and security of baby
- Recognise risk factors in childbearing and take appropriate action including responsiveness to obstetric emergencies

- Provide appropriate care to women once they have given birth
- Explain lactation and techniques for positioning and attachment of the baby during the first feed.

ASSESSING PRE-REGISTRATION STUDENT MIDWIVES AND GRADING CLINICAL COMPETENCIES

The practice setting is where students learn under direct supervision and become competent through hands-on care of women and their families through the pregnancy journey, and later through indirect supervision. In 2009 the NMC introduced mandatory grading of clinical practice within the midwifery curricula, divided into four domains and five essential skill clusters (ESC). The performance of the student and assessment of clinical skill acquisition is graded by their practice assessor in the practice setting.

Prior to the introduction of mandatory grading several HEIs across the UK would have embedded some form of grading for midwifery practice within their curricula. The current midwifery programmes across the UK provide the student with several tools to have at their disposal to monitor their learning and progress and evidence of achievement of competence at appropriate stages of the training programme. Some of these documents include:

- Ongoing Record of Achievement (ORA)
- Competency Log book and Essential Skills Clusters (ESCs)
- European Union Directives.

The assessment and grading of students' clinical performance and achievement is complex. A variety of methods are used to grade practice, including:

- Objective structured clinical examination (OSCE)
- Grading tools/grids
- Triad (or tripartite) assessment.

Grading tools/grids can be developed with explicit descriptions of students' performance for the assessment against three or four grades to measure and quantify a grade for attainment. In accordance with the NMC (2009) it is only the midwifery mentors' grades that are of any significance as that is where attainment of clinical skill and competence is recognised. The OSCE and Triad is often graded in partnership between the academic midwifery team and midwifery practice assessors, either at the HEI or in the practice setting.

The concepts of how best to grade practice, by whom and how much of this grade contributes towards the degree classification is unclear within the NMC documentation and is therefore open to interpretation by each HEI within the UK, as found by Fisher et al. (2017) for example. See Table 8.1 for a snapshot of a proforma that is used at one UK university for grading a competency that has been actioned from the NMC (2009) SOP for a first-year midwifery student.

Table 8.1 Grading a competency for a first-year midwifery student

Criterion statement	0 FAIL Clear	1 FAIL Marginal	2 PASS Satisfactory	3 PASS Good	4 PASS Very good	5 PASS Excellent
Perceives deviations from the norm and seeks appropriate help	Unable to interpret clinical findings and therefore fails to seek any help	Requires assistance to identify a deviation from the norm and fails to seek appropriate help	Identifies deviations from the norm and from whom to seek assistance	Recognises deviations from the norm and seeks appropriate help	Recognises deviations from the norm, discusses the significance and seeks appropriate help	Recognises deviations from the norm, discusses the significance and the implications for midwifery practice. Seeks appropriate help
Communicates effectively with women	Fails to communicate effectively with women	Demonstrates limited communication skills with women	Communicates effectively with women most of the time	Communicates effectively throughout this episode of care	Able to use all levels of communication effectively	Communicates effectively at all levels and suggests ways of improving communication
...	...	...	...	...	...	...

Similarly, the setting and environment of the grading of practice – be it in the practice setting or a proxy practice, such as a portfolio or through simulation – is also undefined by the NMC. Grading of practice allows for recognition of merit beyond a binary system of pass/fail (Andre, 2000) and reflects a value and decision made on performance.

CHALLENGES IN THE PRACTICE SETTING AND THEIR EFFECTS ON PRACTICE SUPERVISION

At the end of every practice placement throughout the three-year BSc (Hons) Degree leading to professional registration as a midwife, students are invited to evaluate their experience. Usually, several opportunities are afforded to students during their three-year programme to provide feedback on the practice supervisor and practice assessor. This is usually during contact with the link lecturer/academic in practice, or with the personal tutor, in module evaluation where clinical placements are a feature and in end-of-year online feedback.

This combined with the end-of-programme evaluation always yields constructive feedback and shines a light on areas of good practice and areas of poor practice in practice supervision. The majority of students report having 'good, effective' supervision with a nominated practice assessor for the required 40% of supervision. Themes emerge from evaluations and conversations with students when asked to report areas of good practice supervision, which tend to include those identified in the box below.

AREAS OF GOOD PRACTICE SUPERVISION IDENTIFIED BY MIDWIFERY STUDENTS

Practice supervisors who:

- Listen to the student's anxiety about learning and converging theory and practice
- Value the student's attempts at creating 'learning contracts' and taking responsibility for their learning
- Provide constructive feedback with 'tips' on how to improve and develop knowledge and clinical skills
- Praise achievements made in the acquisition of new clinical skills/competencies
- Incorporate the 'check and challenge' process
- Empower students by listening to their potential concerns in relation to practice supervision, and manage them effectively before escalating to other practice supervisors, link lecturer or personal tutor.

Subsequent to evaluations by students, and as an incentive and for the purpose of the clinician's own professional portfolio, at some HEIs the Lead Midwifery

Academic sends letters of commendation and praise to practice supervisors that students have rated as champions in the process of practice supervision.

The following section considers some of the main challenges related to student midwives and practice supervision. Some of the most common challenges are that increasing time pressures on midwifery staff delivering care, clinical environments becoming more complex, and lack of time for students have a negative effect on the student experience. Lack of continuity of supervision often compounds this and results in perceptions of poor practice supervision, as also found by research conducted by Bradshaw et al. (2013). Common problems associated with poor practice supervision and assessment that students report in evaluations include:

- Lack of continuity in practice supervision
- Increased number of midwife practice supervisors over a short period of time
- Being supervised on an increasing number of shifts by newly qualified midwives
- Practice supervisors who avoid taking full responsibility for students
- Lack of knowledge and skills related to guideline recommendations from practice supervisors
- Practice assessors reluctant to sign attainment of competencies as 'pass'
- Lack of time for supervisor and student to meet during the clinical shift.

Lack of continuity in the practice setting causes student midwives to raise concerns and complain that they have not been able to have their SOP or competencies signed off at differing stages of their placement. This potentially can inhibit the student from progressing, as it appears that they have not met the required standards at set points of the programme. It stands to reason that this will cause unnecessary stress in the student especially if they have been exposed and engaged in the care of women and their babies, and feel that they have achieved the required competency. This can lead to frustration not only for the student but also for the practice assessor.

For practice assessors, the responsibility of confirming attainment of competency and proficiency at all stages of the programme leading to registration is fundamental. However, as the demands and pressures of delivering high standards of care are of paramount importance it may be that the midwife has been compromised with time during a working shift and has not had sufficient time to complete the student's documentation.

Working in a professional environment in the practice setting often involves time constraints, and at the same time students and practice supervisors have competing demands. Therefore, every effort needs to be made to have some protected time with the student midwife to support and facilitate learning in practice settings and fulfil the NMC requirements for the programme's end.

In a study undertaken by Richmond (2006) to review the perceptions and experience of midwives in their role as mentors in two NHS Trust hospitals, it emerged that the difficulties and challenges for effective practice learning supervision tend to occur in four categories:

1. lack of time to teach the student during the working day;
2. too much paperwork to complete;
3. problematic students;
4. problems with the practice learning supervisor's self-confidence.

> ## REFLECTION POINT 8.3:   RESOLVING DIFFICULTIES AND CHALLENGES OF PRACTICE SUPERVISION
>
> Think of the categories of challenges identified above, and either make some notes, or discuss with a peer how such difficulties and challenges can be averted or resolved.

The majority of midwives are able to absorb the role of practice supervisor into their working role, but strategies need to be in place within the practice setting to support practice supervisors in their role especially since there is an onus on midwives to undertake more clinical teaching.

Consequently, short video files can be compiled through collaboration between midwife practice supervisors, academics and learning technologists, which can capture in the safe environment of a clinical skills laboratory at the HEI examples of positive and negative student–supervisor/–educator relationships. These files can be used as vignettes to aid supervisor and assessor preparation, and demonstrate to students what they should avoid, and the standards to aspire to during their three-year programme.

Furthermore, alongside the inbuilt mechanisms within the HEI for student feedback and student representative meetings, several actions can be taken to resolve the challenges of practice supervision and address those that student midwives tend to voice, including:

- Planned regular meetings in the practice setting with link lecturers and practice supervisors (if and when available)
- Practice supervisor and practice assessor updates in the practice setting delivered by a link lecturer
- Sharing of good practice and discussions on how to provide quality practice supervision that demonstrates compassion towards students
- In conjunction with a Practice Development Midwife, establish partnerships in practice supervision where several midwives from different bands and clinical areas are matched with a group of students
- Practice supervisor champion roles emerging from the clinical setting to act as the key link between students and link lecturers.
- Development of a 'Check and Challenge' (explained shortly) proforma
- Dates of link lecturer visits in advance with contact details for both practice supervisors and students

At times, during an end-of-programme student evaluation, students indicate that although whilst on duty, and at every opportunity the Head of Midwifery (HoM) meets with them and enquires about their progress, they feel unable to raise concerns or complain about practice supervision. As a direct response, the academic team and the HoM can design a proforma known as 'Check and Challenge' (McCalmont and Lees, 2015), that can be used to monitor practice supervision, enquire about the student experience and protect the supervisor–student relationship.

Over time the 'Check and Challenge' process by the HoM or other senior midwives in practice can become integrated and valued by practice supervisors and students, according to McCalmont and Lees (2015). This tool enables supervisors of learning to be challenged by a professional and not the student, and has no repercussions on either party involved, as each role and individual is respected and valued, and encouraged to maintain a high-quality performance in the best interest of the students and women in their care.

Whilst a plethora of examples can be cited to demonstrate good and effective practice learning supervision, case studies related to the challenges or barriers to supervision of learning can be used to explore how problems can be avoided and how knowledge, skills and professionalism can be passed on to students.

CASE STUDY 8.2:   CONCERNS RELATED TO A SECOND-YEAR STUDENT MIDWIFE

Jenny is in her second year of the BSc (Hons) Degree midwifery programme. Practice supervisors have raised concerns about her limited engagement with pregnant women and inappropriate communication skills. Practice supervisors with the support of the link lecturer have been monitoring her engagement throughout year one of the programme where she has been signed off as meeting her competencies by a nominated midwife practice assessor while on placement. The practice supervisors and the nominated practice assessor felt that Jenny had met the competencies as a novice and provided her with further specific learning points at the end of her first year. However, as Jenny progresses into the second year of her training, practice supervisors from a different clinical placement raise the same concerns and she fails to meet the desired outcomes at the next point of progression.

Identify the range of actions that can be taken to support Jenny so that she can achieve the required practice competencies.

Following a tripartite discussion with the practice supervisor, student and link lecturer, a plan of action could be agreed to provide Jenny with the opportunity to succeed. Table 8.2 illustrates the actions that could be agreed to support Jenny achieve the required practice competencies.

Table 8.2   Support for Jenny to achieve required practice competencies

	ACTION PLAN (Failing student)	
Practice supervisor	**Universal goals**	**Link lecturer**
Monitoring competencies	Collaborative agreement to support the student	Design a personal development plan (PDP)
Exposure to clinical experiences	Agreed and achievable targets	Additional reading
Consistency of practice supervisors	Regular meetings in the practice setting with practice supervisor, student and link lecturer	Additional guided studies for area that require attention
Completion of logbook, ESCs and European (EU) Directives		Create formative opportunities in the clinical skills laboratory to rehearse skills
Regular meetings between practice assessor and student	Additional formative assessments for acquisition of clinical skills	Video recording in the clinical skills laboratory to enhance communication skills
	Constructive feedback	One-to-one episodes of care with feedback on performance and development of underpinning knowledge in the clinical setting
		Support from link lecturer and personal tutor

Other tools that are used to monitor the performance of an underperforming student include: Check and Challenge proforma, learning contract, bespoke formative activities to support learning in the practice setting. Figure 8.2 outlines the potential outcomes for the student following provision of an environment that is conducive to learning, and within an agreed length of time.

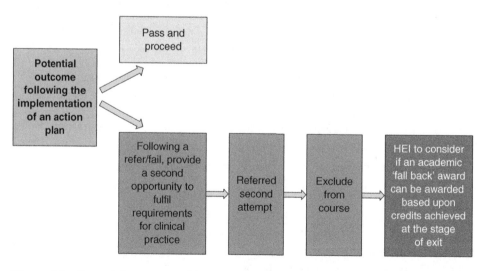

Figure 8.2   Potential outcomes for a student who fails a competency

It takes courage to fail a student, and it is well documented that assessors have previously been reluctant to fail students as they perceive it as a direct reflection on themselves and their performance, and are often anxious about managing the student's reaction (Black et al., 2014). However, it is evident that having the courage to initiate difficult conversations and provide clear, honest, constructive written and verbal feedback is at the core of managing an underperforming student (Duffy, 2013), as discussed in detail in Chapter 7.

RECOMMENDATIONS FOR EFFECTIVE MIDWIFERY PRACTICE EDUCATION

- Continue to prepare student midwives to be fit-for-practice at the point of registration.
- Midwives and managers to consider having 'supported learning time' during practice placement not only to support the student in attaining clinical competence, but also to complete the relevant documentary evidence of progress and achievement.
- Where possible to provide continuity of practice learning supervision.
- Clinical staff must be cognisant of the additional pressure on a newly qualified midwife to automatically take up the role of practice supervisor relatively soon after qualifying.
- Maintain close relationships and communication links between the practice supervisors, practice assessors, academic team and student.
- Continue with the 'Check and Challenge' process.
- Practice supervisors and link lecturers to be supportive and offer appropriate guidance to the next generation of midwives.

SUPPORT FOR PRACTICE SUPERVISORS, PRACTICE EDUCATORS, PRACTICE ASSESSORS

With the relatively wide-ranging problematic situations cited in this chapter, one solution is the support mechanisms that are available to practice supervisors, practice educators and practice assessors. A number of support avenues are identified in some detail in Chapter 7 of this book, mainly related to managing underachieving students, including PEF/CHEF, link lecturer, etc.

CHAPTER SUMMARY

While focusing on the supervision of allied health profession and midwifery students during practice placement, and the assessment of competencies, this chapter has explored key aspects of practice education requirements for AHP students, with specific focus on paramedic students' practice education requirements, the second half of the chapter determining the practice education requirements for student midwives. It consequently addressed the HCPC's standards of proficiency for allied health professionals and the competencies to be achieved by students during practice education, with particular focus on paramedic students' practice competence. Then the chapter examined the midwifery standards of proficiency and competencies, and the assessing and grading of pre-registration student midwives' clinical practice. Some of the issues related to both allied health profession and midwifery students were also discussed.

FURTHER OPTIONAL READING

1. For the justification of student paramedics gaining practice experience in a wide range of care settings in addition to ambulances, see:

    - Jennings, K. and Rae, A. (2016) 'Opportunities for paramedic practice-based education', *Journal of Paramedic Practice*, 8(4): 174–175.

2. For details related to paramedic pre-registration programmes, see:

    - College of Paramedics (2015) *Paramedic Curriculum Guidance*. Bridgewater: College of Paramedics.

3. For recent research on assessing student midwives, see:

    - Newton, J., Taylor, R.M. and Crighton, L. (2017) 'A mixed-methods study exploring sign-off mentorship practices in relation to Nursing and Midwifery Council Standards', *Journal of Clinical Nursing*, 26(19–20): 3056–3066.

To access further resources related to this chapter, visit **https://study.sagepub.com/gopee4e** where a range of learning and teaching materials are provided.

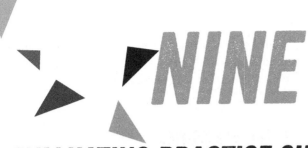

EVALUATING PRACTICE SUPERVISION, AND CONTINUING PROFESSIONAL DEVELOPMENT FOR SUPERVISORS AND ASSESSORS

INTRODUCTION

Having explored a range of components that should make supervision of practice-based learning and practice assessment of healthcare students effective, safe and of high quality, this chapter asks how we know for sure that these activities do actually fulfil the purposes for which we engage in them, and competently. How valuable are our activities for our students? Consequently, this chapter focuses on the evaluation role of practice supervisors and practice assessors.

Evaluation can be a satisfying experience when we receive positive feedback on our teaching, be it practice-based or classroom-based, and if it identifies components for further improvement. Evaluation of practice learning entails healthcare professionals self-monitoring the effectiveness and quality of all their supervision of learning activities. Evaluation information thus forms the basis for progressive learning, and thereby potentially also contributes to the supervisor's own continuing professional development (CPD).

The chapter therefore examines reasons for evaluating practice learning supervision and practice assessment activities, and the general nature of the concept evaluation, which it does by addressing:

- precisely why we evaluate, what evaluation is, and what practice supervisors and practice assessors evaluate
- who should be involved
- how to evaluate, including frameworks for evaluation
- what to do with the evaluation data
- practice supervisors' and practice assessors' CPD, including revalidation.

These areas are discussed in relation to practice supervisors' practice-based facilitation of learning and continuous assessment of competence roles, and to university-based undergraduate and postgraduate course delivery.

CHAPTER OBJECTIVES

1. Identify and elaborate on a number of reasons for evaluating practice learning supervision activities such as facilitation of learning and assessment of competence.
2. Explain the nature and various features of evaluation, and who is involved in evaluating practice learning supervision activities.
3. Identify different ways of evaluating clinically based and academically based teaching and assessment.
4. Justify the action that should be taken following evaluation and the likely difficulties and opportunities.
5. Explain how the challenges encountered by practice supervisors and practice assessors are also opportunities for professional development, as well as for meeting the requirement for continuing learning and updating.

WHY EVALUATE PRACTICE LEARNING SUPERVISION AND PRACTICE ASSESSOR ACTIVITIES?

The reason for evaluating practice-based supervision of learning activities is that it is logical to do so to check that our actions are, and remain, beneficial to learners and effective. Healthcare registrants engage in evaluation of care and treatment continually when on duty, and therefore it is not an unfamiliar activity, as it is also a pre-registration SOP to be achieved (e.g. NMC, 2018b, Platform 4). Previously, the NMC (2008) identified 'Evaluation of learning' as a key domain of supporting learning in practice settings, which included mentors being receptive to students' evaluation of placement-based learning, engaging in self- and peer-evaluation to facilitate professional and personal development, etc.

ACTIVITY 9.1   WHY EVALUATE?

Other than evaluation of learning being a required activity, consider for yourself the question why we should evaluate what we do in the course of our duties. Then consider what we can do with the information obtained from evaluations. Make notes of your thoughts on this.

As noted above, evaluation is an activity that we engage in quite frequently, formally and informally, and at times without realising that we are doing so. Thus, with the problem-solving approach to health and social care, we engage in assessment of service users' health problems, plan of care and interventions, and implementation, and continuously evaluate their effect. More widely, systematic approaches to most novel ventures entail evaluation of the plans implemented and decisions about any action that needs to be taken subsequent to evaluation.

There are a number of reasons for evaluation. If practice supervisors do not evaluate how well they are fulfilling their supervisory activities, then they are taking for granted that their actions meet their learners' learning needs. They are assuming that learners are satisfied with the learning provided, and that they are fulfilling their roles effectively. Formal evaluations provide evidence of the effectiveness of our activities, and often reveal unexpected findings, as the impressions of the recipients of the practice supervision might be different from those anticipated by the supervisor.

In addition to identifying improvement points for subsequent supervisory activities, further reasons for evaluating practice supervision and practice assessment are:

- To anticipate likely problem areas and take preventive actions
- To gauge whether the student's learning is pitched at the appropriate level and in appropriate detail
- For continuing self-monitoring of competence in professional practice, which is often a requirement of employment, and a component of annual development and performance review
- It is a component of the practice setting's quality assurance mechanism
- To gauge progress made
- It is professional 'good practice'.

Evaluation performed for the purposes of quality assurance can be done through looking at structures (for example, resources), processes, procedures, standards and consistency. It is performed for quality enhancement, which is for improvement through change and development. Evaluation can reveal any problematic aspects and which concerned the individual or group of students most, and it can identify areas of confusion or misunderstanding. Consequently, when problematic areas are uncovered, they also present opportunities for improvement, for creativity, and for novel structures and activities to be suggested and instituted.

Four reasons for evaluation can be identified, namely:

1. Evaluation for knowledge – to identify areas of deficiency in care or teaching provision so that action can be taken to rectify the deficiency.
2. Evaluation for development – for engaging in educational or training activities based on evaluation results, and thereby growth and improvement for practice supervisors, team members and the organisation.
3. Evaluation for accountability – to ensure that duties have been performed as required.
4. Evaluation for management – that is, evaluation conducted as a management activity, with a view to identifying and resourcing any professional development requirement.

For university courses, course directors and module leaders evaluate to identify problems being encountered or foreseen by the students on the education programme, and to solve those problems, or avert them in future. At times, what is seen as an issue by students just needs further explaining or justifying.

Before evaluation of any activity, it is important to ascertain what the purposes of the activity are. Thus, if we are evaluating our teaching session, what were the specific aims of the session? The purpose of the teaching will have been to arm the recipient with relevant knowledge and to develop competence, and the purpose of the evaluation will be to check if this has happened. In view of the above-mentioned four reasons for evaluation, consider whether you evaluate your teaching for the purposes of accountability, to receive suggestions and explore associated ideas for the further development of your supervision of learning activities, or as a management exercise?

ACTIVITY 9.2   CAN EVALUATION OF TEACHING IMPROVE LEARNING?

Focusing on the practice supervisor's teaching role, consider the evaluation of teaching that you have experienced, and identify at least two ways in which you can improve your teaching to enhance learning for your learners.

Healthcare course lecturers are required to evaluate their teaching and act on the evaluation data. As for practice supervisors, following evaluation of teaching in the practice setting, the practice supervisor can follow up the teaching component by reflecting on their teaching. Subsequently, further reading materials or information to help rectify or supplement students' learning needs can be offered. Lecturers can arrange further teaching sessions on topics suggested in the evaluation information and can also adjust their subsequent teaching with a view to connecting more fully with the learner's learning needs.

Practice assessors also self-evaluate their assessment activities. At the university, lecturers often evaluate their structured lessons, be it a knowledge base component, or teaching a healthcare skill in the skills laboratory. They also evaluate how fit for purpose the modules and courses that they lead are.

As noted in Chapter 8, at the end of each practice placement, students are asked to evaluate the placement, often by the healthcare team in the practice setting, and always by the university. Practice supervisors can ask students to evaluate 'spoke' visits, or they may ask the student to engage in reflective write-ups that the practice supervisor will subsequently read. All HEIs have their own placement evaluation forms and criteria which students are now invited to complete electronically. Moreover, the RCN (2017a: 15–20) provides a comprehensive list of items for consideration when evaluating practice placements

WHAT IS 'EVALUATION'?

Evaluation is a key component of a systematic approach to care and treatment, and is also an inherent facet of care pathways.

ACTIVITY 9.3 WHAT DOES THE TERM 'EVALUATION' ITSELF MEAN?

Make brief notes on what you understand by the word 'evaluation'. What is it about?

Evaluation of the effectiveness of care given is important, as the goal of providing care is to restore health, and we need to know if this has been achieved. The term *evaluation* originates from the French word *evaluer*, meaning to work out the numerical value of something. In current usage in English, to evaluate means to judge or appraise the quality, value or worth of something (Brookes and O'Neill, 2017: 307). Various definitions of evaluation have been offered by interested parties over the years. For instance, Roberts et al. (2001) indicate that evaluation is essentially about making judgements about the value and worth of something against explicit, justifiable and appropriate criteria.

Thus, evaluation is the process of systematically collecting and analysing information in order to establish objective knowledge based on firm evidence. Furthermore, evaluation is also used as an empirical tool in the form of a research method involving in-depth exploration of the component being evaluated through data collection and analysis (Guba and Lincoln, 1989).

REFLECTION POINT 9.1:   WHAT DO WE EVALUATE?

When evaluating care in clinical practice, exactly what is it that we evaluate, and what are the different ways in which evaluation information is obtained?

Evaluation of care plans and goals is obviously to determine the effectiveness of the plans, which can be supplemented by feedback from the service user. Other terms that tend to have similar or overlapping meanings with evaluation are monitoring, quality appraisal and assessment. The term 'assessment', however, has distinct and specific meanings in healthcare, referring to assessment of patients' health problems and to assessing learners' competence. Thus, assessment usually refers to the collection of data against set criteria. It is therefore objective. Evaluation, on the other hand, refers to the values and personal judgement on whether action taken enabled the achievement of specified goals.

Returning to evaluation of practice supervision, this can also be public evaluation or private evaluation, external or internal, continuous or episodic/intermittent and final or interim (refers to timescale). Moreover, evaluation can be case-specific or generalised/holistic or analytical (see box for a brief explanation of these modes and types of evaluation).

WHO EVALUATES WHAT?

Public evaluation	Open evaluation of an activity by others
Private evaluation	Self-evaluation by the person who performed the teaching, for instance
External evaluation	Evaluation by others outside the organisation
Internal evaluation	Evaluation by departments or individuals inside the organisation
Continuous evaluation	Ongoing evaluation
Episodic/intermittent evaluation	Evaluation at set or specific times
Interim/final evaluation	Evaluation at the end of one or a series of activities
Case-specific evaluation	In-depth evaluation of one particular instance of an activity
Generalised (or holistic) evaluation	Inviting and gaining overall impressions
Analytical evaluation	Detailed evaluation, may include numerical data

Furthermore, evaluation can be quantitative or qualitative, formative or summative, formal or informal. Generally, for new topic areas, qualitative evaluation is likely to elicit data that can enable further development of the topic. For more established topic areas, quantitative data are sought to monitor or ascertain the likely ongoing effectiveness of the activity.

As for formative and summative evaluation, formative evaluation of care is a continuous activity, the frequency of which is adjusted according to the dependency level of the patient/service user, or to the criticality of their condition. With some service users who require longer-term care, or those in the community, evaluation may be recorded at longer intervals at specific set periods. Summative evaluations are conducted at end points, i.e. retrospectively, for example evaluation of a practice placement experience or a module.

Evaluation is also one of the four stages of the regular development review process of healthcare professionals identified in the *NHS KSF* (DH, 2004; NHS Employers, 2010). The first stage is the joint review of the individual's work against the demands of the post. This is in the context of the six core dimensions of healthcare work. The second is the personal development planning stage (PDP), the third is the learning and development stage, and the fourth is the evaluation stage. At the evaluation stage, the individual:

- reflects on the effectiveness of their learning and development of their knowledge and skills
- identifies how their learning has improved the application of their learning to their post
- feeds back to the organisation on how the learning and development can be improved.

In the context of evaluating practice supervision, this chapter addresses all the above aspects of evaluation except evaluation as a research method. Having examined why we need to evaluate practice supervision and practice assessor activities and exactly what evaluation is, it is also important to consider who evaluates before moving on to how practice supervisors evaluate their practice supervision.

WHO EVALUATES TEACHING AND LEARNING?

As mentioned earlier, evaluation can take different forms (see the box above titled 'Who evaluates what?'). Formative evaluation of practice-based teaching and learning is conducted through informal and formal mechanisms. It is a micro-level evaluation that practice supervisors perform informally when teaching clinical interventions, either in the clinical area or in university settings. It is a valuable internal mechanism for monitoring one's own competence through a continuous process of observation and sensory feedback.

There is also the formal evaluation mechanism that requires more concrete evidence to be gathered and reproduced when required. Formal evaluation mechanisms can manifest patterns of good or poor teaching delivery. These formal evaluation exercises take place periodically and allow scrutiny of the quality of theoretical and clinical learning. For instance, during the practice placement, the student also

> ### REFLECTION POINT 9.2: EVALUATION OF TEACHING IN THE PRACTICE SETTING
>
> Who, in your experience, evaluates the effectiveness of teaching, both planned and informal or opportunistic, in the health and social care setting?

engages in a continuous process of informal evaluation of the extent to which the practice setting is also an effective learning environment.

In general, it is the recipient of the teaching, that is, the learner, who is best placed to evaluate the effectiveness of the teaching. The result of the teaching will usually emerge as the knowledge and skill acquired by the learner and is ultimately reflected in the quality of care they deliver to service users. In addition to the practice supervisor and practice assessor engaging in self-evaluation or self-monitoring the quality of their work-based teaching and assessment, quality and effectiveness can also be ascertained through peer evaluation.

Generally, there are at least two parties interested in the quality of a service or education provision: the provider, and the consumer or user (who is at times referred to as the customer). The consumers of practice supervision activities are the students on practice placement, and the university whose students they supervise, as well as healthcare service users.

ACTIVITY 9.4   WHO IS INTERESTED IN THE EVALUATION OF HEALTHCARE COURSES?

Think of all personnel and agencies that you feel are likely to be interested in the effectiveness and quality of healthcare courses at universities, and jot down specifically who they are.

The quality of healthcare courses is of interest to both purchasers and consumers of the provision. Purchasers of education are generally students who directly or indirectly pay course fees. NHS trusts may be regular purchasers of certain post-registration courses. The quality of courses is also of interest to ward managers and other qualified colleagues directly dealing with students and who have certain expectations of them during and after the course; also the public who expect expert professional care.

In the context of purchasing NHS healthcare courses, the funding for this until 2016 emanated from the Department of Health, which through Health Education England (HEE) and Local Education and Training Boards (LETBs) was responsible for the training and education of NHS doctors, dentists, nurses and all healthcare professionals, and thereby ensured the supply of the local health and care workforce (HEE, 2017b; British Medical Association, 2017). LETBs' role still includes identifying local priorities for education and training, and they hold and allocate funding for the provision of education and training.

Another source of funding for healthcare professionals' education is through Local Workforce Action Boards (LWABs) (e.g. Yorkshire and the Humber, 2017), whose remit is to support the work of Sustainability and Transformation Plans (STP) as new models of healthcare provision initiated by NHS England (2017b).

However, as professional learning takes place in clinical as well as university settings, learning is a partnership agreement between healthcare providers, education providers and students to enable learning that ultimately benefits service users' health.

Other stakeholders interested in the quality of educational provision are the HEI's internal audit mechanisms, and externally the QAA, the NMC, HCPC and other regulatory bodies. Other universities who specialise in education in the subject being evaluated might also be involved, usually by invitation.

A number of ways of evaluating education programmes and the various agencies (for example the QAA) who are involved in evaluating learning, teaching and assessment are discussed shortly.

HOW PRACTICE SUPERVISORS EVALUATE LEARNING PROVISION

Having ascertained why we evaluate, what evaluation is and who evaluates, this section explores the different ways in which evaluation is conducted and performed. As noted above, evaluation data can be obtained informally and formally. Informal evaluation can be performed by:

- direct observation of the general state or appearance of a patient or situation
- direct observation of a class or group of students
- casual in-class evaluation
- anecdotal accounts
- information leaks through the 'grapevine' (the organisation's informal sub-groups)
- casual quasi-social conversation
- monitoring whether instructions are being followed.

Formal evaluation can be conducted by:

- student surveys – national or local (i.e. at own university)
- module and course evaluation questionnaires
- asking the patient directly (or electronically, if this facility is available)
- measurements and pathology laboratory results
- focus groups.

The evaluation tools used, however, need to be 'fit for purpose', rather than just convenient tools that might be valid ones. 'Fit for purpose' means exactly what the term states, that is, the evaluation mechanism has to be appropriate for the activity being evaluated, and the criteria in the tool relevant and comprehensive. Furthermore, evaluation can also be conducted by individual professionals, by clinical teams or at the organisational level.

Quantitative and qualitative evaluation information can be obtained through the use of structured or semi-structured forms with selected headings. Such information can also be obtained through verbal or written means. Teaching sessions in practice settings can be evaluated from a number of viewpoints or conducted in various ways. As an internal evaluation mechanism, the teacher (i.e. the practice supervisor) can decide which evaluation tool or model is the most appropriate to gain the necessary information. Some of these tools are identified in the box.

METHODS OF EVALUATION OF TEACHING IN THE PRACTICE SETTING

- General discussion at the end of the session
- Verbal feedback – requested/volunteered
- Verbal question and answers
- Feedback from the university, probably through link lecturers or PEFs from the particular module leader
- Feedback from colleagues or peers, witness statements
- Quiz – on paper/verbal
- Observing how other teachers teach the skill
- Self-evaluation/reflection
- Using questionnaire(s)
- Observing/monitoring clinical skill performance – direct and indirect
- Continuous monitoring of student's general clinical competence and motivation to learn
- Checking whether objectives are being met
- Reflection/reflective account
- A short multiple-choice-type test
- Discussing booklet of competencies
- Asking the student to teach others, e.g. a patient or junior staff
- Service user feedback
- Using evaluation form(s)

However, evaluation is not always a favoured exercise as, according to Handy (1989), the highest quality service is not easily achieved, since it needs the right equipment, the right people and the right environment, which might not always be fully available. It elicits opinions from all interested parties, who might also set new personal or organisational goals for changing educational provision.

EVALUATING LEARNING USING MODELS OF EVALUATION

There are several published or internally designed frameworks for evaluation that individuals or organisations can use for evaluating the quality of learning provision systematically. Maxwell's (1984) six elements or dimensions of quality is one of them.

The six dimensions are: accessibility, acceptability and appropriateness (3 As); and efficiency, effectiveness and equity (3 Es).

Healthcare course providers can develop their own criteria using Maxwell's model for formal evaluation of quality of learning by asking questions related to each of the six dimensions, such as whether the provision was appropriate or efficient. The education provider that aims and claims to offer a quality service should meet all these criteria. Some manage to do so explicitly, while others may be at different stages of development.

Yet another useful model or framework for evaluation is the popular Donabedian (1988) one of quality assurance using standard statements, and structure, process and outcome criteria, which is also adopted by Moore (2015). This model was also discussed in the context of practice development in Chapter 5, and the evaluator may choose to evaluate all three components, or only the process component, or outcome.

Practice supervisors, nurse lecturers and other education facilitators can use the Donabedian model to evaluate their learning facilitation. However, university modules and courses are generally evaluated using items under standard headings such as teaching, assessment and feedback, academic support, organisation and management, resources, personal development, and any other comments.

Yet another model of evaluation, which is also utilised as a strategy for management of change, as noted in Chapter 5, is the P-D-S-A (Plan–Do–Study–Act) cycle (Institute of Healthcare Improvement, 2017). Van Eps et al. (2006) demonstrate the use of an adaptation of the framework referred to as 'Plan–Do–Check–Act' to evaluate a practice assessor programme. Action research can also be similarly utilised.

Two examples of evaluation in healthcare are (1) evaluation of practice-based learning by Logue (2017) and (2) evaluation of a preceptorship programme by Forde-Johnston (2017). In the first example, qualitative information was gathered from students on placement which suggested a variety of influences on how students develop clinical competence during their pre-registration programme.

EVALUATING PROFESSIONAL HEALTHCARE COURSES

It is partly pertinent for practice supervisors and practice assessors to have some knowledge of ways in which university-based healthcare courses are monitored by external organisations, such as the NMC and the QAA. The documents, which include the CQC's review of care provision sites where students are allocated for practice placements, contain the criteria by which the quality of profession-based courses are monitored and are as follows:

Care Quality Commission (2017) *CQC Fundamental Standards*. Available at: www.qcs.co.uk/useful-guides/quick-start-guide-fundamental-standards/

EVALUATING PRACTICE PLACEMENTS

Standards of teaching in practice settings are closely related to the quality of service user care, to the quality of student supervision and the expertise of practice supervisors. For students' learning experiences during placements, the student may be asked informally at the end of the placement how good and useful they feel that the placement has been, maybe at the same time as the final interview at the end of the placement, or they may be given an evaluation form to complete after the final interview. On returning to the university for lectures after the placement, they are asked to complete a practice placement evaluation form, electronically or on paper, along with further verbal evaluation.

The written placement evaluation form asks students to give feedback on various aspects of the experience, such as whether they had adequate preparation for the placement and were given an orientation on the first day of placement. They may be asked to comment on whether nominated practice supervisors had been identified, whether their learning needs and placement objectives were agreed in good time, a range of learning opportunities identified, feedback on performance of clinical skills given, how often they worked with their practice supervisor, and whether evidence-based practice was prevalent. There could also be questions on the amount and nature of personal support available.

However, it is noteworthy that since modules of course evaluation have moved from anonymous paper copies to electronic form, the return rates have been very low. Chan et al.'s (2017) study of student evaluations revealed that students are dubious about completing evaluation forms because they indicate that electronic versions contravene anonymity, that is the university will have some way of identifying which student made negative comments or identified weaknesses in the module or course delivery.

Evaluation information on the quality of the learning experience is imparted to the placement areas by the university afterwards. Practice supervisors may have obtained qualitative evaluation information from the student prior to the end of the placement. Placement evaluations also form a basis for communication between professionals in practice settings and university lecturers, and an additional benefit of the process is that training and development needs of clinical staff can be identified both for more effective clinical care and for more competent practice supervision. Problems reported after the placement are generally investigated by PEFs and CHEFs.

As indicated in Chapter 4 of this book, you are strongly encouraged to take a close look at the latest completed educational audit form for your workplace, which might reassure you that it constitutes a sound learning environment, but also for your own ideas about student placement in the setting.

EVALUATION OF ASSESSMENTS

Practice assessors perform numerous assessments of competencies in this role. How are the quality and efficacy of assessments they perform monitored? Practice assessors' professional judgement comes into play to some extent, as they have to be able to justify the decisions they make about each student's competence, in that the responsibility normally lies with the practice assessor to seek all information relevant to assessments so that their pass/fail decisions are as well-informed as can be.

Furthermore, if a student feels that the result of an assessment was unfair or incorrect, then they can appeal following appropriate procedures. This is usually only for the conduct of the assessment and any technical or practical interference during the assessment, but not against the professional judgement of the practice assessor.

Practice assessors' accountability has a major role to play in ensuring that their own knowledge and competence in assessing students remains up-to-date, valid and reliable. This can be achieved by:

- discussions on practice assessor update study days regarding, say, intra-assessor and inter-assessor reliability
- consulting link lecturer, PEF and/or senior colleague (e.g. ward sister).

Ways of achieving intra-assessor reliability were examined in Chapter 7, and grading practice was discussed in Chapter 8.

ISSUES RELATED TO EVALUATIONS AND PROFESSIONAL DEVELOPMENT OPPORTUNITIES

Accurate evaluation is a complex skill to acquire, especially if making subsequent changes is anticipated. It is also at times an uncomfortable exercise as it may reveal unanticipated or perceived flaws, depending on the evaluator's own state of mind and general outlook. There might be other biased views stated or practical problems related to evaluation of teaching highlighted, and issues of whether the teaching should be clinically-based or classroom-based.

Following on from these observations, the remainder of this chapter explores problems and the possible consequences of evaluations, and then the overall CPD needs of practice supervisors and practice assessors. Practice supervisors and practice assessors as lifelong learners, as well as the use of professional development plans are also discussed.

As indicated throughout this book, the practice supervision role of health professionals has various facets. Consequently, each facet involves a set of activities in itself which requires relevant knowledge and competence. To ascertain how well each role is being performed, practice supervisors self-monitor their performance, and also obtain comments from their students, peers and their own clinical supervisors. How much and how comprehensively do practice supervisors do this, and what do they do with the data obtained?

Mostly, this is not an issue because, as accountable professionals, practice supervisors and practice assessors continually endeavour to rectify any weakness in their performance and knowledge, and strive to improve their practice at all times. However, there can be problems with the evaluation of these roles.

REFLECTION POINT 9.3:   ISSUES WITH EVALUATION

What do you feel are the likely problems associated with evaluation of the practice supervision role?

A possible problem area or danger related to the evaluation of a teaching session (practice or knowledge based) is that the criticisms of one's earlier teaching sessions may give the impression that you are not quite cut out for teaching. Despite this, teaching is one of the competencies of all qualified nurses and, like many other skills, can be learned and subsequently mastered with ample practice. It is also usually one of the items in healthcare professionals' job descriptions, at times worded as 'contribute to professional development of other staff'. On self-evaluation of their practice supervision functions – referred to by Rogers and Horrocks (2010) as post-hoc evaluation – they may encounter weaknesses that they may or may not wish to reveal to others, and choose to rectify themselves by trial and error, or published guidance.

Practice placement evaluations could also highlight serious problems with practice supervision, as was found by Phillips et al. (2000), for instance, that might not prove easy to resolve. The practice supervisor needs to be able to differentiate between progress and levels and speed of attainment by learners. All learners may be making progress, but they could be achieving at different levels, depending on their educational background, efforts and time for study, and learning opportunities. Some of the likely problems of evaluation are as follows:

- Raising certain points that are aimed at influencing peers' opinions.
- Just one incident could colour statements about the whole placement experience, session or module.
- The teacher may be a perfectionist and may feel very disappointed if any weakness is pointed out.
- Points identified by students might not be seen as positive statements.
- Evaluation comments may be seen as 'some you win, some you lose', and no action taken on suggested weaknesses.
- The person might genuinely not appreciate the weaknesses pointed out.
- Difficult to be entirely objective.

Evaluative research on student assessment has sporadically identified problems of students not being fit for practice at the point of registration, because at times in the past mentors had awarded a pass to students on their practice competencies without full evidence of their competence (e.g. Duffy, 2003, 2016). Furthermore, university deans of nursing have indicated that there was 'evidence that students on placements are under extreme pressure' (Duffin, 2005: 4). Subsequently, the NMC (2010a) responded by allocating up to 300 of the 2300 hours of practice learning to be achieved within simulated learning environments, such as in skills laboratories, but also emphasised the need for 'protected time' between supervisors of learning and the student (referred to as 'supported learning time' by the NMC [2018a]).

Nonetheless, recent research conducted by King's College London (2014) concluded that there were growing and conflicting pressures on staff time that could affect the efficacy of supervision of learning, and also called for a coherent strategy that included practice supervision type programmes incorporating the recommendations of the Willis (RCN, 2012) report (e.g. practice learning must be equitably resourced across healthcare professions [2012: 42]), as well as revalidation.

STUDENTS RAISING CONCERNS – PROCESSES AND OUTCOMES

As noted in Chapter 8 and also earlier in this chapter under 'Evaluating practice placements', on returning to the university following a practice placement, some students may voice concerns in relation to aspects of the placement. This therefore forms a basis for further communication between university staff and staff in the practice setting and can result in the development needs of clinical staff being identified.

Students of course do not have to wait till the end of the placement to raise concerns. However, when a conflict situation is reported, this can be due to misunderstandings between the two parties or to deficient communication.

REFLECTION POINT 9.4:   STUDENTS VOICING CONCERNS

From your knowledge of dissatisfaction or complaints that students have voiced either directly in your presence or reported by others, what are the various avenues or media, informal and formal, that students are likely to use to voice their dissatisfaction?

Dedicating just a few minutes to identify the various ways in which students offload their concerns reveals several powerful ways of doing so, but there are also some misleading avenues. It may well be that students at times just 'have a moan' with their close friends with regard to what they were unhappy about in relation to the placement, and the matter goes no further. Alternatively, students can report their concerns through various channels, such as:

- at workshops held by the PEF during the placement
- at post-placement evaluation, as mentioned earlier in this chapter
- to their university personal tutor or link lecturer
- through the Student Union department at the university
- at organised termly Student Forums at the University.

Some students even resort to social media (such as Facebook). Others may even venture to mention their concerns at QAA or NMC periodic reviews, when students are invited to meet reviewers to comment on their programmes of study. The NMC (2018c: 6) re-emphasises the point that students should be able to raise concerns or complaints 'without fear of adverse consequences'.

The NMC (2015b) publication *Raising Concerns* and the NMC's (2015a) code (professional standards of practice) provide guidance for qualified nurses and midwives on raising concerns, albeit at the level of broad principles that can be applied as felt appropriate in each situation. They also include information on legal protection to whistleblowers and information on organisations that nurses and midwives can go to for further advice.

In a review of 23 research papers on support for health professionals who raise concerns related to quality of care, Milligan et al. (2017) deduced that students are fully aware of the need to report concerns, but they fear there could be negative repercussions on their practice assessment results if they do so, especially as they are unclear about how, when and to whom students should report. However, the NMC (2015c) also indicates that students who raise concerns are protected by legislation.

As just indicated, evaluation of practice supervision activities is likely to highlight areas that are problematic or those that warrant further development. The practice supervisor also has a duty to be up-to-date in all aspects of practice supervision. Thus, of necessity, practice supervisors, have to engage in ongoing learning and continuing professional development in relation to all their roles or dimensions. So, what is continuing professional development (CPD) and what is ongoing or lifelong learning, and how do practice supervisors participate in these?

CONTINUING PROFESSIONAL DEVELOPMENT FOR SUPERVISORS AND ASSESSORS

Career development avenues for healthcare professionals have been identified by the Department of Health in the past, but for those who support practice-based learning, the NMC (2008) identified a simple four-stage registrants' role on a continuum that generally progresses as follows:

  1.Nurse or Midwife > 2. Mentor > 3. Practice Teacher > 4. (Qualified) Teacher

Intercalated between these qualification-based positions are likely to be various education facilitation and assessor of competence roles, such as preceptor, practice assessor, supervisor of practice learning for healthcare professionals on specialist practice courses, clinical instructor, clinical education coordinator and lecturer–practitioner, and then to nurse lecturer maybe and beyond. These various stages constitute practice supervisors' and practice assessors' own ongoing professional development.

  Therefore, this final section on supervision and student assessment focuses on the scope of their CPD needs as well as requirements. It suggests that, in addition to continuing to develop their own health or social care practice knowledge and competence, a likely progression for nurses and midwives' teaching roles can therefore develop as illustrated in Figure 9.1.

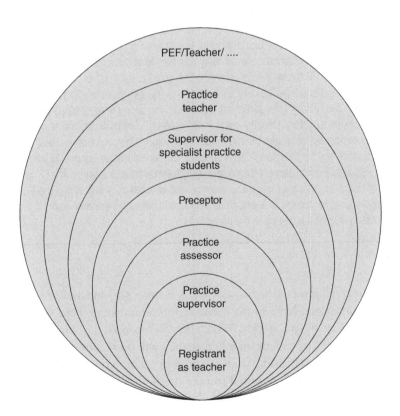

Figure 9.1   Progressive development of the registrant's teaching role

For the practice teacher role, those who have had educational preparation for supporting learning have to be further educationally prepared for supporting practice-based learning for students on specialist practice courses, including those on SCPHN programmes. Gopee (2010) elucidates in detail how practice teachers can fulfil their role effectively with the support of underpinning knowledge base and skills in practice-based teaching and student assessment, along with their clinical expertise.

A brief case study of a registrant on an earlier mentor course who went on to become a qualified 'Teacher' just a few years later is as follows.

CASE STUDY 9.1:   CAREER PROGRESSION FROM MENTOR TO NURSE LECTURER

Straight after qualifying as an RN, Kelly took up a post as a community nurse as she felt that in the community setting she would be in a better position to provide holistic care, see patients' health improve in their own home settings, and also advise on preventing health problems recurring. This in turn enabled Kelly to build good relationships with patients and families, and Kelly felt it was also a very rewarding job.

A condition of the post was that Kelly would have to attend the NMC approved mentor course in a year's time because students were regularly on practice placement with the community team. While on the mentor course, Kelly was alerted to the availability of opportunities to teach student nurses in the university setting, which could entail teaching specific clinical skills for a few pre-agreed hours periodically. On further enquiry, approximately three years later, Kelly negotiated with the university to participate in co-teaching taking manual blood pressure in the university's skills laboratory. Despite some initial anxiety, Kelly realised that she enjoyed imparting this clinical skill to student nurses. On further taking up such opportunities, Kelly finally acquired a place on the postgraduate certificate in higher education course. Eighteen months after her successful completion of the course, Kelly took up an appointment at a UK university's Faculty of Health as a lecturer in clinical practice and simulation, and is loving the experience, and is also hoping to engage in research on simulated learning in the very near future, as well as completing a Master's degree in the same field.

Attending supervision updates and as well as being a self-directed lifelong learning healthcare professional have so far been the more immediate next steps in professionals' careers (e.g. NMC, 2018c; DH, 2010). Professional development of practice supervisors is partly dependent on whether they will be required to progress to the practice assessor role assessing students on their achievement of NMC SOP. The practice supervisor may be required to take on the preceptor role for newly qualified RNs or RMs who are new to the clinical specialism (the preceptor role was discussed in some detail in Chapter 1). They might benefit from the availability of clinical supervision. Practice supervisors and practice assessors may also be required to facilitate learning and to assess competence for RNs on post-qualifying clinical short courses. Naturally, they will need to hold the same post-qualifying short-course qualification themselves in the first place. However, to facilitate learning and assessing students on specialist or advanced practice educational programmes, they will need to hold the particular specialist or advanced practice qualification themselves, and also have successfully completed an NMC approved, HEI-based practice teacher course.

Regarding development of specialist practitioners, however, research conducted by Barton (2006) exploring the experiences of doctors supervising learning for students on nurse practitioner courses, concluded that medical clinical educators experience conflict in that as the students acquire new clinical skills and roles, this also amounts to the supervisors feeling that their traditional medical authority is being challenged. This led to a renegotiation of professional boundaries between nurse practitioners and doctors.

Nevertheless, before moving on to these roles, the practice supervisor needs to continue to develop the supervision of learning skills and knowledge, and keep up-to-date with the latest developments in all aspects of their post. Furthermore, self-evaluation, along with personal research and clinical audits, can highlight issues that can present opportunities for further development for practice supervisors and practice assessors.

In relation to healthcare professionals' own ongoing professional development, a brief overview of what continuing professional development and lifelong learning are is provided next in this chapter, and is followed by specific CPD requirements, including revalidation.

THEORIES OF CONTINUING PROFESSIONAL DEVELOPMENT

Continuing professional development (CPD) is a concept that is an inherent component of lifelong learning and is defined by the HCPC (2012: 1) as 'a range of learning activities through which health professionals maintain and develop throughout their career to ensure that they retain their capacity to practise safely, effectively and legally within their evolving scope of practice'. The definition may sound like a directive from the regulatory body, but for responsible professionals, which healthcare professionals are, CPD is a career-associated attitude of mind, which in turn requires proactive planning and actions, as well as personal decision-making.

At the practical level, Wallace (1999: 28) sees CPD as a 'term given to the learning which takes place in a professional's career after the point of qualification and/or registration'. However CPD is intentional learning in addition to incidental learning in healthcare settings.

Organisations tend to implement one or other of two main approaches to CPD: the sanction model or the benefit model. The employing or regulatory organisation that uses the sanction model tends to penalise the individual for not engaging in the need-related CPD. However, the organisation utilising the benefit model does not threaten with sanctions but reinforces and, where possible, rewards individuals for voluntary or suggested CPD.

Alternatively, Wallace (1999) separates CPD into statutory, mandatory and permissive types. Statutory CPD is that which is undertaken as a result of statute or legislation. Mandatory CPD has a similar meaning, in that it is instigated by an official command or instruction by an authority (such as the NMC) and is therefore compulsory. Wallace identifies the mandatory CPD model as one that suggests that CPD is a mandate by employers or regulatory bodies which has to be executed but no penalty is attached directly to the individual if not fulfilled.

Permissive CPD is the type of CPD in which the individual has choice, and, in this context, research by Lee (2011: 390) revealed that although learning needs are often identified through appraisal and personal development planning, it is CPD based on the 'individual personal drive and enthusiasm of practitioners' that results in contributing to implementing change in clinical practice, while policy-driven factors and national health targets are secondary.

Another perspective on CPD is suggested by Hegarty (2017) as the concept of care practitioners being able to 'demonstrate maintenance of competence' or continuing clinical competence. The concept extends the notion of CPD to practitioners specifically being able to prove their competence when required, whether it is by spot-check or a supervision requirement. Furthermore, Clark et al.'s (2015) research concludes that a well-established positive and supportive organisational culture with the aim of improving healthcare service user care is crucial for CPD to be effective.

CONTINUING LEARNING AND REVALIDATION FOR REGISTRANTS

Most healthcare professions or regulatory bodies have instituted some form of sanction or mandatory model of CPD. The NMC (2015d), for instance, indicates that to meet revalidation requirements, every practising nurse and midwife must have evidence of having undertaken a minimum of 35 hours of CPD, amongst other requirements, that is relevant to their practice during every three-year cycle, to be able to renew their registration. The registrant must also have worked in some capacity by virtue of their professional qualification during the previous three years for a minimum of 450 hours. The GMC and HCPC have similar requirements.

Despite the mandatory nature of revalidation, it seems reasonable to expect healthcare professionals to tread a planned career route, or rewarding vocation, by continually ensuring that their practice is evidence-based, and of the safest and highest quality that they can provide. CPD thus reflects a proactive and responsible approach to one's own professional learning and practice-related research (with small r or big R). It thereby also involves an attitude to life and work that allows for creativity in one's professional activities.

The CPD for meeting revalidation requirements has to be in relevant areas of practice and can be in one or more of the key components of healthcare interventions, aptly categorised in the *NHS KSF* (DH, 2004) as the six core dimensions – as noted in Chapter 5 – and apply to all NHS employees (except doctors, dentists and some board-level managers).

The *NHS KSF* also identifies 24 specific dimensions under *health and well-being, estates and facilities, information and knowledge* and *general*, which apply to some but not all jobs in the NHS. More specific details on each of these dimensions of healthcare interventions are presented in the *NHS KSF* document.

However, registrants are required by the NMC, HCPC, GMC and other regulatory bodies to accumulate evidence of having engaged in a predetermined amount of learning activity for revalidation purposes. The CPD advocated by the NMC is the minimum requirement for safe and competent practice, but it is recognised that the practitioner generally engages in substantially more learning than this minimum.

Relevant university-based courses may meet quite a few of the NMC requirements. Additionally, self-directed or peer-learning can also easily contribute to these requirements. Self-directed learning is explained in detail in Chapter 2 under andragogy and the work of Knowles (2015) and Rogers and Horrocks (2010). Peer learning is also well documented, in particular in the context of human and social capital (see, for instance, Gopee, 2002a).

Numerous healthcare reports and problematic incidents indicate that healthcare registrants need to be receptive to new learning all the time (e.g. Francis, 2013). Continuing learning is also a feature of healthcare professionalism, which has been converted into policy and requirements by healthcare regulatory bodies (e.g. GMC), and is known as revalidation. Revalidation has become a requirement for different professions at different times, and for nurses and midwives from 2015.

Having become effective from April 2016, and replacing the previous requirements for renewal of healthcare professionals' registration with the NMC set out in the preceding Post Registration Education and Practice Standards, the NMC (2015d: 3 – updated March 2017) indicates that 'revalidation' is the process that allows registrants to maintain their registration with the NMC by demonstrating their continued ability to practise safely and effectively, and by a continuous process of learning that registrants need to engage with throughout their career.

Registrants need to demonstrate this ability every three years (in addition to paying an annual fee to the NMC) by compiling the following evidence:

1. 450 practice hours or 900 hours if revalidating as both nurse and midwife
2. 35 hours of continuing professional development (of which 20 must be participatory learning)
3. Five pieces of practice-related feedback

4. Five written reflective accounts
5. Reflective discussion
6. Health and character
7. Professional indemnity arrangement
8. Confirmation from a NMC confirmer.

Each item of evidence has to be cross-referenced against themes of the NMC's (2015a) code of practice. Practice supervisors have to meet revalidation requirements themselves, and, when appropriate, facilitate other registrants to meet theirs. Both the NMC and subsequent publications in professional journals elaborate on ways in which revalidation requirements can be met (e.g. Middleton and Llewellyn, 2016; Jolly et al., 2017). For ample details on ways in which revalidation requirements can be met, see 'Revalidation' on the NMC's or HCPC's website.

UPDATE SESSIONS FOR PRACTICE SUPERVISORS AND PRACTICE ASSESSORS

In addition to educational preparation for the practice supervisor and practice assessor roles, as well as meeting revalidation requirements, it is helpful for both to attend regular updates related to these roles. Annual update sessions should include the opportunity to meet and explore assessment and supervision issues with other supervisors and assessors (face-to-face) and explore as a group the validity and reliability of judgements made when assessing practice in challenging circumstances'.

ACTIVITY 9.5   REGULAR UPDATES FOR SUPERVISORS AND ASSESSORS

Following completion of a practice supervisor or practice assessor preparation course, you need to be aware of your own CPD as a registrant and a learning facilitator. Consider how you can keep yourself up-to-date with new developments in professional knowledge and competence within your profession in relation to both clinical practice and supervision of learning. Discuss this with a colleague or your clinical supervisor.

What would practice supervisors and practice assessors themselves wish to see covered in the update study days?

Practice supervisors' and practice assessors' update events are usually one-day or half-day events, conducted by PEFs/CHEFs within the healthcare trust premises or at universities. At the update sessions, issues related to reliability and validity of assessments should always be discussed so that a certain level of parity is achieved in the locality or, better still, examined in small-group workshops, which could include group activities to explore the exact ways in which intra- and inter-assessor reliability is achieved and monitored. The NMC (2008) made some suggestions of activities to include on annual update study days, such as ensuring:

- knowledge of current NMC approved programmes
- discussion on the implications of changes to NMC requirements
- opportunity to discuss issues related to supervision of practice-based learning, assessment of competence and fitness for safe and effective practice.

Support mechanisms available for dealing with 'failing students' could be explored, as well as any new NMC rules and guidelines related to supervision of learning and student assessment in practice, and their implications. Practice supervisors and practice assessors should be prepared to provide evidence to their employers and NMC quality assurance agents of how they have maintained and developed their knowledge, skills and competence in student supervision,

Some healthcare trusts conduct workshops to facilitate building and presentation of portfolio evidence of supervision of practice-based learning activities (for example, Gover, 2010). In such workshops, attendees can work in groups to identify a range of activities that comprise items that are pertinent evidence of supervision of leaning activities. In addition to attending updating sessions, evidence could also include annual performance review objectives, achievement of personal development plans (PDP) objectives, evaluation or feedback from any related presentations (in-house, or at local or national conferences), any EBP initiative implemented or disseminated, etc.

PRACTICE SUPERVISORS AS ROLE MODELS OF LIFELONG LEARNING

To be a role model for learners, practice supervisors need to be lifelong learners in both professional practice and in supervision of learning. Lifelong learning has been examined with intense attention in university education departments for some time, and in relation to healthcare professionals' CPD for a couple of decades. The NMC (2004b: 3) sees lifelong learning as 'more than simply keeping up to date … (but also incorporate) an enquiring approach to nursing and midwifery', implying a state of mind that is enthusiastic about delivering the highest standard of care.

_____ **ACTIVITY 9.6   WHY LIFELONG LEARNING?** _____

List as many reasons as you can think of for healthcare professionals being required to be lifelong learners. How can healthcare professionals achieve lifelong learning? What are the probable problems with lifelong learning?

The NMC (2004b) provides several reasons for healthcare professionals being lifelong learners, including increasing technological advances in treatment and care, and expanding roles. Furthermore, lifelong learning differs from lifelong education in that, while lifelong education refers to learning activities directed by established education institutions and that normally lead to a qualification, lifelong learning refers to all avenues of learning – formal, informal and incidental.

Practice supervisors continue to learn and become even more effective through attending formal updating events after successfully completing the initial educational preparation programme to become a practice supervisor and, informally, through consulting and advising colleagues such as during peer-supervision, as well as by incidental learning. This means that the healthcare registrant not only has a responsibility to facilitate the learning of others, but also to continue learning themselves.

The learning activity undertaken is of course also based on self-assessment, and members of healthcare professions need to be responsible for identifying their own learning needs. Indeed, the NMC's (2015a) code of professional standards states that as registrants we must keep our knowledge and competence up to date through regular learning and professional development activities (Clause 22.3). Thus, healthcare professions explicitly either dictate or encourage all registrants to continue the process of learning, asking us to reflect on and question the ways in which we deliver care, to engage in continuing development of our competence and to improve our performance.

Furthermore, de la Harpe and Radloff (2000) explored the characteristics of lifelong learners, and found that they have:

- self-knowledge, self-confidence and persistence
- a positive view of the value of learning
- good self-management skills, such as being well organised and managing time effectively, knowing when and how to seek help and when to collaborate with peers
- motivation to learn
- positive feelings about themselves as learners
- the ability to manage their feelings during highs and lows of learning
- developed a set of learning strategies (e.g. when to dedicate time to study and where to learn; and skills such as note-taking and summarising).

Other known characteristics can be added to the above list such as external motivators and situational support. Moreover, a study of lifelong learning in nursing by Davis et al. (2014) identified several other characteristics of lifelong learners, the most common ones of which include: enjoys learning, creates time for learning, reflective, asks questions and tracks down answers.

As to a systematic approach to facilitating lifelong learning, Gopee (2005) concluded from a qualitative study of nurses' perceptions of lifelong learning that a

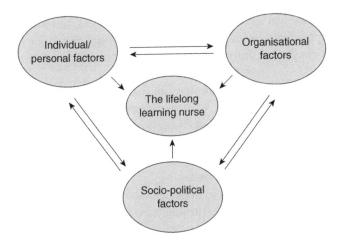

Figure 9.2   A conceptual framework for lifelong learning in nursing

Source: Gopee (2005)

model (or framework) of lifelong learning in healthcare comprises three groups of factors, as presented in Figure 9.2. In brief, these are:

- *organisational factors* (e.g. time and release from work to attend CPD courses, work-based learning)
- *socio-political factors* (e.g. social group influences in practice settings, clinical supervision)
- *individual factors* (the healthcare professional's professionalism, learning as a natural human activity).

The above-mentioned characteristics of lifelong learners are obviously 'individual factors', and as for the other two groups of factors identified by Gopee, naturally, there are numerous ways in which healthcare professionals can and do engage in CPD and lifelong learning, which range from university-based degree-awarding courses or modules, informal much shorter trust-based study days and workshops, to self-directed learning.

ORGANISATIONAL SUPPORT WITH CONTINUING LEARNING

Usually, all university–healthcare trust partnerships already have an infrastructure of support for professionals in supervisory or assessment roles. Such support implies a network of personnel and other resources that can be accessed to discuss and sound out the decisions that they are about to make on their student's performance of clinical skills, or to consult. Support is also available from peers and colleagues within their practice setting or department, and also from PEFs, link teachers and the student's personal tutor, which invariably results in further learning. Further support can be gained through professional networks, some of which are formed informally at conferences, and when exploring issues at regular update study days.

Clinical supervision is another mechanism that practice supervisors and practice assessors can draw on for regular structured support and for identifying learning. However, one of the key sources of such support for CPD is the PEF team, and the study days and workshops that they offer. Lecturers who teach on the practice assessor and similar courses at the partner university, as well as reflective practice, are other modes of support mechanisms.

Various sources of funding have been available for all registrants to undertake CPD related to their employment, although the funding has usually been meagre. Health Education England is the organisation that has taken responsibility for education, training and CPD of healthcare staff since April 2013, which is delivered via LETBs as noted earlier in this chapter. For further details see *Liberating the NHS: Developing the Healthcare Workforce from Design to Delivery* (DH, 2012c) at the HEE website and subsequent documents.

PERSONAL DEVELOPMENT PLANS

Systematic CPD and lifelong learning for health and social care professionals can also be effectively supported through the utilisation of Personal Development Plans (PDPs). PDPs have been advocated for a number of years in the UK through key NHS and education policy documents such as *The Dearing Report* (NCIHE, 1997), *NHS KSF* (DH, 2004) and *Personal Development Planning: Guidance for Institutional Policy and Practice in Higher Education* (QAA, 2009). The *NHS KSF* advocates the use of PDPs by all NHS healthcare professionals for their professional development throughout their careers. Other than education and health policies, influential writers on self- and staff management such as Lancer et al. (2016) also advocate the use of PDPs.

PDPs provide individuals with the opportunity to focus attention on their career aspirations and are a mechanism for recording and reviewing career decisions periodically. However, PDPs should not be part of the annual performance and development review (PDR) (or appraisal) process, which is a managerial activity more focused on work productivity. They are however powerful agreements that can be stored locally, or preferably by the employee only (i.e. are not centrally recorded). PDPs are nevertheless, a component of an effective learning organisation (a concept discussed in Chapter 4).

A PDP is also often an NMC requirement for reinstatement to the professional register where a registrant's competence has been in question, and it suggests that, in future, PDPs can be easily linked to revalidation. However, a PDP is not a punitive activity, as it can be beneficially utilised in conjunction with annual development and performance reviews (e.g. Liefer, 2002). It is feasible to implement PDPs so that they are discussed as part of annual development reviews, with only an agreed selection of objectives being incorporated into the performance review and the remaining PDP objectives being supported by clinical supervision.

The QAA (2009: 2) defines a PDP as 'a structured and supported process undertaken by a learner to reflect upon their own learning, performance and/or achievement and to plan for their personal, educational and career development'. Thus, PDPs can be separated as either personal or professional development, except that for most individuals these two components are either intertwined or experienced on a continuum in day-to-day activities. An example of a PDP for practice supervisors – which has been constructed from prevailing guidance and other literature on the topic, and can be constituted in landscape or portrait format – is presented in Template 9.1.

The two development needs mentioned in Template 9.1 are part of the education component of nurses' and midwives' roles, other components being clinical practice, research and management, as noted at the beginning of Chapter 3. Various components of required knowledge and competence can be acquired through in-house and in-service training, but for paid time for study, funding and support from managers for HEI-based courses, this can be an issue (Liefer, 2002; RCN, 2012 [Willis Report]) and therefore needs forward planning.

CHAPTER SUMMARY

This chapter has provided a comprehensive analysis of evaluation of the whole range of practice supervisor and practice assessor activities, and having completed this chapter you will have examined:

- Why we should evaluate the effectiveness with which practice supervisors facilitate learning and engage in continuous assessment, while they also fulfil other roles.
- What evaluation is, i.e. the nature and various aspects of evaluation, and who evaluates the practice supervisor's teaching activities.
- Different ways of evaluating clinically based and academically based teaching and assessment; and how practice supervisors evaluate learning provision and assessments during practice placements. The use of models of evaluation, including heeding the findings of audits by external organisations such as the QAA and NMC.
- The likely problems of evaluation, the results of evaluations, issues ensuing from them, related consequences and subsequent actions that can be taken.
- The opportunities and scope for ongoing learning arising from the results of evaluations, practice learning for RNs on specialist practice courses, and the

Template 9.1 A professional development plan

Name: .... [Other relevant details, e.g. clinical supervisor's name]

Objective and development need/interest	Relevant dimension of my work and career	Hours required and date objective to be achieved	What will I do to achieve this development need/interest? Resources and support required	How will I apply this learning to my work?	How will I know I have completed the development activity successfully?	How will I share this learning with relevant others?
1. Establish supported learning time for practice supervision	Teaching learners	One hour every week, achieve by end of learner's practice placement	Off-duty planned in advance. Team members aware. Two alternative protected times identified each week	Spend the protected time focusing on practice supervision activities. Monitor and record use of protected time	An appropriate record of practice supervision activities	Item on team meeting agenda. Present at local conference
2. Develop teaching skills further	......	......	......	......	......	......

requirement for continuing professional development in one's practice supervisor role, ways of meeting NMC revalidation requirements, as well as the practice supervisor as a lifelong learner.

FURTHER OPTIONAL READING

1. Kirkpatrick and Kirkpatrick's (2006) framework for evaluating training and education programmes is available from internet websites, where they provide variable insights into this model, but a more thorough account is provided in the Kirkpatrick and Kirkpatrick book. Implementation of the model is also discussed in the context of practice teaching in the *Practice Teaching in Healthcare* (Gopee, 2010) book.

   - Kirkpatrick, D.L. and Kirkpatrick, J.D. (2006) *Evaluating Training Programs: The Four Levels*, 3rd edn. San Francisco, CA: Berrett-Koehler Publishers.

2. For a current textbook explaining learning supervision, see:

   - Johnson, E. A. (2017) *Working Together in Clinical Supervision – A Guide for Supervisors and Supervisees*. New York, Momentum Press Health.

To access further resources related to this chapter, visit **https://study.sagepub.com/gopee4e** where a range of learning and teaching materials are provided.

FURTHER THOUGHTS – A JOURNEY JUST BEGINNING

Teaching transforms careers and lives. The practice learning supervisor or practice educator role gives you permission to teach and impart your knowledge and care intervention skills to learners and colleagues. It is a career-long journey, whether it's to do with facilitating learning for learners of one's own healthcare profession, or of allied health professions, medical students, associates or healthcare assistants. On the one hand, it is a journey that begins soon after your preceptee status ends. One of the strengths of nursing, midwifery and SCPHNs is the holistic approach that other healthcare professionals intend, endeavour and at times succeed in taking in their day-to-day practice. Some clinical settings have students all the time, others occasionally but always have learners, but the actions that learning supervisors and mentors take stay in the minds of healthcare professionals for several years, as they shape their careers and quality of care for health or social care service users. The practice learning supervisor's actions are therefore seminal in shaping the attitudes of practitioners for years to come.

On the other hand, as Rogers and Freiberg (1994: 375) indicate, 'not all journeys are trouble-free … but the process alone makes us a bit wiser. Gaining wisdom comes not with time or age, but from living the challenges of life, learning from our mistakes, and building on experiences.' This book on supervision of learning was designed to achieve the objectives outlined in the introductory section, which are predominantly to examine the knowledge and understanding necessary for effective and mutually beneficial person-centred practice, partly based on standards for supervision of learning and assessment (e.g. (NMC, 2018a). The knowledge and skills that you develop can be built upon by further pursuing opportunities for imparting knowledge and skills. They could play a significant role along your career path, be it as a much more senior clinical practitioner or in part- or full-time educational roles. What are the next steps that you will take to facilitate and supervise learning as you further develop your expertise by seizing the multifarious opportunities that will come your way from now on?

GLOSSARY

academic assessor Assigned to collate and confirm student achievement of proficiencies and programme outcomes in the academic environment for each part of the programme

action research Scientifically designed research that is conducted while in the process of implementing a new activity or a change

andragogy An approach to teaching adults that is different from teaching children and adolescents whereby the teacher takes a facilitator of learning role, rather than being an authoritarian who has all the knowledge and the answers to all issues

clinical (or care) intervention Any action taken by healthcare professionals to improve the health of patients or service users, or to enhance their health and prevent health problems

clinical learning environment (CLE) The practice setting as an environment where learning occurs amongst staff and students, which is valued and encouraged, along with effective care delivery. The term is used interchangeably with 'practice learning environment'

Collaborative Learning in Practice (CLiP) A novel model of nursing and midwifery mentorship, whereby the clinical educator supports, coaches and mentors learners, and is available to actively contribute to the ward learning environment; and also acts as a source of expert advice in such circumstances as when students are struggling to pass their practice competencies

competency The skill and associated practical knowledge required to perform a clinical intervention

educational audit An audit that is normally conducted jointly by senior staff in a practice setting and a university academic to ensure the practice setting is suitable for healthcare students' practice placement as part of their professional learning

ethical competence Refers to the ability of the healthcare professional to deliver safe and effective care that is based on full accountability, and whose practice and social behaviour are based on the principles of ethics and on moral values such as doing good, demonstrating respect for human rights and dignity, etc.

evidence-based practice (EBP) Practice that is based on evidence, which can be research evidence

facilitation of learning An idea that is different from the term teaching in that it signifies a practice-based teacher or lecturer structuring activities that enable students to learn by themselves, as individuals or in groups. The concept can be applied to acquiring healthcare knowledge base, as well as to clinical competencies

forcefield analysis An analysis that applies to a proposed change, and entails identifying the factors that are indicating the need for the change, and also factors that are hindering the implementation of the change

healthcare organisations NHS Acute Trusts, primary care, private hospitals, nursing homes, clinical commissioning groups, etc., involved in the provision of care and treatment

healthcare provider Healthcare organisations in the public or independent sector that directly provide care and treatment to individuals with health problems

informal learning Learning that occurs ad hoc, often based on seizing learning opportunities as they arise

intuitive knowledge Refers to personal and professional knowledge that is based on intuition and sensing, but which may not have an underpinning of demonstrable reasoning or scientific evidence on which the knowledge is based

learning pathway A structured plan of learning based on patients' or service users' journeys through health and/or social care

link lecturer A university lecturer who singly or as part of a team of lecturers is the named academic contact whom staff in specific practice settings can contact for information, clarification, etc., about student matters

patients or service users The two terms are used interchangeably to signify anyone who uses or receives health or social care from care provision organisations

person-centred care Is an approach to practice that is holistic and underpinned by such values as respect for the person, for individuals' rights, and a culture of empowerment for the patient

practice assessor Healthcare professional who is assigned for the conduct of students' practice assessments to confirm student achievement of practice objectives and proficiencies, and whose assessment decisions are also informed by comments sought and received from practice supervisors

practice learning Learning that occurs during practice placements

practice setting Any NHS or independent sector setting where health and/or social care is provided in accordance with Department of Health and Social Care guidelines

practice supervisor A registered health or social care professional who supports and supervises learning in practice in line with their competence (also referred to as practice learning supervisor in this textbook)

practice teacher A specialist or advanced practice nurse who has successfully completed a course in preparation for the role of supervising registered nurses (RNs) who are students on specialist or advanced practice courses

preceptorship A role allocated to an appropriately qualified and experienced healthcare professional for the supervision of the professional development of a newly qualified registrant in the practice setting

pre-registration This term is used interchangeably with pre-qualifying and pre-service professional education to signify health or social care profession students' education programmes that lead to students becoming eligible to have their names entered on the NMC or HCPC professional registers

registrants Refers to qualified healthcare professionals on either the Nursing and Midwifery Council's (NMC) or Health and Care Professions Council's (HCPC) professional register

supernumerary status Health profession students are deemed supernumerary if they are not part of the paid workforce in a practice setting, but are expected to engage in learning healthcare knowledge and skills by participating in care of patients or service users

REFERENCES

Academy of Medical Royal Colleges (2017) *Joint Professions' Statement*. Available at: www. aomrc.org.uk/wp-content/uploads/2017/10/JOINT-PROFESSIONS-STATEMENT-111018.pdf (accessed 4 November 2017).

Adam, D. and Taylor, R. (2014) 'Compassionate care: Empowering students through nurse education', *Nurse Education Today*, 34(9): 1242–1245.

Adelman-Mullally, T., Mulder, C.K., McCarter-Spalding, D.E., Hagler, D.A., Gaberson, K.B., Hanner, M.B., Oermann, M.H., Speakman, E.T., Yoder-Wise, P.S. and Young, P.K. (2013) 'The clinical nurse educator as leader', *Nurse Education in Practice*, 13(1): 29–34.

Agnew, T. (2018) 'New Standards will prepare students for the rigours of modern nursing', *Nursing Standard*, 33(1): 14–17.

Amy, A.H. (2008) 'Leaders as facilitators of individual and organizational learning', *Leadership & Organizational Development*, 29(3): 212–234.

An, D. and Carr, M. (2017) 'Learning styles theory fails to explain learning and achievement: Recommendations for alternative approaches', *Personality and Individual Differences*, 116: 410–416.

Anderson, A., Cant, R. and Hood, K. (2014) 'Measuring students' perceptions of inter-professional clinical placements: Development of the Inter-professional Clinical Placement Learning Environment Inventory', *Nurse Education in Practice*, 14(5): 518–524.

Anderson, E.E. (2009) 'Learning pathways in contemporary primary care settings – student nurses' views', *Nurse Education Today*, 29(8): 835–839.

Anderson, I. (2016) 'Identifying different learning styles to enhance the learning experience', *Nursing Standard*, 31(7): 53–61.

Anderson, L.W., Krathwohl, D.R. and Airasian, P.W. (2014) *A Taxonomy for Learning, Teaching, and Assessing: A Revision of Bloom's Taxonomy of Educational Objectives*. Harlow: Pearson Education Limited.

Andre, K. (2000) 'Grading student clinical practice performance: The Australian perspective', *Nurse Education Today*, 20(8): 672–679.

Andrews, M., Brewer, M., Buchan, T., Denne, A., Hammond, J., Hardy, G., Jacobs, L., McKenzie, L. and West, S. (2010) 'Implementation and sustainability of the nursing and midwifery standards for mentoring in the UK', *Nurse Education in Practice*, 10(5): 251–255.

Argyle, M. (1994) *The Psychology of Interpersonal Behaviour*, 5th edn. London: Penguin.

Armitage, E. (2010) 'Role of paramedic mentors in an evolving profession', *Journal of Paramedic Practice*, 2(1): 26–31.

Ashenafi, M.M. (2017) 'Peer-assessment in higher education – twenty-first-century practices, challenges and the way forward', *Assessment & Evaluation in Higher Education*, 42(2): 226–251.

Assessment Reform Group (for Nuffield Foundation) (2002) *Assessment of Learning: 10 Principles*. Available at: https://www.aaia.org.uk/content/uploads/2010/06/Assessment-for-Learning-10-principles.pdf (accessed 20 June 2018).

Association of Ambulance Chief Executives and Joint Royal Colleges Ambulance Liaison Committee (2016) *UK Ambulance Services Clinical Practice Guidelines 2016*. London: Class Publishing.

Ausubel, D., Novak, J. and Hanesian, H. (1978) *Educational Psychology: A Cognitive View*. New York: Rinehart & Winston.

Ballantyne, H. (2017) 'Undertaking effective handovers in the healthcare setting', *Nursing Standard*, 31(45): 53–61.

Bandura, A. (1996) *Social Learning Theory*. Harlow, UK: Pearson.

Bandura, A. (1997) *Self-Efficacy: The Exercise of Control*. New York: W.H. Freeman.

Barnett, J.E. (2008) 'Mentoring, boundaries, and multiple relationships: Opportunities and challenges', *Mentoring & Tutoring: Partnership in Learning*, 16(1): 3–16.

Baron, S. (2009) 'Evaluating the patient journey approach to ensure health care is centred on patients', *Nursing Times*, 105(22): 20–23.

Barr, H. (2003) 'Inter-professional issues and work-based learning', in J. Burton and N. Jackson (eds), *Work-Based Learning in Primary Care*. Oxford: Radcliffe Medical.

Barton, T.D. (2006) 'Clinical mentoring of nurse practitioners: The doctors' experience', *British Journal of Nursing*, 15(15): 820–824.

Bear, S. and Jones, G. (2016) 'Students as protégés – factors that lead to success', *Journal of Management Education*, 41(1): 146–168.

Benner, P. (2001) *From Novice to Expert: Excellence and Power in Clinical Nursing Practice*. London: Addison-Wesley.

Bennett, S., Mohr, J., Deal, K.H. and Hwang, J. (2012) 'Supervisor attachment, supervisory working alliance, and affect in social work field instruction', *Research on Social Work Practice*, 23(2): 199–209.

Berger, P. and Luckmann, T. (1967) *The Social Construction of Reality*. Middlesex: Penguin Books.

Bergsteiner, H., Avery, G.C. and Neumann, R. (2010) 'Kolb's experiential learning model: Critique from a modelling perspective', *Studies in Continuing Education*, 32(1): 29–46.

Biggs, J. and Tang, C. (2011) *Teaching for Quality Learning at University*, 4th edn. Maidenhead: Open University Press.

Bijol, V., Byrne-Dugan, C.J. and Hoenig, M.P. (2015) 'Medical student web-based formative assessment tool for renal pathology', *Medical Education Online*, 20(1): 26765. Available at: https://www.ncbi.nlm.nih.gov/m/pubmed/28229680/?i=4&from=/28277691/related#fft (accessed 22 March 2018).

Billay, D.B. and Yonge, O. (2004) 'Contributing to the theory development of preceptorship', *Nurse Education Today*, 24(7): 566–574.

Black, S., Curzio, J. and Terry, L. (2014) 'Failing a student nurse: A new horizon of moral courage', *Nursing Ethics*, 21(2): 224–238.

Bloom, B. (ed.) (1956) *Taxonomy of Educational Objectives: The Classification of Educational Goals, Handbook One: Cognitive Domain*. London: Longman.

Boitel, C.R. and Fromm, L.R. (2014) 'Defining signature pedagogy in social work education: Learning theory and the learning contract', *Journal of Social Work Education*, 50(4): 608–622.

Bondy, K.N. (1983) 'Criterion-referenced definitions for rating scales in clinical evaluation', *Journal of Nursing Education*, 22(9): 376–382.

Boud, D. (2016) *Enhancing Learning Through Self-assessment*. London: Routledge.

Boud, D., Keogh, R. and Walker, D. (eds) (2005 digital print) *Reflection: Turning Experience into Learning*. London: Kogan Page.

Bowker, P., French, D., Atkin, S.L., Patmore, J.E., Walton, C. and Aye, M. (2005) 'Financing a diabetes network: Care pathway based costing model for Type 1 diabetes mellitus', *Diabetic Medicine*, 23(Supp. 2): 107.

Bradshaw, C., Noonan, M., Barry, M. and Atkinson, S. (2013) 'Working and learning: Post-registration student midwives' experience of the competency assessment process', *Midwifery*, 29(5): 519–525.

Bray, L. and Nettleton, P. (2007) 'Assessor or mentor? Role confusion in professional education', *Nurse Education Today*, 27(8): 848–855.

Bray, L., O'Brien, M.R., Kirton, J., Zubairu, K. and Christiansen, A. (2014) 'The role of professional education in developing compassionate practitioners: A mixed methods study exploring the perceptions of health professionals and pre-registration students', *Nurse Education Today*, 34(3): 480–486.

British Association for Counselling and Psychotherapy (2016) *Ethical Framework for the Counselling Professions*. Available at: www.bacp.co.uk/events/learning_programmes/ethical_framework/documents/ethical_framework.pdf (accessed 1 May 2017).

British Medical Association (2012) *What is the European Working Time Directive?* Available at: www.bma.org.uk/advice/employment/working-hours/ewtd (accessed 20 August 2017).

British Medical Association (2017) *Deaneries and LETBs – What are the Core Functions of LETBs?* Available at: www.bma.org.uk/advice/career/applying-for-training/find-your-deanery (accessed 26 September 2017).

Brooke, J. and Ham, A. (2003) 'Coaching managers to become better team leaders', *Strategic Communication Management (SCM)*, 7(2): 4–27.

Brookes, I. and O'Neill, M. (eds) (2017) *Collins English Dictionary*, 2nd edn. Glasgow: HarperCollins Publishers.

Brown, J., Bullock, D. and Grossberg, S. (1999) 'How the basal ganglia use parallel excitatory and inhibitory learning pathways to selectively respond to unexpected rewarding cues', *Journal of Neuroscience*, 19(23): 10502–10511.

Brown, L. (2005) 'Ethics in clinical education', in M. Rose and D. Best (eds), *Transforming Practice through Clinical Education, Professional Supervision and Mentoring*. Edinburgh: Elsevier Churchill Livingstone.

Brown, T., Williams, B., McKenna, L., Palermo, C., McCall, L., Roller, L., Hewitt, L., Molloy, L., Baird, M. and Aldabah, L. (2011) 'Practice education learning environments: The mismatch between perceived and preferred expectations of undergraduate health science students', *Nurse Education Today*, 31(8): e22–e28.

Bruner, J. (1960) *The Process of Education*. Cambridge, MA: Harvard University Press.

Bryar, R.M. and Griffiths, J.M. (eds) (2003) *Practice Development in Community Nursing*. London: Arnold.

Buring, S.M., Bhushan, A., Broeseker, A., Conway, S., Duncan-Hewitt, W., Hansen, L. and Westberg, S. (2009) 'Inter-professional education: Definitions, student competencies, and guidelines for implementation', *American Journal of Pharmaceutical Education*, 73(4): 59.

Campbell, C. and Evans, P. (2016) 'Reciprocal benefits, legacy and risk: Applying Ellinger and Bostrom's model of line manager role identity as facilitators of learning', *European Journal of Training and Development*, 40(2): 74–89.

Care Quality Commission (2017) *CQC Fundamental Standards*. Available at: www.qcs.co.uk/useful-guides/quick-start-guide-fundamental-standards/ (accessed 17 April 2018).

Carlisle, C., Calman, L. and Ibbotson, T. (2009) 'Practice-based learning: The role of practice education facilitators in supporting mentors', *Nurse Education Today*, 29(7): 715–721.

Carlson, E. and Idvall, E. (2014) 'Nursing students' experiences of the clinical learning environment in nursing homes: A questionnaire study using the CLES + T evaluation scale', *Nurse Education Today*, 34(7): 1130–1134.

Carnwell, R., Baker, S., Bellis, M. and Murray, R. (2007) 'Managerial perceptions of mentor, lecturer practitioner and link tutor roles', *Nurse Education Today*, 27(8): 923–932.

Carper, B. (1978) 'Fundamental patterns of knowing in nursing', *Advances in Nursing Science*, 1(1): 13–23.

Centre for Policy on Ageing (2014) *The Effectiveness of Care Pathways in Health and Social Care*. Available at: www.ageuk.org.uk/Documents/EN-GB/For-professionals/Research/CPA-Effectiveness_of_care_pathways.pdf?dtrk=true (accessed 4 January 2018).

Centre for the Advancement of Inter-professional Education (2016) *CAIPE Inter-professional Education Guidelines 2016*. Available at: CAIPEInterprofessionalEducationGuidelines 2016.pdf (accessed 22 June 2018)

Centre for the Advancement of Inter-professional Education (2017) *CAIPE Inter-professional Education Guidelines*. Available at: www.caipe.org/resources/publications/caipe-publications/caipe-2017-interprofessional-education-guidelines-barr-h-ford-j-gray-r-helme-m-hutchings-m-low-h-machin-reeves-s (accessed 2 November 2017).

Chan, Z.C.Y., Stanley, D.J., Meadus, R.J. and Chien, W.T. (2017) 'A qualitative study on feedback provided by students in nurse education', *Nurse Education Today, 55*: 128–133.

Chartered Institute of Personnel and Development (2017) *What are Coaching and Mentoring?* Available at: www.cipd.co.uk/knowledge/fundamentals/people/development/coaching-mentoring-factsheet#6995 (accessed 13 January 2018).

Chartered Society of Physiotherapy (2011) *Physiotherapy Framework: Putting Physiotherapy Behaviours, Values, Knowledge and Skills into Practice*. Available at: http://esp.freshtester.co.uk/cms/wp-content/uploads/2015/09/physiotherapy_framework_condensed_updated_Sept_2013.pdf (accessed 5 May 2017).

Chartered Society of Physiotherapy (2017) *Learning and Development Principles*. Available at: www.csp.org.uk/professional-union/careers-development/career-physiotherapy/learning-principles (accessed 17 March 2017).

Choe, K., Park, S. and Yoo, S.Y. (2014) 'Effects of constructivist teaching methods on bioethics education for nursing students: A quasi-experimental study', *Nurse Education Today, 34*(5): 848–853.

Choi, Y., Kim, J.Y. and Yoo, T. (2016) 'A study on the effect of learning organisation readiness on employees' quality commitment: The moderating effect of leader–member exchange', *Total Quality Management & Business Excellence, 27*(3–4): 325–338.

Clark, E., Draper, J. and Rogers, J. (2015) 'Illuminating the process: Enhancing the impact of continuing professional education on practice', *Nurse Education Today, 35*(2): 388–394.

Clark, J.M., Maben, J. and Jones, K. (1997) 'Project 2000. Perception of the philosophy and practice of nursing: Preparation for practice', *Journal of Advanced Nursing, 26*(2): 246–256.

Cleak, H. and Smith, D. (2012) 'Student satisfaction with models of field placement supervision', *Australian Social Work, 65*(2): 243–258.

Cochrane Collaboration (2017) *What is a Systematic Review?* Available at: http://consumers.cochrane.org/what-systematic-review (accessed 24 May 2017).

Coleman, M. and Glover, D. (2010) *Educational Leadership and Management*. Maidenhead: Open University Press.

College of Operating Department Practitioners (2009) *Standards, Recommendations and Guidance for Mentors and Practice Placements: Supporting Pre-Registration Education in Operating Department Practice Provision*. Available at: www.uos.ac.uk/content/odp-mentoring-requirements (accessed 1 May 2017).

College of Social Work (2013) *Practice Educator Professional Standards for Social Work*. Available at: http://cdn.basw.co.uk/upload/basw_105938-8.pdf (accessed 1 May 2017).

Connor, M. and Pokora, J. (2012) *Coaching and Mentoring at Work: Developing Effective Practice*, 2nd edn. Maidenhead: Open University Press.

Council of Deans of Health (2017a) *Apprenticeships in Nursing and The Allied Health Professions – Briefing Paper Version 4*. Available at: www.councilofdeans.org.uk/wp-content/uploads/2016/08/Apprenticeships-paper-version-4-January-2017.pdf (accessed 19 November 2017).

Council of Deans of Health (2017b) *Online Practice Assessment and Evaluation (PARE) Project*. Available at: https://councilofdeans.org.uk/case-study/online-practice-assessment-evaluation-pare-project/ (accessed 2 October 2017).

Crombie, A., Brindley, J., Harris, D., Marks-Maran, D. and Thompson, T.M. (2013) 'Factors that enhance rates of completion: What makes students stay?', *Nurse Education Today*, 33(11): 1282–1287.

Cross, K.D. (1996) 'An analysis of the concept facilitation', *Nurse Education Today*, 16(5): 350–355.

Currie, K., Biggam, J., Palmer, J. and Corcoranm, T. (2012) 'Participants' engagement with and reactions to the use of on-line action learning sets to support advanced nursing role development', *Nurse Education Today*, 32(3): 267–272.

Curtis, K., Horton, K. and Smith, P. (2012) 'Student nurse socialisation in compassionate practice: A Grounded Theory study', *Nurse Education Today*, 32(7): 790–795.

Curzon, L.B. and Tummons, J. (2013) *Teaching in Further Education: An Outline of Principles and Practice*, 7th edn. London: Bloomsbury Academic.

Daloz, L.A. (1989) *Effective Teaching and Mentoring: Realizing the Transformational Power of Adult Learning Experiences*. San Francisco, CA: Jossey-Bass.

Darling, L.A.W. (1984) 'What do nurses want in a mentor?', *Journal of Nursing Administration*, 14(10): 42–44.

Darling, L.A.W. (1985) 'What to do about toxic mentors?', *Journal of Nursing Administration*, 15(5): 43–44.

Davies, S. and Priestley, M.J. (2006) 'A reflective evaluation of patient handover practices', *Nursing Standard*, 20(21): 49–52.

Davis, L., Taylor, H. and Reyes, H. (2014) 'Lifelong learning in nursing: A Delphi study', *Nurse Education Today*, 34(3): 441–445.

de la Harpe, B. and Radloff, A. (2000) 'Informed teachers and learners: The importance of assessing the characteristics needed for lifelong learning', *Studies in Continuing Education*, 22(2): 169–182.

de Luc, K. (2000) 'Care pathways: An evaluation of their effectiveness', *Journal of Advanced Nursing*, 32(2): 485–496.

DeBrew, J.K. and Lewallen, L.P. (2014) 'To pass or to fail? Understanding the factors considered by faculty in the clinical evaluation of nursing students', *Nurse Education Today*, 34(4): 631–636.

Department of Education & Department of Health (2016) *0 to 25 SEND Code of Practice: A guide for health professionals*. Available at https://assets.publishing.service.gov.uk/governement/uploads/system/uploads/attachment_data_file/502913/Health_Professional_Guide_to_the_Send_Code_of_Practice.pdf (accessed 18 June 2018).

Department of Health (2001) *Placements in Focus: Guidance for Education in Practice for Health Care Professions*. Available at: http://webarchive.nationalarchives.gov.uk/+/www.dh.gov.uk/en/Publicationsandstatistics/Publications/PublicationsPolicyAndGuidance/DH_4009511 (accessed 28 August 2017).

Department of Health (2002) *Liberating the Talents: Helping Primary Care Trusts and Nurses to Deliver the NHS Plan*. Available at: http://webarchive.nationalarchives.gov.uk/+/www.dh.gov.uk/en/Publicationsandstatistics/Publications/PublicationsPolicyAndGuidance/DH_4007473 (accessed 17 January 2018).

Department of Health (2004) *The NHS Knowledge and Skills Framework (NHS KSF) and the Development Review Process*. Available at: http://webarchive.nationalarchives.gov.uk/+/www.dh.gov.uk/en/Publicationsandstatistics/Publications/PublicationsPolicyAndGuidance/DH_4090843 (accessed 16 August 2017).

Department of Health (2007) *Patient Pathways: What is a Patient Pathway?* Available at: http://webarchive.nationalarchives.gov.uk/+/www.dh.gov.uk/en/Healthcare/Primarycare/Treatmentcentres/DH_4097263 (accessed 15 September 2017).

Department of Health (2008) *Towards a Framework for Post-Registration Nursing Careers: Consultation Response Report*. Available at: http://aape.org.uk/wp-content/uploads/2015/02/Mod-nursing-careers-consultation-rep-230708.pdf (accessed 17 January 2018).

Department of Health (2010) *Preceptorship Framework for Newly Registered Nurses, Midwives and Allied Health Professionals*. Available at: http://webarchive.nationalarchives.gov.uk/+/http://www.dh.gov.uk/en/Publications and statistics/Publications/PublicationsPolicyAndGuidance/DH_\\4074 (accessed 22 June 2018).

Department of Health (2012a) *Health and Social Care Act 2012*. Available at: www.legislation.gov.uk/ukpga/2012/7/contents/enacted (accessed 12 January 2018).

Department of Health (2012b) *Compassion in Practice: Nursing, Midwifery and Care Staff: Our Vision and Strategy*. Available at: www.england.nhs.uk/wp-content/uploads/2012/12/compassion-in-practice.pdf. (accessed 12 August 2017).

Department of Health (2012c) *Liberating the NHS: Developing the Healthcare Workforce from Design to Delivery*. Available at: www.gov.uk/government/publications/developing-the-healthcare-workforce-from-design-to-delivery (accessed 16 January 2018).

Department of Health (2013) *Education Outcomes Framework for Healthcare Workforce*. Available at: www.gov.uk/government/publications/education-outcomes-framework-for-healthcare-workforce (accessed 2 August 2017).

Department of Health (2015) *The NHS Constitution for England and Accompanying Documents*. Available at: www.gov.uk/government/collections/nhs-constitution-for-england-resources (accessed 12 August 2017).

Department of Health (2016a) *NHS Outcomes Framework 2016 to 2017*. Available at: www.gov.uk/government/publications/nhs-outcomes-framework-2016-to-2017 (accessed 26 January 2018).

Department of Health (2016b) *Health Education England Mandate 2016 to 2017*. Available at: www.gov.uk/government/publications/hee-mandate-2016-to-2017 (accessed 29 January 2018).

Department of Health and Children (Dublin) (2010) *A Review of Practice Development in Nursing and Midwifery in the Republic of Ireland and the Development of a Strategic Framework*. Available at: http://health.gov.ie/wp-content/uploads/2014/03/review_practice-development_nursing_midwifery.pdf (accessed 11 October 2017).

Dixon-Woods, M., Baker, R., Charles, K., Dawson, J., Jerzembek, G., Martin, G., McCarthy, I., McKee, L., Minion, J., Ozieranski, P., Willars, J., Wilkie, P. and West, M. (2014) 'Culture and behaviour in the English National Health Service: Overview of lessons from a large multimethod study', *BMJ Quality and Safety*, 23: 106–115.

Donabedian, A. (1988) 'The quality of care: How can it be assessed?', *American Journal of Public Health*, 260(12): 1743–1748.

Donaldson, J.H. and Carter, D. (2005) 'The value of role modelling: Perceptions of undergraduate and diploma nursing (adult) students', *Nurse Education in Practice*, 5(6): 353–359.

Dougherty, L., Lister, S. and West-Oram, A. (eds) (2015) *The Royal Marsden Hospital Manual of Clinical Nursing Procedures (Royal Marsden Manual Series)*, 9th edn. Oxford: Wiley-Blackwell.

du Toit-Brits, C. and Van Zyl, C. (2017) 'Self-directed learning characteristics: Making learning personal, empowering and successful', *Africa Education Review*, 14(3–4): 122–141.

Duane, B.T. and Satre, M.E. (2014) 'Utilizing constructivism learning theory in collaborative testing as a creative strategy to promote essential nursing skills', *Nurse Education Today*, 34(1): 31–34.

Duers, L.E. (2017) 'The learner as co-creator: A new peer review and self-assessment feedback form created by student nurses', *Nurse Education Today*, 58: 47–52.

Duffin, C. (2005) 'Pre-registration education to undergo major review', *Nursing Standard*, 19(26): 4.

Duffy, K. (2003) *Failing Students: A Qualitative Study of Factors that Influence the Decisions Regarding Assessment of Students' Competence in Practice*. Available at: https://pdfs.semanticscholar.org/4f28/68c6a3d66bcedb8ea079b0d19ec87bbe6148.pdf (accessed 3 October 2017).

Duffy, K. (2013) 'Providing constructive feedback to students during mentoring', *Nursing Standard*, 27(31): 50–56.

Duffy, K. (2016) *Failure to Fail – A Systematic Review of Where We Are Now*. Available at: www.rcn.org.uk/professional-development/research-and-innovation/research-events/rcn-2016-research-conference (accessed 27 April 2017).

Education and Training Foundation (2018) *Diploma in Education and Training*. Available at: https://www.feadvice.org.uk/i-want-work-fe-skills-sector/i-want-be-teacher-fe-skills/teaching-qualifications-fe-skills-sector/level15 (accessed 29 May 2018).

Elkan, R. and Robinson, J. (1995) 'Project 2000: A review of published research', *Journal of Advanced Nursing*, 22(2): 386–392.

Eller, L.S., Lev, E.L. and Feurer, A. (2014) 'Key components of an effective mentoring relationship: A qualitative study', *Nurse Education Today*, 34(5): 815–820.

Embo, M., Driessen, E., Valcke, M. and van der Vleuten, C.P.M (2014) 'A framework to facilitate self-directed learning, assessment and supervision in midwifery practice: A qualitative study of supervisors' perceptions', *Nurse Education in Practice*, 14(4): 441–446.

Encyclopaedia Britannica, Inc. (2018) *Herbartianisn – Education*. Available at: www.britannica.com/topic/Herbartianism (accessed 26 January 2018).

Equality Challenge Unit (2012) *Equality Act 2010: Implications for Colleges and HEIs*. Available at: http://www.ecu.ac.uk/publications/equality-act-2010-revised/ (accessed 20 March 2018).

European Parliament and The Council (2013) *Directive 2013/55/EU (amendment of European Union Directive 2005/36/EC)*. Available at: http://eur-lex.europa.eu/legal-content/EN/ALL/?uri=celex%3A32013L0055 (accessed 13 September 2017).

Evans, D. (2003) 'Hierarchy of evidence: A framework for ranking evidence evaluating healthcare interventions', *Journal of Clinical Nursing*, 12(1): 77–84.

Falender, C.A. (2014) 'Clinical supervision in a competency-based era', *South African Journal of Psychology*, 44 (1): 6–17.

Faugier, J. (2005a) 'Reality check', *Nursing Standard*, 19(19): 14–15.

Faugier, J. (2005b) 'Developing a new generation of nurse entrepreneurs', *Nursing Standard*, 19(30): 49–53.

FE News – Further Education College & Training Provider Magazine (2016) *Apprenticeship Standard: Registered Nurse Degree Apprenticeship Approved for Delivery*. Available at: www.fenews.co.uk/sector-news/13886-apprenticeship-standard-registered-nurse-degree-apprenticeship-approved-for-delivery (accessed 25 May 2017).

Fernandez, N., Dory, V., Ste-Marie, L., Chaput, M., Charlin, B. and Boucher, A. (2012) 'Varying conceptions of competence: An analysis of how health sciences educators define competence', *Medical Education*, 46(4): 357–365.

Field, J. (1999) 'Participation under the magnifying glass', *Adults Learning*, 11(3): 10–13.

Finnerty, G. and Collington, V. (2013) 'Practical coaching by mentors: Student midwives' perceptions', *Nurse Education in Practice*, 13(6): 573–577.

Fish, J., Baillie, L., Sykes, S., Barclay, J., Case, D., Crussell, J., O'Brien, M., Icheku, V., Humphries, P., Thompson, S. and Mitchell, J. (2016) 'An evaluation of the implementation of the Pan London Practice Assessment Document (PLPAD) for pre-registration nursing in London (9 London Universities)', NET2016 – 27th International Networking for Healthcare Education Conference. Available at: www.jillrogersassociates.co.uk/images/stories/NET_conf_pdfs/g1%20ecp%20theme%20abstract%20booklet.compressed.pdf (accessed 17 Feb 2017).

Fisher, M., Way, S., Chenery-Morris, S., Jackson, J. and Bower, H. (2017) 'Core principles to reduce current variations that exist in grading of midwifery practice in the United Kingdom', *Nurse Education in Practice*, 23(March 2017): 54–60.

Fitts, P.M. and Posner, M.I. (1973) *Human Performance*. London: Prentice-Hall.

Fleming, S., Mckee, G. and Huntley-Moore, S. (2011) 'Undergraduate nursing students' learning styles: A longitudinal study', *Nurse Education Today*, 31(5): 444–449.

Forde-Johnston, C. (2017) 'Developing and evaluating a foundation preceptorship programme for newly qualified nurses', *Nursing Standard*, 31(42): 42–52.

Foronda, C., MacWilliams, B. and McArthur, E. (2016) 'Inter-professional communication in healthcare: An integrative review', *Nurse Education in Practice*, 19(July 2016): 36–40.

Foster, H., Ooms, A. and Marks-Maran, D. (2015) 'Nursing students' expectations and experiences of mentorship', *Nurse Education Today*, 35(1): 18–24.

Francis, R. (2013) *Report of the Mid Staffordshire NHS Foundation Trust Public Inquiry (Francis Report)*. Available at: http://webarchive.nationalarchives.gov.uk/20150407084952/www.midstaffspublicinquiry.com/sites/default/files/report/Volume%201.pdf (accessed 15 August 2017).

Frazer, K., Connolly, M., Naughton, C. and Kow, V. (2014) 'Identifying clinical learning needs using structured group feedback: First-year evaluation of pre-registration nursing and midwifery degree programmes', *Nurse Education Today*, 34(7): 1104–1108.

Freire, P. (1996) *Pedagogy of the Oppressed*. London: Penguin.

Fretwell, J.E. (1980) 'An inquiry into the ward learning environment', *Nursing Times*, 76(16): 69–75.

Furness, S. and Gilligan, P. (2004) 'Fit for purpose: Issues from practice placements, practice teaching and assessment of students' practice', *Social Work Education*, 23(4): 465–479.

Gagné, R.M., Wager, W.W., Golas, K.C. and Keller, J.M. (2005) *Principles of Instructional Design*, 5th edn. Belmont (USA): Wadsworth Publishing.

Gainsbury, S. (2010) 'Mentors passing students despite doubts over ability', *Nursing Times*, 106(16): 1–3.

Garbett, R. and McCormack, B. (2002) 'A concept analysis of practice development', *Journal of Research in Nursing*, 7(2): 87–100.

Garside, J.R and Nhemachena, J.Z.Z. (2013) 'A concept analysis of competence and its transition in nursing', *Nurse Education Today*, 33(5): 541–545.

Garside, J., Nhemachena, J.Z.Z, Williams, J. and Topping, A. (2009) 'Repositioning assessment: Giving students the "choice" of assessment methods', *Nurse Education in Practice*, 9(2): 141–148.

General Medical Council (2013) *Good Medical Practice*. Available at: www.gmc-uk.org/static/documents/content/GMP_.pdf (accessed 26 September 2017).

Gibbs, G. (1988) *Improving the Quality of Student Learning*. Bristol: Technical Education Services.

Gilmour, J.A., Kopeiki, A. and Douché, J. (2007) 'Student nurses as peer-mentors: Collegiality in practice', *Nurse Education in Practice*, 7(1): 36–43.

Godlee, F. (2014) 'Evidence based medicine: Flawed system but still the best we've got' (Editorial), *BMJ*, 348(7942): g440.

Goldsmith, J., Clarke, B. and Cross, S. (2009) 'The art of learning to teach inter-professionally', *Practice Nursing*, 20(8): 414–416.

Gopee, N. (2000) 'Self-assessment and the concept of the lifelong learning nurse', *British Journal of Nursing*, 9(11): 724–729.

Gopee, N. (2001) 'The role of peer assessment and peer review in nursing', *British Journal of Nursing*, 10(2): 115–121.

Gopee, N. (2002a) 'Human and social capital as facilitators of lifelong learning in nursing', *Nurse Education Today*, 22(8): 608–616.

Gopee, N. (2002b) 'Demonstrating critical analysis in academic assignments', *Nursing Standard*, 16(35): 45–52.

Gopee, N. (2005) 'Facilitating the implementation of lifelong learning in nursing', *British Journal of Nursing*, 14(14): 761–767.

Gopee, N. (2010) *Practice Teaching in Healthcare*. London: Sage Publications.

Gopee, N. and Deane, M. (2013) 'Strategies for successful academic writing: Institutional and non-institutional support for students', *Nurse Education Today*, 33(12): 1624–1631.

Gopee, N. and Galloway, J. (2017) *Leadership and Management in Healthcare*, 3rd edn. London: Sage Publications.

Gopee, N., Tyrell, A., Raven, S., Thomas, K. and Hari, T. (2004) 'Effective clinical learning in primary care settings', *Nursing Standard*, 18(37): 33–37.

GOV.UK (2018) *Definition of Disability under the Equality Act 2010*. Available at: www.gov.uk/definition-of-disability-under-equality-act-2010 (accessed 26 January 2018).

Gover, S. (2010) 'Triennial review workshops facilitated by practice education facilitators', paper presented at Royal College of Nursing Education Forum 'Partners in Practice' Conference, 26–27 February, Blackpool.

Gratrix, L. and Barrett, D. (2017) 'Desperately seeking consistency: Student nurses' experiences and expectations of academic supervision', *Nurse Education Today*, 48(January 2017): 7–12.

Gray, J.A.M. (2001) *Evidence-Based Health Care: How to Make Policy and Management Decisions*, 2nd edn. Edinburgh: Churchill Livingstone.

Gray, M.A. and Smith, L.N. (2000) 'The qualities of an effective mentor from the student nurse's perspective: Findings from a longitudinal qualitative study', *Journal of Advanced Nursing*, 32(6): 1542–1549.

Guba, E.G. and Lincoln, Y.S. (1989) *Fourth Generation Evaluation*. London: Sage.

Gustafsson, M., Blomberg, K. and Holmefur, M. (2015) 'Test-retest reliability of the Clinical Learning Environment, Supervision and Nurse Teacher (CLES + T) scale', *Nurse Education in Practice*, 15(4): 253–257.

Hall, K.M., Draper, R.J., Smith, L.K. and Bullough, Jr, R.V. (2008) 'More than a place to teach: Exploring the perceptions of the roles and responsibilities of mentor teachers', *Mentoring & Tutoring: Partnership in Learning*, 16(3): 328–345.

Hallin, K. and Danielson, E. (2009) 'Being a personal preceptor for nursing students: Registered nurses' experiences before and after introduction of a preceptor model', *Journal of Advanced Nursing*, 65(1): 161–174.

Handy, C. (1989) *Age of Unreason*. London: Business Books.

Hauer, K.E., Oza, S.K., Kogan, J.R., Stankiewicz, C.A., Stenfors-Hayes, T., Cate, O.T., Batt, J. and O'Sullivan, P.S. (2015) 'How clinical supervisors develop trust in their trainees: A qualitative study', *Medical Education*, 49(8): 783–795.

Hawkins, P. and Shohet, R. (2012) *Supervision in the Helping Professions*, 4th edn. Milton Keynes: Open University Press.

Haycock-Stuart, E., Donaghy, E. and Darbyshire, C. (2016) 'Involving users and carers in the assessment of preregistration nursing students' clinical nursing practice: A strategy for patient empowerment and quality improvement?' *Journal of Clinical Nursing*, 25(13–14): 2052–2065.

Health and Care Professions Council (2012) *Your Guide to Our Standards for Continuing Professional Development*. Available at: www.hcpc-uk.org/assets/documents/10003B70Yourguidetoourstandardsofcontinuingprofessionaldevelopment.pdf (accessed 16 August 2017).

Health and Care Professions Council (2013) *Standards of Proficiency – Physiotherapists*. Available at: www.hpc-uk.org/assets/documents/10000DBCStandards_of_Proficiency_Physiotherapists.pdf (accessed 4 April 2017).

Health and Care Professions Council (2014a) *Standards of Proficiency – Paramedics*. Available at: www.hpc-uk.org/assets/documents/1000051CStandards_of_Proficiency_Paramedics.pdf (accessed 28 July 2017).

Health and Care Professions Council (2014b) *Standards of Proficiency – Operating Department Practitioners*. Available at: www.hpc-uk.org/assets/documents/10000514Standards_of_Proficiency_ODP.pdf (accessed 30 May 2017).

Health and Care Professions Council (2016) *Standards of Conduct, Performance and Ethics*. Available at: www.hcpc-uk.org/publications/index.asp?id=38#publicationSearchResults (accessed 15 February 2017).

Health and Care Professions Council (2017a) *Standards of Education and Training*. Available at: www.hpc-uk.org/assets/documents/10000BCF46345Educ-Train-SOPA5_v2.pdf (accessed 4 July 2017).

Health and Care Professions Council (2017b) *About Us*. Available at: www.hpc-uk.org/aboutus/ (accessed 1 May 2017).

Health Education East of England (2014) *Collaborative Learning in Practice (CLiP) for Pre-registration Nursing Students*. Available at: https://hee.nhs.uk/sites/default/files/documents/CLiP-Paper-final-version-Sept-14.pdf (accessed 7 April 2017).

Health Education England (2014) *Values Based Recruitment Framework*. Available at: www.hee.nhs.uk/sites/default/files/documents/VBR_Framework%20March%202016.pdf (accessed 28 August 2017).

Health Education England (2015) *Mentor Toolkit*. Available at: www.valuesbasedmentorship.co.uk/the-toolkit.html (accessed 20 April 2017).

Health Education England (2017a) *Nursing Associate Curriculum Framework*. Available at: www.hee.nhs.uk/sites/default/files/documents/Nursing%20Associate%20Curriculum%20Framework%20Feb2017.pdf (accessed 29 August 2017).

Health Education England (2017b) *Our Leaders and Structure*. Available at: www.hee.nhs.uk/about-us/how-we-work/our-leaders-structure (accessed 12 August 2017).

Hean, S., Clark, J.M., Adams, K., Humphris, D. and Lathlean, J. (2006) 'Being seen by others as we see ourselves: The congruence between the in-group and outgroup perceptions of health and social care students', *Learning in Health and Social Care*, 5(1): 10–22.

Heaslip, V. and Scammell, J.M.E. (2012) 'Failing underperforming students: The role of grading in practice assessment', *Nurse Education in Practice*, 12(2): 95–100.

Hegarty, J. (2017) 'Schema to demonstrate maintenance of professional competence for Nurses and Midwives: Results of a National Mixed Methods Study presented at NET2017 conference'. Available at: www.heacademy.ac.uk/knowledge-hub/schema-demonstrate-maintenance-professional-competence-nurses-and-midwives-results (accessed 16 March 2018).

Heirs, B. and Farrell, P. (1986) *The Professional Decision Thinker*. London: Sidgwick & Jackson.

Helminen, K., Johnson, M., Isoaho, H., Turunrn, H. and Tossavainen, K. (2017) 'Final assessment of nursing students in clinical practice: Perspectives of nursing teachers, students and mentors', *Journal of Clinical Nursing*, 26 (23–24): 4795–4803.

Henderson, A., Creedy, D., Boorman, R., Cooke, M. and Walker, R. (2010) 'Development and psychometric testing of the Clinical Learning Organisational Culture Survey (CLOCS)', *Nurse Education Today*, 30(7): 598–602.

Henderson, A., Cooke, M., Creedy, D.K. and Walker, R. (2012) 'Nursing students' perceptions of learning in practice environments: A review', *Nurse Education Today*, 32(3): 299–302.

Henricson, M., Fridlund, B., Martensson, J. and Hedberg, B. (2018) 'The validation of the Supervision of Thesis Questionnaire (STQ)', *Nurse Education Today*, 65 (2018): 11–16.

Heron, J. (2009) *Helping the Client – A Creative Practical Guide*, 5th edn. London: Sage Publications.

Heyns, T., Botma, Y. and Van Rensburg, G. (2017) 'A creative analysis of the role of practice development facilitators in a critical care environment', *Health SA Gesondheid*, 22(December): 105–111.

Hinton, J. (2009) 'Mentorship: The experiences of a tutor in a pre-registration operating department practice education programme', *Journal of Perioperative Practice*, 19(7): 221–224.

Hodgson, A.K. and Scanlan, J.M. (2013) 'A concept analysis of mentoring in nursing leadership', *Open Journal of Nursing*, 3: 389–394.

Holland, K. and Lauder, W. (2012) 'A review of evidence for the practice learning environment: Enhancing the context for nursing and midwifery care in Scotland', *Nurse Education in Practice*, 12(1): 60–64.

Holt, J., Coates, C., Cotterill, D., Eastburn, S., Laxton, J., Young, C. and Mistry, H. (2010) 'Identifying common competences in health and social care: An example of multi-institutional and inter-professional working', *Nurse Education Today*, 30(3): 264–270.

Honey, P. and Mumford, A. (2000) *The Learning Styles Helper's Guide*. Maidenhead: Peter Honey.

Hood, K., Cant, R., Baulch, J., Gilbee, A., Leech, M., Anderson, A. and Davies, K. (2014) 'Prior experience of inter-professional learning enhances undergraduate nursing and healthcare students' professional identity and attitudes to teamwork', *Nurse Education in Practice*, 14(2): 117–122.

Houghton, T. (2016) 'Assessment and accountability: Part 2 – managing failing students', *Nursing Standard*, 30(41): 41–49.

Hughes, C. (1999) 'The dire in self-directed learning', *Adults Learning*, 11(2): 7–9.

Hughes, L.J., Mitchell, M. and Johnston, A.N.B (2016) '"Failure to fail" in nursing – A catch phrase or a real issue? A systematic integrative literature review', *Nurse Education in Practice*, 20(September): 54–63.

Hughes, S.J. and Quinn, F.M. (2013) *Quinn's Principles and Practice of Nurse Education*, 6th edn. Andover: Cengage Learning EMEA.

Hunt, J. (1997) 'Towards evidence-based practice', *Nursing Management*, 4(2): 14–17.

Hunt, L.A., McGee, P., Gutteridge, R. and Hughes, M. (2012) 'Assessment of nurses in practice: A comparison of theoretical and practical assessment results in England', *Nurse Education Today*, 32(4): 351–355.

Hunt, L.A., McGee, P., Gutteridge, R. and Hughes, M. (2016) 'Manipulating mentors' assessment decisions: Do underperforming student nurses use coercive strategies to influence mentor's practical assessment decisions?' *Nurse Education in Practice*, 20(September): 154–162.

Hutchison, T. and Cochrane, J. (2014) 'A phenomenological study into the impact of the sign-off mentor in the acute hospital setting', *Nurse Education Today*, 34(6): 1029–1033.

Institute for Apprenticeships (2016a, updated May 2017) *Apprenticeship Standard: Registered Nurse Degree Apprenticeship (Approved for Delivery)*. Available at: www.gov.uk/government/publications/apprenticeship-standard-registered-nurse-degree-apprenticeship (accessed 4 September 2017).

Institute for Apprenticeships (2016b, updated May 2017) *Non-integrated Degree Apprenticeship Standard – Registered Nurse – Assessment Plan*. Available at: www.gov.uk/government/uploads/system/uploads/attachment_data/file/613261/Degree_Nursing_EPA.pdf (accessed 3 September 2017).

Institute for Apprenticeships (2017) *Apprenticeship Standard: Registered Nurse Degree Apprenticeship (Approved for Delivery)*. Available at: www.gov.uk/government/publications/apprenticeship-standard-registered-nurse-degree-apprenticeship (accessed 20 March 2018).

Institute of Directors (2014) *Coaching*. Available at: www.iod.com/training/bespoke-training/coaching (accessed 30 December 2017).

Institute of Healthcare Improvement (2017) *Plan–Do–Study–Act (PDSA) Worksheet*. Available at: www.ihi.org/resources/Pages/Tools/PlanDoStudyActWorksheet.aspx (accessed 14 August 2017).

Irving, S., Millins, M. and Milman, E. (2016) 'Introducing the UK Ambulance Services Clinical Practice Guidelines 2016', *Journal of Paramedic Practice*, 8(2): 68–69.

Jack, K., Hamshire, C. and Chambers, A. (2017) 'The influence of role models in undergraduate nurse education', *Journal of Clinical Nursing*, 26(23–24): 4707–4715.

Jarvis, P. (2010) *Adult Education and Lifelong Learning Theory and Practice*, 4th edn. New York: Routledge.

Jayasekara, R., Smith, C., Hall, C., Rankin, E., Smith, M., Visvanathan, V. and Friebe, T. (2018) 'The effectiveness of clinical education models for undergraduate nursing programs: A systematic review', *Nurse Education in Practice*, 29 (March 2018): 116–126.

Jeffs, T. (2003) 'Quest for knowledge begins with a recognition of shared ignorance', *Adults Learning*, 14(6): 28.

Jervis, A. and Tilki, M. (2011) 'Why are nurse mentors failing to fail student nurses who do not meet clinical performance standards?' *British Journal of Nursing*, 20(9): 582–587.

Johansson, U., Kaila, P., Ahlner-Elmqvist, M., Leksell, J. and Isoaho, H. (2010) 'Clinical learning environment, supervision and nurse teacher evaluation scale: Psychometric evaluation of the Swedish version', *Journal of Advanced Nursing*, 66(9): 2085–2093.

Johnson, E.A. (2017) *Working Together in Clinical Supervision – A Guide for Supervisors and Supervisees*. New York, Momentum Press Health.

Joint Royal Colleges Ambulance Liaison Committee & Association of Ambulance Chief Executives (2017) *UK Ambulance Services Clinical Practice Guidelines 2016*. Available at: https://aace.org.uk/clinical-practice-guidelines/ (accessed 28 July 2017).

Jokelainen, M., Turunen, H., Tossavainen, K., Jamookeeah, D. and Coco, K. (2011) 'A systematic review of mentoring nursing students in clinical placements', *Journal of Clinical Nursing*, 20(19–20): 2854–2867.

Jolly, S.N., Hyatt, S.A., Dadge, J.R. and Summerhill, K. (2017) 'Using mentor activities to assist nurses and midwives with their revalidation requirements', *Nursing Standard*, 31(20): 45–52.

Jones, P., Comber, J. and Conboy, A. (2012) 'The art and science of mentorship in action', *Journal of Paramedic Practice*, 4(8): 474–479.

Joyce, B., Calhoun, E. and Hopkins, D. (2009) *Models of Learning: Tools for Teaching*, 3rd edn. Maidenhead: Open University Press.

Kelton, M.F. (2014) 'Clinical coaching – An innovative role to improve marginal nursing students' clinical practice', *Nurse Education in Practice*, 14(6): 709–713.

Kendall-Raynor, P. (2007) 'Nurse cleared in supervision case is to face NMC', *Nursing Standard*, 21(17): 9.

Kerry, T. and Mayes, A.S. (eds) (1995) *Issues in Mentoring*. London: Routledge/Open University.

Kilminster, S.M., Jolly, B.C., Grant, J. and Cottrell, D. (2007) 'AMEE Guide No. 27: Effective educational and clinical supervision', *Medical Teacher*, 29(1): 2–19. Also available at: https://www.researchgate.net/publication/6297076_AMEE_Guide_N_27_Effective_educational_and_clinical_supervision (accessed 3 May 2018).

King's College London (National Nursing Research Unit) (2014) *Sustaining and Assuring the Quality of Student Nurse Mentorship: What are the Challenges?* Available at: www.kcl.ac.uk/nursing/research/nnru/policy/By-Issue-Number/Policy-Issue-43.pdf (accessed 26 September 2017).

Kirkham, L.A. (2018) 'Exploring the use of high-fidelity simulation training to enhance clinical skills', *Nursing Standard*, 32(24): 44–53.

Knowles, M.S. (2015) *The Adult Learner: The Definitive Classic in Adult Education and Human Resource Development*, 8th edn. London: Routledge.

Koffka, K. (1935) *Principles of Gestalt Psychology*. Available at: https://archive.org/details/in.ernet.dli.2015.7888 (accessed 19 November 2017).

Kohler, W. (1925) 'The mentality of apes', in E. Smith, S. Nolen-Hoeksema and B. Fredrickson (eds) (2003) *Atkinson and Hilgard's Introduction to Psychology*, 14th edn. London: Thomson/Wadsworth.

Kolb, D.A. (2014) *Experiential Learning: Experience as the Source of Learning and Development*, 2nd edn. New Jersey (US): Pearson FT Press.

Kopp, P. (2001) 'Fit for practice – 6.1: what is evidence-based practice?', *Nursing Times*, 97 (22): 47–50.

Kouzes, J.M. and Posner, B.Z. (2012) *The Leadership Challenge*, 5th edn. San Francisco, CA: Jossey-Bass.

Kramer, M. (1974) *Reality Shock: Why Nurses Leave Nursing*. St Louis, MO: Mosby.

Krathwohl, D.R. (2002) 'A revision of Bloom's Taxonomy: An overview', *Theory into Practice*, 41(4): 212–218.

Krathwohl, D.R., Bloom, B.S., Masia, B.B. (1964) *Taxonomy of Educational Objectives; The Classification of Educational Goals. Handbook II: The Affective Domain*. New York: Longman, Green.

Krathwohl, D., Bloom, B. and Masia, B. (1999) *A Taxonomy of Educational Objectives: The Classification of Education Goals, Handbook 2: Affective Domain*, 2nd edn. Harlow: Longman.

Kumar, S., Osborne, K., and Lehmann, T. (2015) 'Clinical supervision of allied health professional in country South Australia: A mixed methods pilot study'. *Australian Journal of Rural Health*, 23(5): 265–271.

Lafave, M.R. and Katz, L. (2014) 'Validity and reliability of the Standardized Orthopedic Assessment Tool (SOAT): A variation of the traditional objective structured clinical examination', *Journal of Athletic Training*, 49(3): 373–380.

Lait, J., Suter, E. and Deutschlander, S. (2011) 'Inter-professional mentoring: Enhancing students' clinical learning', *Nurse Education in Practice*, 11(3): 211–215.

Lakasing, E. and Francis, H. (2005) 'The crisis in student mentorship', *Primary Health Care*, 15(4): 40–41.

Lancer, N., Megginson, D. and Clutterbuck, D. (2016) *Techniques for Coaching and Mentoring*, 2nd edn. London: Routledge.

Lane, M. (2014) 'Student perceptions in relation to paramedic educator (ped) roles', *Journal of Paramedic Practice*, 6(4): 194–199.

Lankshear, A. (1990) 'Failure to fail: The teacher's dilemma', *Nursing Standard*, 4(20): 35–37.

Lavender, R.J.B. (2017) 'What can dyslexic paramedic students teach us about mentoring? A case study', *Journal of Paramedic Practice*, 9(5): 202–206.

Lee, N. (2011) 'An evaluation of CPD learning and impact upon positive practice change', *Nurse Education Today*, 31(4): 390–395.

Leggat, S.G., Balding, C. and Schiftan, D. (2014) 'Developing clinical leaders: The impact of an action learning mentoring programme for advanced practice nurses', *Journal of Clinical Nursing*, 24(11/12): 1576–1584.

Lester, S. and Costley, C. (2010) 'Work-based learning at higher education level: Value, practice and critique', *Studies in Higher Education*, 35(5): 561–575.

Liefer, D. (2002) 'Do you have a plan?', *Nursing Standard*, 16(41): 14–17.

Lindberg, J.B., Hunter, M.L. and Kruszewski, A.Z. (1998) *Introduction to Nursing: Concepts, Issues and Opportunities*, 3rd edn. Philadelphia, PA: Lippincott.

Lindquist, I., Engardt, M., Garnham, L., Poland, F. and Richardson, B. (2006) 'Development pathways in learning to be a physiotherapist', *Physiotherapy Research International*, 11(3): 129–139.

Lockeman, K.S., Appelbaum, N.P., Dow, A.W., Orr, S., Huff, T.A., Hogan, C.J. and Queen, B.A. (2017) 'The effect of an inter-professional simulation-based education program on perceptions and stereotypes of nursing and medical students: A quasi-experimental study', *Nurse Education Today*, 58(November): 32–37.

Logue, N.C. (2017) 'Evaluating practice-based learning', *Journal of Nursing Education*, 56(3): 131–138.

Lunyk-Child, O.L., Crooks, D., Ellis, P.J., Ofosu, C., O'Mara, L. and Rideout, E. (2001) 'Self-directed learning: Faculty and student perceptions', *Journal of Nursing Education*, 40(3): 116–123.

Macneil, C. (2001) 'The supervisor as a facilitator of informal learning in work teams', *Journal of Workplace Learning*, 13(1): 246–253.

Mallik, M. and McGowan, B. (2007) 'Issues in practice-based learning in nursing in the United Kingdom and the Republic of Ireland: Results from a multi-professional scoping exercise', *Nurse Education Today*, 27(1): 52–59.

Marks-Maran, D., Ooms, A., Tapping, J., Muir, J., Phillips, S. and Burke, L. (2013) 'A preceptorship programme for newly qualified nurses: a study of preceptees' perceptions', *Nurse Education Today*, 33(11): 1428–1434.

Marshall, J.E. (2012) 'Developing midwifery practice through work-based learning: An exploratory study', *Nurse Education in Practice*, 12(5): 273–278.

Marton, F., Hounsell, D. and Entwistle, N. (eds) (1997) *The Experience of Learning*, 2nd edn. Edinburgh: Scottish Academic Press.

Maslow, A.H. (1987) *Motivation and Personality*, 3rd edn. London: Harper & Row.

Maxwell, R.J. (1984) 'Quality assurance in health care', *British Medical Journal*, 288(6428): 1470–1472.

Maynard, S.P., Mertz, L.K.P. and Fortune, A.E. (2015) 'Off-site supervision in social work education: What makes it work?', *Journal of Social Work Education*, 51(3): 519–534.

McCalmont, C. and Lees, S. (2015) 'Care and compassion count: Support student midwives in practice', in S. Byram and S. Downe (eds), *The Roar Behind the Silence: Why Kindness, Compassion and Respect Matter in Maternity Care*. London: Martin Ltd. Chapter 27.

McCarthy, B. and Murphy, S. (2008) 'Assessing undergraduate nursing students in clinical practice: Do preceptors use assessment strategies?', *Nurse Education Today*, 28(3): 301–313.

McCarthy, S., O'Raghallaigh, P., Woodworth, S., Lim, Y.L., Kenny, L.C. and Adam, F. (2016) 'An integrated patient journey mapping tool for embedding quality in healthcare service reform', *Journal of Decision Systems*, 25(sup1): 354–368.

McCormack, B., Manley, K. and Titchen, A. (2013) *Practice Development in Nursing and Healthcare*. Oxford: Wiley-Blackwell.

McGivney, V. (2003) *Adult Learning Pathways: Through Routes or Cul-de-Sacs?*. Leicester: National Institute of Adult Continuing Education.

McGregor, D. (1987) *The Human Side of Enterprise*. London: Penguin.

McKimm, J., Jollie, C. and Hatter, M. (2007) *Mentoring: Theory and Practice*. Available at: www.faculty.londondeanery.ac.uk/e-learning/feedback/files/Mentoring_Theory_and_Practice.pdf (accessed 29 December 2017).

McLeod, F., Jamison, C. and Treasure, K. (2018) 'Promoting interprofessional learning and enhancing the pre-registration student experience through reciprocal cross professional peer tutoring', *Nurse Education Today*, 64 (2018): 190–195.

Mead, D. (2011) 'Views of nurse mentors about their role', *Nursing Management*, 18(6): 18–23.

Megginson, D., Clutterbuck, D., Garvey, B., Stokes, P. and Garrett-Harris, R. (2006) *Mentoring in Action: A Practical Guide*. London: Kogan Page.

Middleton, L. and Llewellyn, D. (2016) 'How to record and evidence continuing professional development for revalidation', *Nursing Standard*, 30(44): 42–46.

Millar, L., Conlon, M. and McGirr, D. (2017) 'Students' perspectives of using the hub and spoke model to support and develop learning in practice', *Nursing Standard*, 32(9): 41–49.

Milligan, F., Wareing, M., Preston-Shoot, M., Pappas, Y., Randhawa, G. and Bhandol, J. (2017) 'Supporting nursing, midwifery and allied health professional students to raise concerns with the quality of care: A review of the research literature', *Nurse Education Today*, 57(October): 29–39.

Mikkonen, K., Elo, S., Miettunen, J., Saarikoski, M., Kääriäinen, M. (2017) 'Development and testing of the CALDs and CLES+T scales for international nursing students' clinical learning environments', *Journal of Advanced Nursing*, 73 (8): 1997–2011.

Molle, E.A. and Durham, L.S. (2004) *Lippincott Williams and Wilkins' Administrative Medical Assisting*. New York: Lippincott Williams & Wilkins.

Moniz, T., Arntfield, S., Miller, K., Lingard, L., Watling, C. and Regehr, G. (2015) 'Considerations in the use of reflective writing for student assessment: Issues of reliability and validity', *Medical Education*, 49(9): 901–908.

Mooney, H. (2009) 'Lack of support for nurse entrepreneurs may hold back practice innovation', *Nursing Times*. Available at: www.nursingtimes.net/whats-new-in-nursing/lack-of-support-for-nurse-entrepreneurs-may-hold-back-practice-innovation/1981253. article (accessed 24 April 2014).

Moore, A. (2018) 'Preceptorship scheme aims to give new nurses a flying start', *Nursing Standard*, 32(22): 18–20.

Moore, L. (2010) 'Work-based learning and the role of managers', *Nursing Management*, 17(5): 26–29.

Moore, L. (2015) 'Donabedian's structure-process-outcome quality of care model', *Journal of Trauma and Acute Care Surgery*, 78(6): 1168–1175. Available at: www.ncbi.nlm.nih.gov/pubmed/26151519.

Moore, A. (2017) 'At the vanguard of quality patient care', *Nursing Standard*, 31(28): 22–3.

Morley, D. (2016) 'Applying Wenger's communities of practice theory to placement learning', *Nurse Education Today*, 39(April 2016): 161–162.

Morley, D.A., Wilson, K. and McDermott, J. (2017) 'Changing the practice learning landscape', *Nurse Education in Practice*, 27(November): 169–171.

Mott Macdonald and Nursing and Midwifery Council (2017) *Quality Assurance Handbook – September 2017*. Available at: http://www.nmc.mottmac.com/Portals/0/QA_Handbook_A4%20version_2017-18_FINAL.pdf?ver=2017-09-28-154531-177 (accessed 17 April 2018).

Mulholland, J., Scammell, J., Turnock, C. and Gregg, B. (2006) *Making Practice-Based Learning Work: Final Report*. Newcastle-upon-Tyne: Northumbria University.

Nancarrow, S.A., Wade, R., Moran, A., Coyle, J., Young, J. and Boxall, D. (2014) 'Connecting practice: a practitioner centered model of supervision', *Clinical Governance: An Internation Journal*, 19(3): 235–252.

National Committee of Inquiry into Higher Education (1997) *Higher Education in the Learning Society (The Dearing Report)*. Norwich: HMSO.

National Institute for Health and Care Excellence (2014) *Safe Staffing for Nursing in Adult Inpatient Wards in Acute Hospitals*. Available at: www.nice.org.uk/guidance/sg1 (accessed 31 January 2018).

National Institute for Health and Care Excellence (2017) *NICE Pathways*. Available at: https://pathways.nice.org.uk/ (accessed 28 August 2017).

National Institute for Health Research (2017) *Health Technology Assessment*. Available at: www.nihr.ac.uk/funding-and-support/funding-for-research-studies/funding-programmes/health-technology-assessment/ (accessed 12 August 2017).

Neary, M. (2000) 'Responsive assessment of clinical competence (Part 1)', *Nursing Standard*, 15(9): 34–36.

Nevalainen, M., Lunkka, N. and Suhonen, M. (2018) 'Work-based learning in health care organisations experienced by nursing staff: A systematic review of qualitative studies', *Nurse Education in Practice*, 29 (March 2018): 21–29.

Newton, J.M., Billett, S. and Ockerby, C.M. (2009) 'Journeying through clinical placements: An examination of six student cases', *Nurse Education Today*, 29(6): 630–634.

Newton, J.M., Jolly, B.C., Ockerby, C.M. and Cross, W.M. (2010) 'Clinical learning environment inventory: Factor analysis', *Journal of Advanced Nursing*, 66(6): 1371–1381.

Ng, J.Y. (2014) 'Combining Peyton's four-step approach and Gagne's instructional model in teaching slit-lamp examination', *Perspectives on Medical Education*, 3(6): 480–485.

NHS Education for Scotland (2014) *Practice Education Facilitator and Care Home Education Facilitator*. Available at: www.nes.scot.nhs.uk/media/3037761/pef_chef_report_2014_final.docx (accessed 29 December 2017).

NHS Education for Scotland (2017) *Flying Start NHS*. Available at: https://learn.nes.nhs.scot/735/flying-start-nhs (accessed 29 December 2017).

NHS Employers (2010) *Simplified KSF*. Available at: http://webarchive.nationalarchives.gov.uk/20130513104708/www.nhsemployers.org/PayAndContracts/AgendaForChange/KSF/Simplified-KSF/Pages/SimplifiedKSF.aspx (accessed 21 January 2018).

NHS England (2016) *Leading Change, Adding Value – A Framework for Nursing, Midwifery and Care Staff*. Available at: www.england.nhs.uk/wp-content/uploads/2016/05/nursing-framework.pdf (accessed 14 August 2017).

NHS England (2017a) *A-EQUIP a Model of Clinical Midwifery Supervision*. Available at: https://www.england.nhs.uk/wp-content/upload/2017/04/a-equip-midwifery-supervision-model.pdf (accessed 15 May 2018).

NHS England (2017b) *Next Steps on The NHS Five Year Forward View*. Available at: www.england.nhs.uk/wp-content/uploads/2017/03/NEXT-STEPS-ON-THE-NHS-FIVE-YEAR-FORWARD-VIEW.pdf (accessed 4 October 2017).

NHS England (2017c) *Change Model*. Available at: www.england.nhs.uk/ourwork/qual-clin-lead/sustainableimprovement/change-model/ (accessed 17 September 2017).

NHS England (2018) *Sustainable Improvement Team*. Available at: www.england.nhs.uk/sustainableimprovement/ (accessed 24 January 2018).

NHS England National Quality Board (2014) *How to Ensure the Right People, with the Right Skills, are in the Right Place at the Right Time: A Guide to Establishing Nursing, Midwifery and Care Staffing Capacity and Capability*. Available at: www.england.nhs.uk/wp-content/uploads/2013/11/nqb-how-to-guid.pdf (accessed 26 January 2018).

Nolen-Hoeksema, S., Fredrickson, B., Loftus, G.R., Lutz, C. (2014) *Atkinson and Hilgard's Introduction to Psychology*, 14th edn. Hampshire: Cengage Learning.

Norman, I.J., Watson, R., Murrells, T., Calman, L. and Redfern, S. (2002) 'The validity and reliability of methods to assess the competence to practise of pre-registration nursing and midwifery students', *International Journal of Nursing Studies*, 39(2): 133–145.

Nursing and Midwifery Council (2004a) *Standards of Proficiency for Specialist Community Public Health Nurses*. London: Nursing and Midwifery Council.

Nursing and Midwifery Council (2004b) *Supporting Nurses and Midwives through Lifelong Learning*. London: Nursing and Midwifery Council.

Nursing and Midwifery Council (2006) *Preceptorship Guidelines*, NMC Circular 21/2006. Available at: www.nmc.org.uk/globalassets/siteDocuments/Circulars/2006circulars/NMC-circular-21_2006.pdf (accessed 29 December 2017).

Nursing and Midwifery Council (2007a) *Guidance for the Introduction of the Essential Skills Clusters for Pre-registration Nursing Programmes*. Available at: www.nmc.org.uk/globalassets/sitedocuments/circulars/2007circulars/nmccircular07_2007.pdf (accessed 11 January 2018).

Nursing and Midwifery Council (2007b) *Ensuring Continuity of Practice Assessment through the Ongoing Achievement Record*, NMC Circular 33/2007. Available at: http://resourcelists.rgu.ac.uk/items/91EA454D-6AFC-AAC3-1D8F-320B17C4C890.html (accessed 11 January 2018).

Nursing and Midwifery Council (2008) *Standards to Support Learning and Assessment in Practice*. London: Nursing and Midwifery Council.

Nursing and Midwifery Council (2009) *Standards for Pre-registration Midwifery Education*. Available at: www.nmc.org.uk/globalassets/sitedocuments/standards/nmc-standards-for-preregistration-midwifery-education.pdf (accessed 24 September 2017).

Nursing and Midwifery Council (2010a) *Standards for Pre-registration Nursing Education*. Available at: www.nmc.org.uk/globalassets/sitedocuments/standards/nmc-standards-for-pre-registration-nursing-education.pdf (accessed 21 January 2018).

Nursing and Midwifery Council (2010b) *Sign-Off Mentor Criteria, NMC Circular 05/2010*. Available at: www.nmc.org.uk/globalassets/sitedocuments/circulars/2010circulars/nmccircular05_2010.pdf (accessed 29 December 2017).

Nursing and Midwifery Council (2010c) *Record Keeping: Guidance for Nurses and Midwives*. Available at: www.nmc.org.uk/standards/code/record-keeping (accessed 21 January 2018).

Nursing and Midwifery Council (2015a) *The Code: Professional Standards of Practice and Behaviour for Nurses and Midwives*. Available at: www.nmc.org.uk/globalassets/sitedocuments/nmc-publications/nmc-code.pdf (accessed 14 August 2017).

Nursing and Midwifery Council (2015b) *Raising Concerns: Guidance for Nurses and Midwives*. Available at: www.nmc.org.uk/standards/guidance/raising-concerns-guidance-for-nurses-and-midwives/ (accessed 14 August 2017).

Nursing and Midwifery Council (2015c) *Legal Change Will Protect Nursing and Midwifery Students Who Raise Concerns*. Available at: www.nmc.org.uk/news/press-releases/2015/legal-change-will-protect-nursing-and-midwifery-students-who-raise-concerns/ (accessed 19 September 2017).

Nursing and Midwifery Council (2015d, updated March 2017) *Revalidation – How to Revalidate with the NMC*. Available at: www.nmc.org.uk/globalassets/sitedocuments/revalidation/how-to-revalidate-booklet.pdf (accessed 11 January 2018).

Nursing and Midwifery Council (2016) *Quality Assurance – Ensuring a Safe and Effective Learning Environment*. Available at: www.nmc.org.uk/education/programme-of-change-for-education/quality-assurance/ (accessed 12 February 2017).

Nursing and Midwifery Council (2017a) *Meeting of the Council – To be Held from 10:30am on Wednesday 24 May 2017, Cardiff*. Available at: www.nmc.org.uk/globalassets/sitedocuments/councilpapersanddocuments/council-2017/may-2017-council-papers.pdf?_t_id=1B2M2Y8AsgTpgAmY7PhCfg%3d%3d&_t_q=Apprentice&_t_tags=language%3aen%2csiteid%3ad6891695-0234-463b-bf74-1bfb02644b38&_t_ip=213.122.128.16&_t_hit.id=NMC_Web_Models_Media_DocumentFile/_7333d684-dca1-4831-a1d2-33617632a154&_t_hit.pos=8 (accessed 29 October 2017).

Nursing and Midwifery Council (2017b) *Enabling Professionalism in Nursing and Midwifery Practice*. Available at: www.nmc.org.uk/globalassets/sitedocuments/other-publications/enabling-professionalism.pdf (accessed 10 January 2018).

Nursing and Midwifery Council (2017c) *Quality Assurance Framework – For Nursing and Midwifery Education*. Available at: www.nmc.org.uk/globalassets/sitedocuments/edandqa/nmc-quality-assurance-framework.pdf (accessed 14 September 2017).

Nursing and Midwifery Council (2018a) *Standards for Student Supervision and Assessment*. London, NMC. Available at: https://www.nmc.org.uk/standards-for-education-and-training/standards-for-student-supervisor-and-assessment/ (accessed 18 May 2018).

Nursing and Midwifery Council (2018b) *Future Nurse: Standards of Proficiency for Registered Nurses*. London, NMC. Available at: https://www.nmc.org.uk/globalassets/sitedocuments/education-standards/future-nurse-proficiencies.pdf (accessed 20 May 2018).

Nursing and Midwifery Council (2018c) *Standards Framework for Nursing and Midwifery Education*. London NMC. Available at: https://www.nmc.org.uk/standards-for-education-and-training/standards-framework-for-nursing-and-midwifery-education/ (accessed 20 May 2018).

Nursing and Midwifery Council (2018d) *Standards of Proficiency for Nursing Associates – Draft April 2018*. London: NMC, Available at: https://www.nmc.org.uk/globalassets/sitedocuments/na-consultation/standards-of-proficiency-for-nursing-associates.pdf (accessed 2 June 2018).

Nursing and Midwifery Council (2018e) *Standards for Pre-Registration Nursing Programmes*. London: NMC. Available at: https://www/nmc.org.uk/standards/standards-for-nurses/standards-for-pre-registration-nursing-programmes/ (accessed 20 May 2018).

Nygren. F. and Carlson, E. (2017) 'Preceptors' conceptions of a peer learning model: A phenomenographic study', *Nurse Education Today*, 49 (February 2017): 12–16.

O'Driscoll, M.F., Allan, H.T. and Smith, P.A. (2010) 'Still looking for leadership: who is responsible for student nurses' learning in practice?', *Nurse Education Today*, 30 (3): 212–17.

Ohaja, M., Dunlea, M. and Muldoon, K. (2013) 'Group marking and peer assessment during a group poster presentation: The experiences and views of midwifery students', *Nurse Education in Practice*, 13(5): 466–470.

Olofsson, A., Taube, K. and Ahl, A. (2015) 'Academic achievement of university students with dyslexia', *Dyslexia*, 21(4): 338–349.

Orton, H.D., Prowse, J. and Millen, C. (1993) *Charting the Way to Excellence* (Ward Learning Climate Project). Sheffield: Sheffield Hallam University.

Palfreyman, S., Tod, A. and Doyle, J. (2003) 'Comparing evidence-based practice of nurses and physiotherapists', *British Journal of Nursing*, 12(4): 246–253.

Pallen, N. and Timmins, F. (2002) 'Research-based practice: Myth or reality? A review of the barriers affecting research utilisation in practice', *Nurse Education in Practice*, 2(2): 99–108.

Papastavrou, E., Dimitriadou, M., Tsangari, H. and Andreou, C. (2016) 'Nursing students' satisfaction of the clinical learning environment: A research study', *BMC Nursing*, 15(44): 1–10.

Passmore, H. and Chenery-Morris, S. (2014) 'Exploring the value of the tripartite assessment of students in pre-registration midwifery education: A review of the evidence', *Nurse Education in Practice*, 14(1): 92–97.

Peters, R.S. (1966) *Ethics and Education*. London: George Allen & Unwin.

Peters, R.S. (1973) *The Philosophy of Education* (Oxford Readings in Philosophy). Oxford: Oxford University Press.

Peyton, J.W.R (ed.) (1998) *Teaching and Learning in Medical Practice*. Hertfordshire: Manticore Europe Limited.

Phillips, B.N., Turnbull, B.J. and He, F.X. (2015) 'Assessing readiness for self-directed learning within a non-traditional nursing cohort', *Nurse Education Today*, 35(3): e1–e7.

Phillips, T., Schostak, J. and Tyler, J. (2000) *Practice and Assessment in Nursing and Midwifery: Doing It for Real*. Researching Professional Education Research Series Report. Available at: https://eric.ed.gov/?id=ED463398 (accessed 29 September 2017).

Piaget, J. (1962) 'The stages of intellectual development of the child', in I. Roth (ed.), *Introduction to Psychology*. Milton Keynes: Lawrence Erlbaum Associates Ltd (LEA)/ Open University.

Pla-Campas, G., Arumí-Prat, J., Senye-Mir, A.M. and Ramírez, E. (2016) 'Effect of using formative assessment techniques on students' grades', *Procedia – Social and Behavioral Sciences*, 228(July): 190–195.

Polit, D.F. and Beck, C.T. (2018) *Essentials of Nursing Research: Appraising Evidence for Nursing Practice* (9th edition). London: Lippincott Williams and Wilkins.

Power, A. and Farmer, R. (2017) 'Pre-registration midwifery education: Do learning styles limit or liberate students?' *British Journal of Midwifery*, 25(2): 123–126.

Price, A. and Price, B. (2009) 'Role modelling practice with students on clinical placements', *Nursing Standard*, 24(11): 51–56.

Proctor, B. (2011) 'Training for the supervision alliance – attitude, skills and intention', in J.R. Cutcliffe, K. Hyrkas and J. Fowler (eds), *Routledge Handbook of Clinical Supervision – Fundamental International Themes*. London: Routledge. Chapter 3.

Quality Assurance Agency for Higher Education (2008) *Outcomes from Institutional Audit Second Series: Work-Based and Placement Learning, and Employability*. Available at: www.qaa.ac.uk/publications/information-and-guidance/publication?PubID=150#.WZXIsWZK3IU (accessed 15 September 2017).

Quality Assurance Agency for Higher Education (2009) *Personal Development Planning: Guidance for Institutional Policy and Practice in Higher Education*. Available at: www.qaa.ac.uk/en/Publications/Documents/Personal-development-planning-guidance-for-institutional-policy-and-practice-in-higher-education.pdf (accessed 15 August 2017).

Quality Assurance Agency for Higher Education (2010) *Code of Practice for the Assurance of Academic Quality and Standards in Higher Education, Section 3: Disabled Students*. Available at: www.admin.cam.ac.uk/univ/disability//practice/pdf/qaa.pdf (accessed 26 February 2017).

Quality Assurance Agency for Higher Education (2013) *UK Quality Code for Higher Education – Chapter B6: Assessment of Students and the Recognition of Prior Learning*. Available at: www.qaa.ac.uk/publications/information-and-guidance/uk-quality-code-for-higher-education-chapter-b6-assessment-of-students-and-the-recognition-of-prior-learning1#.WVuTGGZK3IU (accessed 4 July 2017).

Quality Assurance Agency for Higher Education (2014a) *UK Quality Code for Higher Education Part A: Setting and Maintaining Academic Standards: The Frameworks for Higher Education Qualifications of UK Degree-Awarding Bodies (FHEQ)*. Available at: www.qaa.ac.uk/en/Publications/Documents/qualifications-frameworks.pdf (accessed 26 July 2017).

Quality Assurance Agency for Higher Education (2014b) *Higher Education Review: Themes for 2015–16*. Available at: www.qaa.ac.uk/publications/ information-and-guidance/publication?PubID=2859#.WZBlNWZK3IU

Race, P. (2014) *Making Learning Happen: A Guide for Post-Compulsory Education*, 3rd edn. London: Sage Publications.

Ramsden, P. (2003) *Learning to Teach in Higher Education*, 2nd edn. London: Routledge Falmer.

Richmond, H. (2006) 'Mentoring in midwifery', *RCM Midwives Journal*, 9(11): 434–437.

Roberts, P., Priest, H. and Bromage, C. (2001) 'Selecting and utilising data sources to evaluate health care education', *Nurse Researcher*, 8(3): 15–29.

Rogers, A. and Horrocks, H. (2010) *Teaching Adults*, 4th edn. Maidenhead: Open University Press/McGraw-Hill Education.

Rogers, C. (1983) *Freedom to Learn in the 80s*. Columbus, OH: Charles Merrill.

Rogers, C. and Freiberg, H.J. (1994) *Freedom to Learn*, 3rd edn. Upper Saddle River, NJ: Pearson Education.

Rooke, N. (2014) 'An evaluation of nursing and midwifery sign off mentors, new mentors and nurse lecturers' understanding of the sign off mentor role', *Nurse Education in Practice*, 14(1): 43–48.

Rowntree, D. (1987) *Assessing Students: How Shall We Know Them?* London: Kogan Page.

Roxburgh, M., Conlon, M. and Banks, D. (2012) 'Evaluating hub-and-spoke models of practice learning in Scotland, UK: A multiple case study approach', *Nurse Education Today*, 32(7): 782–789.

Royal College of Nursing (2004) *The Future Nurse: Evidence of the Impact of Registered Nurses*. London: Royal College of Nursing.

Royal College of Nursing (2012) *Quality with Compassion: The Future of Nursing Education* (Willis Commission Report). Available at: www.nursingtimes.net/Journals/2012/11/02/j/c/c/Willis-Commission-report-2012.pdf (accessed 17 January 2018).

Royal College of Nursing (2016) *RCN Mentorship Project 2015. From Today's Support in Practice to Tomorrow's Vision for Excellence.* Available at: www.rcn.org.uk/professional-development/publications/pub-005454 (accessed 14 September 2017).

Royal College of Nursing (2017a) *Helping Students Get the Best from Their Practice Placements (A Royal College of Nursing Toolkit)* (3rd edition). London: Royal College of Nursing. Also available at: https://www.rcn.org.uk/professional-development/publications/pub-006035 (accessed 16 March 2018).

Royal College of Nursing (2017b) *RCN Guidance for Mentors of Nursing and Midwifery Students.* Available at: www.rcn.org.uk/professional-development/publications/pub-006133 (accessed 4 October 2017).

Sackett, D.L., Rosenburg, W., Gray, J.M., Haynes, R.B. and Richardson, S.W. (1996) 'Evidence-based medicine: What it is and what it isn't', *BMJ*, 312(7023): 71–72.

Sackett, D.L., Strauss, S.E., Richardson, S.W., Rosenburg, W. and Haynes, R.B. (2000) *Evidence-Based Medicine: How to Practise and Teach EBM*, 2nd edn. Edinburgh: Churchill Livingstone.

Saltie, D. (2017) 'Supervision: A contested space for learning decision making', *Qualitative Social Work*, 16(4): 533–549

Sanders, C.E. (2018) *Lawrence Kohlberg's Stages of Moral Development Psychology.* Available at: www.britannica.com/topic/Lawrence-Kohlbergs-stages-of-moral-development (accessed 12 January 2018).

Scammell, B. (1990) *Communication Skills.* Basingstoke: Macmillan.

Schon, D. (1995) *The Reflective Practitioner: How Professionals Think in Action.* Aldershot: Arena.

Scott, B., Rapson, T., Allibone, L., Hamilton, R., Mambanje, C.S. and Pisaneschi, L. (2017) 'Practice education facilitator roles and their value to NHS organisations', *British Journal of Nursing*, 26(4): 222–227.

Scullion, P. (2002) 'Effective dissemination strategies', *Nurse Researcher: Qualitative Approaches*, 10(1): 65–67.

Scullion, P.A. (2010) 'Models of disability: Their influence in nursing and potential role in challenging discrimination', *Journal of Advanced Nursing*, 66(3): 697–707.

Shivers, E., Hasson, F. and Slater, P. (2017) 'Pre-registration nursing students' quality of practice learning: Clinical learning environment inventory (actual) questionnaire', *Nurse Education Today*, 55(August): 58–64.

Siles-González, J. and Solano-Ruiz, C. (2016) 'Self-assessment, reflection on practice and critical thinking in nursing students', *Nurse Education Today*, 45(October): 132–137.

Simpson, J. and Weiner, E. (1989) *The Oxford English Dictionary*, 2nd edn. Oxford: Oxford University Press.

Sines, D., Harris, D., Firth, J. and Boden, L. (2006) 'Applied leadership: ensuring fitness for practice', *Nursing Management*, 13 (8): 28–31.

Skills for Health (2017) *The Care Certificate Standards.* Available at: www.skillsforhealth.org.uk/standards/item/216-the-care-certificate (accessed 26 May 2017).

Skinner, B.F. (1971) *Beyond Freedom and Dignity.* New York: Alfred Knopf.

Smith, R. and Rennie, D. (2014) 'Evidence based medicine – an oral history (Editorial)', *BMJ*, 348(7942): g371.

Society and College of Radiographers (2018) *Education Approval and Accreditation.* Available at: www.sor.org/career-progression/practice-educators (accessed 13 January 2018).

Spouse, J. (2001) 'Bridging theory and practice in the supervisory relationship: A socio-cultural perspective', *Journal of Advanced Nursing*, 33(4): 512–522.

Steinaker, N.W. and Bell, M.R. (1979) *The Experiential Learning: A New Approach to Teaching and Learning.* New York: Academic Press.

Stewart, K.R. and Hand, K.I. (2017) 'SBAR, communication, and patient safety: An integrated literature review', *MEDSURG Nursing*, 26(5): 297–305.

Stickley, T. (2011) 'From SOLER to SURETY for effective non-verbal communication', *Nurse Education in Practice*, 11(6): 395–398.

Stickley, T., Stacey, G., Pollock, K., Smith, A., Betinis, J. and Fairbank, S. (2010) 'The practice assessment of student nurses by people who use mental health services', *Nurse Education Today*, 30(1): 20–25.

Tanner, K. (2014) 'Increasing objectivity in the assessment of interpersonal skills and attitude', *Journal of Paramedic Practice*, 6(11): 566–571.

Tee, S.R., Owens, K., Plowright, S., Ramnath, P., Rourke, S., James, C. and Bayliss, J. (2010) 'Being reasonable: Supporting disabled nursing students in practice', *Nurse Education in Practice*, 10 (4): 216–21.

Thiroux, J. and Krasemann, K. (2014) *Ethics, Theory and Practice*, 11th edn. Harlow: Pearson Education Limited.

Thomas, M. and Westwood, N. (2016) 'Student experience of hub and spoke model of placement allocation – An evaluative study', *Nurse Education Today*, 46 (November): 24–28.

Thompson, C., McCaughan, D., Cullum, N., Sheldon, T. and Raynor, P. (2002) 'The value of research in clinical decision-making', *Nursing Times*, 98(42): 30–34.

Titchen, A. (2003) 'The practice development diamond', Paper presented at the RCN Annual International Nursing Research Conference, 10–12 April, UMIST, Manchester.

Tweed, A., Graber, R. and Wang, M. (2010) 'Assessing trainee clinical psychologists' clinical competence', *Psychology Learning and Teaching*, 9(2): 50–60.

University of St Andrews (2017) *Learning Agreement.* Available at: www.st-andrews.ac.uk/studyabroad/outgoingstudents/academicinformation/learningagreement/ (accessed 21 November 2017).

van Eps, M., Cooke, M., Creedy, D. and Walker, R. (2006) 'Student evaluations of a year-long mentorship program: A quality improvement initiative', *Nurse Education Today*, 26(6): 519–524.

van Wijngaarden, J.D.H., Dirks, M., Dippel, D.W.J., Minkman, M. and Niessen, L.W. (2006) 'Towards effective and efficient care pathways: Thrombolysis in acute ischaemic stroke', *Qjm*, 99(4): 267–272.

VARK Learning Limited (2017) *The VARK Questionnaire.* Available at: http://vark-learn.com/the-vark-questionnaire/ (accessed 20 November 2017).

Vinales, J.J. (2015) 'Exploring failure to fail in pre-registration nursing', *British Journal of Nursing*, 24(5): 284–288.

Viney, R. and McKimm, J. (2010) 'Mentoring', *British Journal of Hospital Medicine*, 71(2): 106–109.

Walia, S. and Marks-Maran, D. (2014) 'Leadership development through action learning sets: An evaluation study', *Nurse Education in Practice*, 14(6): 612–619.

Wallace, M. (1999) *Lifelong Learning: PREP in Action.* Edinburgh: Churchill Livingstone.

Ward, L., Fenton, K. and Maher, L. (2010) 'The high impact actions for nursing and midwifery 3: Staying safe, preventing falls', *Nursing Times*, 106(29): 12–13.

Warne, T., Johansson, U., Papastavrou, E., Tichelaar, E., Tomietto, M., Van den Bossche, K., Moreno, M.F.V. and Saarikoski, V.M. (2010) 'An exploration of the clinical learning experience of nursing students in nine European countries', *Nurse Education Today*, 30(8): 809–815.

Waskett, C. (2010) 'Clinical supervision using the 4S model 1: Considering the structure and setting it up', *Nursing Times*, 106(16): 12–14.

Webb, C. and Shakespeare, P. (2008) 'Judgements about mentoring relationships in nurse education', *Nurse Education Today*, 28(5): 563–571.

Webber, E. (2017) *Building Successful Communities of Practice*. London: Blurb.

Wenger, E. (2000) *Communities of Practice: Learning, Meaning and Identity*. Cambridge: Cambridge University Press.

White, J. (2007) 'Supporting nursing students with dyslexia in clinical practice', *Nursing Standard*, 21(19): 35–42.

Whiting, V.R. and de Janasz, S.C. (2004) 'Mentoring in the 21st century: Using the internet to build skills and networks', *Journal of Management Education*, 28(3): 275–293.

Wilkinson, J.E., Rushmer, R.K. and Davies, H.T.O. (2004) 'Clinical governance and the learning organization', *Journal of Nursing Management*, 12(2): 105–113.

Williams, B., Perillo, S. and Brown, T. (2015a) 'What are the factors of organisational culture in health care settings that act as barriers to the implementation of evidence-based practice? A scoping review', *Nurse Education Today*, 35(2): e34–e41.

Williams, B., Hardy, K. and McKenna, L. (2015b) 'Near-peer teaching in paramedic education: Results from 2011 to 2013', *Medical Science Educator*, 25(2): 149–156.

Williamson, G. (2009) 'Student support on placement: The student experience and staff perceptions of the implementation of placement development team', The 2009 RCN International Nursing Research Conference: Book of Abstracts (Section 9.1.3): 107.

Wood, S. (2005) 'The experiences of a group of pre-registration mental health nursing students', *Nurse Education Today*, 25(3): 189–96.

Yang, K., Nisbet, G. and McAllister, L. (2017) 'Students' experiences and perceptions of inter-professional supervision on placement', *International Journal of Practice-based Learning in Health and Social Care*, 5(2): 1–18.

Yorkshire and the Humber & Health Education England (2017) *Local Workforce Action Boards*. Available at: https://hee.nhs.uk/hee-your-area/yorkshire-humber/about-us/local-workforce-action-boards-0 (accessed 15 August 2017).

Young, P., Moore, E., Griffiths, G., Raine, R., Stewart, R., Cownie, M. and Frutos-Perez, M. (2010) 'Help is just a text away: The use of short message service texting to provide an additional means of support for health care students during practice placements', *Nurse Education Today*, 30(2): 118–123.

INDEX

Made in the USA
Columbia, SC
09 October 2018